Manual of Contact Lens Prescribing and Fitting with CD-ROM

Manual of Contact Lens Prescribing and Fitting with CD-ROM

Second Edition

Edited by

Milton M. Hom, O.D., F.A.A.O.
Private Practice, Azusa, California

CD-ROM designed by
Milton M. Hom, O.D., F.A.A.O.

and

Adrian S. Bruce, B.Sc.Optom., Ph.D., F.A.A.O.
Senior Fellow, Department of Optometry and Vision Science, University of Melbourne, Melbourne, Victoria, Australia; Senior Optometrist, Victorian College of Optometry, Melbourne

Forewords by
Rodger T. Kame, O.D., F.A.A.O.
Associate Professor, Adjunct Faculty, Southern California College of Optometry, Fullerton

and

Edward S. Bennett, O.D., M.S.Ed.
Associate Professor of Optometry and Chief, Contact Lens Service, University of Missouri–St. Louis School of Optometry, St. Louis

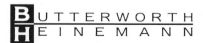

BUTTERWORTH
HEINEMANN

Boston   Oxford   Auckland   Johannesburg   Melbourne   New Delhi

Recognizing the importance of preserving what has been written, Butterworth–Heinemann prints its books on acid-free paper whenever possible.

 Butterworth–Heinemann supports the efforts of American Forests and the Global ReLeaf program in its campaign for the betterment of trees, forests, and our environment.

Library of Congress Cataloging-in-Publication Data

Manual of contact lens prescribing and fitting with CD-ROM / edited by Milton M. Hom ; forewords by Rodger T. Kame and Edward S. Bennett.— 2nd ed.
  p. cm.
  Includes bibliographical references and index.
  ISBN 0-7506-7215-3 (alk. paper)
    1. Contact lenses—Handbooks, manuals, etc. I. Hom, Milton M.

 RE977.C6 M257 2000
 617.7'523—dc21

                                                                    00-037948

British Library Cataloguing-in-Publication Data
A catalogue record for this book is available from the British Library.

The publisher offers special discounts on bulk orders of this book.
For information, please contact:

Manager of Special Sales
Butterworth–Heinemann
225 Wildwood Avenue
Woburn, MA 01801-2041
Tel: 781-904-2500
Fax: 781-904-2620

For information on all Butterworth–Heinemann medical publications available,
contact our World Wide Web home page at: http://www.bh.com

10 9 8 7 6 5 4 3 2 1

Printed in the United States of America

This book is dedicated to my family,
Jill, Jennifer, and Zachary Hom;
and to my parents, Milton and Norma Hom

Contents

Contributing Authors

Christine L. K. Astin, B.Sc., M.Phil. (London), F.C.Optom., D.C.L.P., F.A.A.O.
Sessional Lecturer in Vision Science, Aston University, Birmingham; Senior
Optometrist, Department of Ophthalmology, Birmingham Heartlands Hospital,
Birmingham, England

Adrian S. Bruce, B.Sc.Optom., Ph.D., F.A.A.O.
Senior Fellow, Department of Optometry and Vision Science, University of
Melbourne, Melbourne, Victoria, Australia; Senior Optometrist, Victorian College
of Optometry, Melbourne

Shelley I. Cutler, O.D., F.A.A.O.
Adjunct Faculty and Consultant to the Contact Lens Department, Pennsylvania
College of Optometry, Philadelphia

Michael D. DePaolis, O.D.
Adjunct Faculty, Pennsylvania College of Optometry, Philadelphia; Clinical Associate,
Department of Ophthalmology, University of Rochester School of Medicine and
Dentistry and Strong Memorial Hospital, Rochester, New York

Timothy B. Edrington, O.D., M.S.
Professor of Optometry and Chief, Cornea and Contact Lens Service, Southern
California College of Optometry, Fullerton

Milton M. Hom, O.D., F.A.A.O.
Private Practice, Azusa, California

Rodger T. Kame, O.D., F.A.A.O.
Associate Professor, Adjunct Faculty, Southern California College of Optometry, Fullerton

Simon A. Little, Ph.D., M.Sc., M.C.Optom., F.A.A.O., F.B.D.O.
Private Practice, West Yorkshire, England; Former Lecturer in Optometry, University
of Manchester Institute of Science and Technology, Manchester, England

Harue J. Marsden, O.D., M.S.
Assistant Professor, Department of Cornea and Contact Lens, Southern California
College of Optometry, Fullerton

John Mountford, Dip.App.Sc., F.A.A.O., F.V.C.O., F.C.L.S.
Visiting Lecturer in Optometry, Queensland University of Technology and University of New South Wales, Australia; Visiting Contact Lens Specialist, Royal Brisbane Hospital, Brisbane, Australia

Arlene A. Orehek, O.D.
Clinical Associate, Halpern Eye Associates, Dover, Delaware; Adjunct Faculty, Pennsylvania College of Optometry, Philadelphia

Jerry R. Paugh, O.D., Ph.D., F.A.A.O.
Technical Advisor, Allergen Inc., Irvine, California

Joseph P. Shovlin, O.D.
Clinical Associate, Northeastern Eye Institute, Scranton, Pennsylvania; Adjunct Faculty, Pennsylvania College of Optometry, Philadelphia

Ronald Watanabe, O.D.
Associate Professor, Department of Clinical Skills and Practice, New England College of Optometry, Boston

Foreword

One of the most effective clinical learning techniques is the grand rounds format. The *Manual of Contact Lens Prescribing and Fitting, Second Edition,* with its remarkable CD-ROM feature, enables the clinician to observe important dynamics of fluorescein pattern interpretation through the advantage of instantaneous observation. Moreover, the CD-ROM feature provides an untiring subject that may be studied even more closely than in the normal clinical grand rounds format.

The addition of the CD-ROM to Dr. Hom's *Manual of Contact Lens Prescribing and Fitting, Second Edition,* makes this the best source available today on clinical contact lenses and should be included in every serious cornea and contact lens clinician's library. The inexperienced aspiring contact lens "expert" will find this especially useful as an excellent learning tool.

Rodger T. Kame

Foreword

As rapid changes occur in eye care today, practitioners desire comprehensive but concise clinical manuals to address their questions about cases encountered in everyday practice. *Manual of Contact Lens Prescribing and Fitting, Second Edition* is a reference manual that is written in a concise, practical outline manner but is comprehensive and should address almost every question an inquisitive practitioner has about a contact lens–related clinical topic. Likewise, management information is presented throughout the book to assist in fitting and problem-solving situations, and numerous clinical pearls are isolated in each chapter to highlight key points.

This manual flows logically from beginning to end, covering basic prefitting topics, rigid lenses, soft lenses, and advanced/specialty topics. The information about contact lens–induced complications, including hypoxia-related, mechanical, and desiccation-based complications, is outstanding. The chapter about the dry-eye patient is very welcome, as this is one of the major challenges experienced on an ongoing basis by contact lens practitioners. The brand names of popular lens materials and care products are used frequently to help the practitioner in determining how to fit and solve problems. Nevertheless, this clinical manual should not be outdated for several years. The chapters on refractive surgery and orthokeratology are especially timely; the former addresses fitting photorefractive keratectomy (PRK) and phototherapeutic keratectomy (PTK) patients in addition to radial keratotomy (RK) patients.

A tremendous addition and an outstanding educational benefit to the second edition of this text is a comprehensive CD-ROM on RGP lenses. With the assistance of Adrian Bruce, this CD-ROM provides different RGP fitting relationships, cases, orthokeratology fitting relationships, as well as bifocal, keratoconic, and post-graft cases and problem solving. Video images are used extensively to show different fitting relationships and, when appropriate, topography maps are provided. This is an invaluable learning aid to practitioners and the quality of the video images—as one would expect from the author—is very good.

Manual of Contact Lens Prescribing and Fitting, Second Edition is a very beneficial reference source on all clinical contact lens topics. Dr. Hom has once again edited a superb text, and I recommend this manual to all practitioners who want to update their clinical knowledge on contact lenses.

Edward S. Bennett

Preface to the Second Edition

Reliance on printed material to learn about prescribing and fitting contact lenses has served us well for many years. Advances in technology, however, now offer new opportunities to enhance learning. As any expert who has tried to teach the fitting of contact lenses can tell you, the use of video offers a far better teaching tool than still pictures.

The second edition of *Manual of Contact Lens Prescribing and Fitting* introduces the first multimedia CD-ROM available in a contact lens book. The CD-ROM fulfills a need unique to optometric practice: understanding the dynamics of fitting rigid contact lenses. The use of video, animation, and morphing help the clinician learn the fundamental skills of movement and positioning that are fundamental to correctly fitting contact lenses. We hope that this approach will help dispel some of the mystery about rigid lens fitting.

The second edition of *Manual of Contact Lens Prescribing and Fitting* features eight new multimedia chapters (see About the CD-ROM). For ease of use, the text of the multimedia chapters is included in the book as Chapters 22–29. There are other significant revisions to the *Manual* as well. In order to keep up with the tremendous progress in the contact lens field in the past three years, material has been added on silicone hydrogel extended wear lenses and other innovations.

We appreciate the kind comments many of you have given us about the first edition. We hope this Second Edition will also further your knowledge and increase your understanding of contact lenses.

We would like to thank Michael G. Harris, Janice M. Jurkis, and the late Roy Rengstorff for initially reviewing the CD-ROM.

We would also like to especially thank Karen Oberheim of Butterworth–Heinemann for her support. Her tireless persistence and vision made this unique project a reality.

M.M.H.
A.B.

Preface to the First Edition

There has been a wealth of excellent books and papers written about contact lenses. As have many of you, I have benefited from studying these great works. This manual's compact format in outline form was purposely designed to make the information more conveniently accessible and easy to look up. It is meant to be a practical chairside book, useful for the contact lens practitioner and student. I also hope that this book and its references will be a guide for finding more information about a particular subject.

I would like to thank the following people for their help in reviewing the manuscript and for their photographic support: Ed Bennett, Adrian Bruce, Tim Edrington, Richard Lindsay, Harue Marsden, Bob Mandell, Joe Shovlin, Nick Stoyan, and Karla Zadnik. I would also like to acknowledge my computer friends for all of their support and help: Paul Tran, Tim Lindquist of Mindset, Bob Bradley, and Todd Weber. Finally, I would like to acknowledge Barbara Murphy, Karen Oberheim, and Butterworth–Heinemann for their patience and support.

M.M.H.

PART I

Basic Concepts

Chapter 1

Anatomy and Physiology

Milton M. Hom

I. **Tear film** provides the necessary optical surface for vision. It also protects the eye, flushes cellular debris and foreign matter, gives the cornea nutrition, and provides wetting for a contact lens. The average volume of the tear film is 5–10 µl ($\frac{1}{10}$–$\frac{1}{5}$ of a drop). It is secreted at 2 µl ($\frac{1}{30}$ of a drop) per minute. Twenty-five percent of the tears secreted are lost by evaporation, and the rest drains into the **nasolacrimal duct** via the **puncta.** The **tear pH** of the open eye is 7.14–7.82, the average being 7.45.[1,2]

   A. The tear film is considered **triphasic,** made up of **three layers**: the oily, or lipid; aqueous; and mucoid, or mucous layers.

      1. The **lipid layer** is secreted by Zeiss, Moll, and meibomian glands in the lids. Tear lipid inhibits evaporation and prevents spillage over the lids. Lipids consist of cholesterol esters, lecithin, fatty acids, free cholesterol, and phospholipids.[1] The lipid layer is normally 0.1–0.2 µl thick. A thicker than normal lipid layer can be detected by viewing interference patterns in the biomicroscope (see Chapters 3 and 16).

      2. The **aqueous layer** is produced by Krause and Wolfring glands, both accessory lacrimal glands. **Basal tears** constitute normal lacrimation; the majority of these tears are produced by the accessory glands. **Reflex tears,** or **stimulated tears,** are the result of excessive lacrimation produced by the lacrimal gland.[3] Reflex tearing can be triggered by a host of factors, including the presence of a foreign body under a contact lens, a bad edge of a contact lens, a torn lens, corneal abrasion, or toxic solution reactions.

      3. The **mucous layer** is produced by Manz's glands, goblet cells, and crypts of Henle. Mucus, or glycoprotein, is a scant 1% of the total aqueous volume. Glycoproteins are rod-shaped, consisting of a protein core and carbohydrate side chain. These molecules have both a polar and nonpolar component. The nonpolar end aligns with the hydrophobic epithelial cells; the polar end attracts water. Some rigid contact lens solutions use the same principle to better wet a hydrophobic lens surface. **Polyvinyl alcohol** uses

3

the same principle for better wetting (see Chapter 9). Poor spreading of mucus results from abnormalities, such as improper blinking and lagophthalmos. Inadequate mucus may result from goblet cell loss, vitamin A deficiency, and chemical burns.[1]

B. **Tear composition** includes electrolytes, vitamin A, and proteins. Other components are glucose, metabolites, and vitamin C.

1. **Electrolytes** in the tears are **sodium** and **chloride** in high concentrations. Bicarbonate, potassium, calcium, magnesium, and manganese ions are also contained in the tear film. Potassium, calcium, and magnesium are needed for corneal epithelium maintenance. Calcium is also involved in hemidesmosome formation. Many times, lens soilage consists of calcium deposition from the tears.[3]

2. **Vitamin A** is present in tears. Vitamin A deficiency is associated with goblet cell loss. Vitamin A has been suggested for dry-eye patients. Topical administration of vitamin A helps combat severely dry eyes.[3]

3. **Sixty protein types** are present in the tear film, including albumin, globulin, and lysozyme. The lacrimal gland produces lysozyme, lactoferrin, and albumin for the tear film. **Albumin** makes up 60% of the tear protein.[2] **Lysozyme** (mucopeptide *N*-acetylmuramyhydralase) comprises 20–40% of the total tear protein. The lytic activity of lysozyme protects the eye and destroys some bacterial cell walls.[1] The immune system is highly dependent on lysozyme.

4. The **immunoglobulins** in the tears are **IgG, IgA, IgM,** and **IgE**. IgG and IgA are the most plentiful in the tear film under normal conditions and defend against infection. IgA is associated with control of the normal flora. IgM appears in severe inflammation. IgE is related to allergies. All of the immunoglobulins are involved in the defense system of the eyes.[4]

C. **Cells** of the tear film include conjunctival, corneal, and keratinized epithelial cells; polymorphonuclear neutrophils; eosinophils; and lymphocytes. Macrophages are present when there is infection. Basophils are more numerous with allergic conjunctivitis.

D. **Osmolarity effects** are based on the electrolytes in the tears. If the tears are more or less concentrated than normal, the sensitive cornea experiences thickness changes. Normal osmotic pressure is equivalent to that created by a 0.9% sodium chloride solution.[2]

1. **Hypotonic** tears are more dilute than normal. More water than usual enters the epithelium, causing swelling and corneal thickening.[1] Hypotonic wetting drops are popular for marginally dry eyes.

2. **Hypertonic** tears are more concentrated than normal tears—water is drawn out of the epithelium, causing thinning.[1] Hypertonic solutions are used to create the same thinning effect on the cornea. In cases of corneal swelling, such as the hydrops seen in kerato-

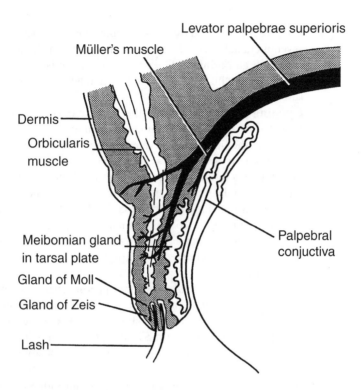

Müller's muscle

Levator palpebrae superioris

Dermis

Orbicularis
muscle

Meibomian gland
in tarsal plate

Gland of Moll

Gland of Zeis

Lash

Palpebral
conjuctiva

FIGURE 1.1   *A cross-section of lid anatomy. (Reprinted with permission from JD Bartlett, GG Melore. Diseases of Eyelids. In JD Bartlett, SD Jaanus [eds], Clinical Ocular Pharmacology [3rd ed]. Boston: Butterworth–Heinemann, 1995;562.)*

conus, **hypertonic ointments** are used to help to draw out the fluid (see Chapter 17).

II. **Lids** have a significant effect on contact lenses. Contact lens positioning, orientation, and movement depend heavily on the eyelids. Understanding the blink dynamics is essential to fit toric as well as bifocal lenses. Much of the tear film also originates from the glands located in the lids.

A. **Lid anatomy** consists of muscles (orbicularis and levator palpebrae superioris), skin (dermis), lashes (cilia), nerves (third nerve), connective tissue (tarsal plates), and glands (Zeiss, Moll, and meibomian) (Figure 1.1).

B. **Blinking** is one of the most important functions of the eyelids related to contact lenses. The upper lid moves downward then upward like a windshield wiper. The lower lid moves in a horizontal, transverse nasal motion. As the upper lid moves downward, the lower lid moves toward the medial canthus. This lid action results in nasal rotation of the prism ballasted lens on blinking.[5]

1. **Closure** is performed by the **orbicularis** muscle innervated by the seventh cranial nerve. The orbicularis has two main portions: the palpebral and orbital.[6] The palpebral portion is used in normal blinking and winking. The orbital portion takes part in forced closure or blepharospasm.[6,7]

2. **Opening** is mostly done by the **levator** muscle, which is innervated by the third cranial nerve. Müller's muscle also helps to elevate the lid. It is innervated by the sympathetic division of the autonomic nervous system.[6,7]

3. **Spontaneous blinking** is known as normal blinking.[6] It should be relaxed, complete, and frequent. **Incomplete blinking** or **infrequent blinking** can create dryness problems for the contact lens patient (see Chapter 16). Sometimes, the upper lid moves only halfway over the cornea, leaving the blink incomplete. At other times blinking is infrequent, occurring less than the optimal 10–15 times per minute.

C. On **downgaze,** the levator relaxes, and the upper lid displaces downward. The lower lid moves up slightly with respect to the lower limbus. A translating bifocal lens such as the Tangent Streak (Fused Kontacts, Kansas City, MO) or Fluoroperm ST (Paragon Vision Sciences, Mesa, Arizona) relies heavily on this movement. Lower lid positioning is very important (see Chapter 18). On **upgaze,** the upper lid is pulled upward by the levator and frontalis muscles. The lower lid shows slight movement.[1] When the eye closes, the globe moves mostly upward and sometimes nasalward to protect the cornea. This is referred to as **Bell's phenomenon.**[6,8]

D. The **palpebral aperture,** or **fissure,** is normally 9–11 mm wide. The size of the patient's fissure has a direct influence on rigid gas-permeable fittings and problem solving. The upper lid normally covers a portion of the superior cornea from 10 to 2 o'clock.[9] A lid attachment fit can be used for this common type of lid configuration. If the lower lid covers a portion of the cornea, resulting in a smaller aperture, the lens must be made smaller to gain the same effect. If the upper lid has no corneal coverage, a lid attachment fit is difficult. A smaller interpalpebral lens would fit better (see Chapter 4).

E. **Glands of Zeis** and **Moll** surround the cilia. Glands of Zeis and Moll and meibomian glands are sebaceous glands that secrete oil. Glands of Moll are modified sweat glands.[7] All three types of glands contribute to the tear film.

F. **Meibomian glands** are located behind the lash line at the junction of the moist and dry parts of the epithelium.[1] There are approximately 25 glands in the upper lid and 20 glands in the lower lid. The meibum, or oil secreted by the meibomian glands, makes up the lipid layer of the tear film. Many times, the meibum is cloudy or insufficient, resulting in poor tear film quality and contact lens problems. Expression of the gland reveals the quality of the meibum (see Chapter 16).

G.   **Tarsal plates** are made of connective tissue and serve as the backbone of the lids. The lashes emerge anterior to the tarsal plate. When the lid is everted for inspection, the lid is folded right above the tarsal plate.[1]

III.   The **cornea** is the main refracting surface of the eye. Contact lens practitioners must have a good understanding of the cornea. The temperature of the cornea is below body temperature, about 37°C.[1] The thickness is approximately 0.52 mm centrally and 0.65 mm peripherally. The average horizontal diameter is 11.7 mm, with a range of 11.0–12.5 mm. The average vertical diameter is 10.6 mm. Under some rigid gas-permeable lens philosophies, visible iris diameter is used to determine lens diameter. Other philosophies, however, do not take corneal diameter into account. **Empirical methods** of fitting rigid gas-permeable lenses assume that sag heights are the same for all corneas. Empirical methods fail when the cornea is large and steep (large sag height) or small and flat (small sag height). Knowledge of the corneal relative size and curvature can help in determining if a potential fitting problem exists.

A.   The **layers of cornea** are epithelium; Bowman's membrane, or anterior limiting membrane; stroma; Descemet's membrane, or posterior limiting membrane; and endothelium (Figure 1.2).

B.   **Epithelium** provides a protective fluid and microorganism barrier. Its surface supplies optical refracting and tear stabilization. Two-thirds of the total eye's refractive power takes place at the anterior corneal surface. The epithelium is 50–60 μm thick and accounts for 10% of corneal thickness. The epithelium is capable of renewing and replicating itself when traumatized (postnatal mitosis). Almost all of the cornea's responses to contact lens wear can be traced to the epithelium.[10]

1.   **Cell layers** consists of five to seven layers of tightly packed cells known as superficial squamous, wing, and basal cells.[1] These are actually all the same type of cell in different stages of life span. The **basement membrane** helps the epithelium attach to Bowman's membrane.[8] **Langerhans' cells** are located in the deep epithelium among the basal cells.

a.   **Superficial epithelium** has numerous irregularities called **microvilli** and **microplicae** along the surface extending into the tear film. Their size is less than ⅒ μm, and they help stabilize the tear film. The villi are covered by the **glycocalyx.** The villi function has capturing pegs that help fix microbes, giving the natural tear defense elements more contact time.[8,11] Contact lens wear causes these structures to diminish in size and number.

b.   **Cell reproduction** and **movement** originate from the basal cells and move anteriorly toward the surface. Reproduction is

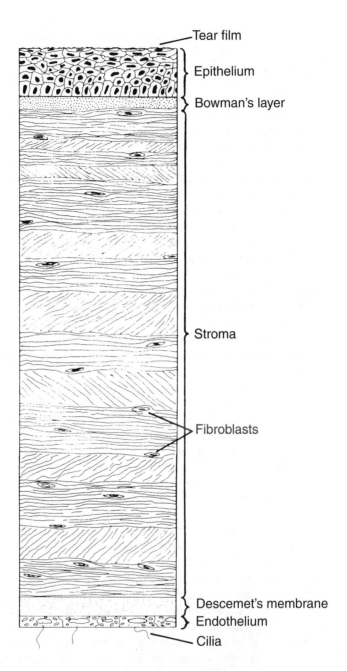

FIGURE 1.2   *Cornea cross-section. (Reprinted with permission from NL Burstein. Ophthalmic Drug Formulations. In JD Bartlett, SD Jaanus [eds], Clinical Ocular Pharmacology [3rd ed]. Boston: Butterworth–Heinemann, 1995;25.)*

greatest at the basal cells and tapers off in the wing cells. Cells also move from peripheral to central cornea. The cells move in a circular swirl-like, or **centripetal,** pattern.[12,13] Additional cells are believed to come from stem cells in the limbus and palisades of Vogt.[9,13] It takes approximately 7 days from the time of formation to exfoliation into the tear film.[1] After the cell emerges from the basal layer, it enlarges as time passes. The newer, younger cells are smaller than the older cells. The presence of predominately large cells in the epithelium indicates some sort of inhibition of the normal sloughing off process. Studies have shown extended-wear lenses prevent normal sloughing because of increased cell sizes.[14] The **X, Y, Z hypothesis** states that the number of cells lost must match the number of cells replaced. A balance is necessary to maintain a healthy epithelium.[12,13]

   c. **Strength** is enhanced by compactness and interdigitated sides of the cells. Cell junctions called **desmosomes** offer additional attachments to adjacent cells. **Hemidesmosomes** attach the cells to the basement membrane from the cells along the basement membrane. The attachment between the cells and basement membrane is not as strong as the attachment between the membrane and stroma. **Gap junctions** facilitate cell-to-cell communications. **Zonula occludens** are located along the superficial squamous cells and act as a fluid barrier.

   d. **Healing** occurs when the epithelium is injured. Mitosis stops, and cells migrate from the periphery to replace lost cells. Mitosis resumes when the cells have covered the injured area.[10] The pseudopodia of neighboring basal cells first cover the damaged area after about 1 hour. Epithelial cells then slide down the walls of the wound and fill the area. Small pinpoint areas of superficial damage clear up in 2–3 hours. Larger denuded areas approximately 2–3 mm in size take about 3 days to recover. Although the area may appear fully healed, contact lens wear can cause sloughing of the epithelial cells, damaging the area again. If the abrasion is deep enough to remove the basement membrane, adequate regeneration may take up to 6 or 7 weeks.[1]

2. **Nerves** are in two plexuses: stromal and epithelial. The epithelium is innervated by the ophthalmic nerve and some fibers from the maxillary division of the trigeminal nerve.[15] The nerve terminals in the epithelium are located deep in the basal cell layer. There are not many nerve endings in the superficial cells, which is why many patients do not feel the symptoms associated with **superficial punctate staining.**[16]

    C. Bowman's membrane, or **anterior limiting membrane,** is a thin layer that ends at the limbus. It is highly resistant to trauma and infection but does not regenerate if traumatized. A damaged Bowman's membrane leaves a scar, or opacity.

    D. Stroma, or **substantia propria,** consists of lamellae made of equally spaced collagen fibrils and **glycosaminoglycans,** or mucopolysaccharides.[17] Ninety percent of the corneal thickness is stroma.[8] The equal spacing of the fibrils is smaller than a wavelength of light and gives the stroma transparency. If the spacing is disrupted by the intake of fluid (**edema**), the cornea loses transparency.[1] **Keratocytes,** or corneal corpuscles, are cells in the stroma that secrete proteoglycans and procollagen.[18]

    E. Descemet's membrane, or **posterior limiting membrane,** serves as the basement membrane for the endothelial cells. It is 10–12 μm thick and elastic. Thickening of this membrane appears as **Hassal-Henle warts**[1] (see Chapter 2).

    F. Endothelium is a single layer of cells that provides much of the corneal metabolism. Cells are attached to Descemet's membrane by hemidesmosomes.[8] The endothelium can be affected by a great deal by contact lens wear.

        1. Polymegethism and **pleomorphism** are changes in cell shape, size, and number. Both of these changes are seen with contact lens wear. Polymegethism and pleomorphism may or may not have an effect on endothelial function (see Chapter 15).

        2. Endothelial blebs are black spots sometimes observed after 20–30 minutes of lens wear. **Hypercapnia,** or carbon dioxide buildup, is believed to be the cause. The increased amount of carbon dioxide reduces corneal pH and subsequently causes the blebs.[19]

    G. Corneal metabolism involves the endothelium and epithelium. Whenever there is interference with metabolism, the cornea clouds, and transparency suffers. The cornea must be kept hydrated at 78% water.

        1. Stromal swelling pressure, or **stromal imbibition pressure,** results from the natural characteristic of the stroma to take on water (Figure 1.3). The glycosaminoglycans in the stroma are hydrophilic and absorb fluid like a gel. The endothelium and epithelium act as **passive barriers** to slow down the water leaking through the cornea. The endothelium and epithelium also actively pump the fluid (water). These active **metabolic pumps** move ions through the cornea. An osmotic pressure is created that moves the water through the cornea. The endothelium accounts for 90% of the metabolic pumping action.[19]

        2. Oxygen and **glucose** are actively used by the metabolic pumps. Without the oxygen and glucose, the cornea cannot maintain proper

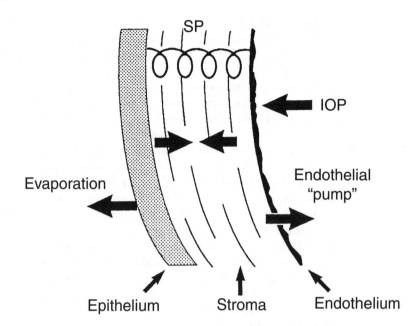

FIGURE 1.3   *Stromal swelling pressure. The stromal swelling pressure (SP) is balanced by the endothelium and epithelial barriers and endothelial metabolic pump system. (IOP = intraocular pressure.) (Reprinted with permission from SD Jaanus. Anti-Edema Drugs. In JD Bartlett, SD Jaanus [eds], Clinical Ocular Pharmacology [3rd ed]. Boston: Butterworth–Heinemann, 1995;370.)*

hydration and edema. The result is swelling. The oxygen demand of the cornea is 9.54 µl/hour/cm^2.[20] Glucose comes mostly from the aqueous humor and is taken up by the endothelium. Glucose is processed by a pathway called **glycolysis** in the mitochondria to yield energy in the form of **adenosine triphosphate (ATP)**. ATP is usable by the metabolic pumps located in the endothelium and epithelium.[21] The net result of glycolysis is two pyruvate molecules and two ATP molecules. The pyruvate molecules are converted to even more ATP through the **citric acid cycle,** or **Krebs' tricarboxylic cycle,** and **oxidative phosphorylation.** Each molecule of glucose nets 38 ATP molecules when oxygen is present.[19] When there is not enough oxygen, only two molecules of ATP are made through the **Embden-Meyerhof** anaerobic glycolysis pathway.[1,21] Lack of oxygen, or **hypoxia,** leads to inefficient metabolic pumping and subsequent corneal edema.

3. **Epithelial edema,** or **Sattler's veil,** results from **lactate** buildup between epithelial cells. **Hypoxia** leads to a buildup of the lactate

waste product. Its formation causes pyruvate to increase, slowing down glycolysis and ATP formation. Lactate buildup is believed to draw water out of cells into the extracellular spaces by osmosis. The increased extracellular space scatters light and causes hazy vision.

4. **Superficial punctate keratitis** resulting from hypoxia is caused by premature desquamation of epithelial cells. The cells are stressed and form gaps that stain. Hypoxia inhibits the healing process involving cell migration and mitosis.

5. **Stromal swelling** usually accompanies epithelial edema. The swelling can be directly correlated with oxygen permeability (Dk/L or Dk/t) when wearing a contact lens. Lower Dk/L or Dk/t have higher amounts of swelling.[19] Reduction of the metabolic pump system can be attributed to hypoxia, acidosis (related to carbon dioxide buildup), and lactate. All of these factors contribute to stromal swelling.[19] **Vertical striae** appear when the stroma contains more than 5% of swelling, and **folds in Descemet's membrane** appear when the stroma contains more than 10% of swelling.[22] The appearance of these conditions can help determine the amount of swelling (see Chapter 15).

6. **Corneal sensitivity** is reduced under hypoxic conditions as seen with polymethyl methacrylate (PMMA) lens wear. Many times with PMMA rehabilitation, the cornea regains lost sensitivity when hypoxia is relieved.[23] Patients who formerly wore PMMA lenses sometimes complain of sensing more foreign body sensations than they sensed before switching to gas-permeable lenses. These patients are usually experiencing increased corneal sensitivity because their eyes are healthier.

7. **Microcysts** and **neovascularization** are other effects of hypoxia (see Chapter 15). **Epithelial thinning** is also seen.

IV. The **limbus** is the transition area between the bulbar conjunctiva, sclera, and cornea. It is considered a safety zone to help maintain corneal stability.[24] There is a great immunologic response in the limbus. The limbal epithelium is approximately 12 layers thick, unlike the corneal epithelium, which has five or six layers.

A. The **vascular arcade,** or **limbal arcade,** is a series of blood vessels within the limbus. **Limbal hyperemia** is increased blood flow and distention of the limbal arcade. A low-grade limbal hyperemia is common with extended lens wearers, especially on awakening.[9] **Vessel penetration** beyond the limbus into the cornea usually indicates active inflammation. A closed-end plexus at the leading edge during vessel penetration into the cornea indicates a nonprogressive state. An open-ended plexus with twiglike, branching projections indicates an active and progressive state. **Vascular pannus** is vascularization and connective tissue deposition beneath the epithelium, commonly in the superior limbus.[25]

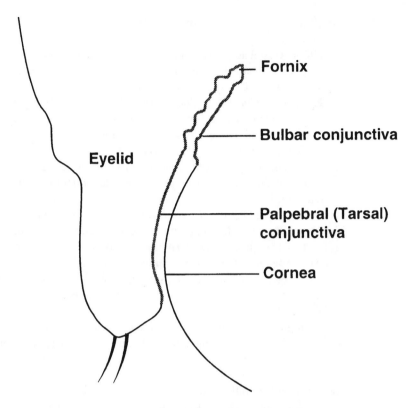

FIGURE 1.4   *The conjunctiva is divided into three sections: palpebral, fornix, and bulbar. (Reprinted with permission from GE Oliver CJ, Quinn, JJ Thimons. Diseases of the Conjunctiva. In JD Bartlett, SD Jaanus [eds], Clinical Ocular Pharmacology [3rd ed]. Boston: Butter-worth–Heinemann, 1995;632.)*

    B. **Immunologic factors** are very active in the highly vascular limbal area.[24] The area is rich with macrophages, neutrophils, mast cells, and immunoglobins.[4] The greatest concentration of **Langerhans' cells** makes the limbus the most immunologically reactive area of the eye. These cells are the most peripheral arm of the immune system and function as the first afferent and last efferent component.[10,26]

  V. The **conjunctiva** is a mucous membrane made up of connective tissue (**substantia propria,** or **stroma**) and epithelium. At the limbus, the conjunctival stroma becomes the palisades of Vogt. The blood supply is through the ophthalmic artery by way of the palpebral arcades and anterior ciliary arteries. It is innervated by branches of the ophthalmic nerve.[27] The conjunctiva consists of three different sections: palpebral, fornix, and bulbar (Figure 1.4).

A. Tear film components are produced in glands and cells residing in the conjunctiva.

1. **Goblet cells** that produce mucus are located in the conjunctiva. The mucous layer of the tear film originates from the goblet cells.[1] Most of the cells are located near the fornix.[26,27]

2. **Epithelial cells** also produce mucus of a different quality. Whenever the eye is stressed, a thicker type of mucus is produced. The thicker epithelial mucus is seen in conditions such as giant papillary conjunctivitis and allergic conjunctivitis.

3. The **accessory glands of Krause** and **Wolfring** are in the deeper layers of the conjunctiva and produce the aqueous layer of the tear film.[1]

B. The **morphology** of the tarsal conjunctiva consists of **papillae** and **follicles.** Clinically, it best appears with lid eversion and fluorescein staining. The tarsal conjunctiva has been categorized as having small or large features, the features being papillae and follicles. Studies have shown that soft contact lenses increase the size and variability of already large papillae and follicles while decreasing the size of already small papillae and follicles.[28]

C. Immunologic cells are numerous in the conjunctiva. Within the substantia propria, there are lymphocytes, lymphoid follicles, neutrophils, plasma cells, and mast cells.

D. Inflammation of the conjunctiva appears as chemosis, hyperemia, discharge or exudate, follicles, and papillae (see Chapter 2).

E. Normal flora are *Staphylococcus epidermidis, Staphylococcus aureus,* and *Corynebacterium.* Other microorganisms seen are *Streptococcus pneumoniae, Haemophilus influenzae, Pseudomonas aeruginosa,* and members of the viridans group of streptococci.[26]

REFERENCES

1. Bier N, Lowther GE. Anatomy and Physiology of the Cornea and Related Structures. In N Bier, GE Lowther (eds), Contact Lens Correction. London: Butterworths, 1977;3–25.

2. Milder B. The Lacrimal Apparatus. In RA Moses (ed), Adler's Physiology of the Eye (7th ed). St. Louis: Mosby, 1981;16–37.

3. Wilson G. Tear Layer Composition and Properties. In ES Bennett, BA Weissman (eds), Clinical Contact Lens Practice. Philadelphia: Lippincott, 1991(1);1–12.

4. Allansmith MR, Ross RN. Immunology of the Anterior Segment. In ES Bennett, BA Weissman (eds), Clinical Contact Lens Practice. Philadelphia: Lippincott, 1991(8);1–6.

5. Doane MG, Gleason WJ. Tear Layer Mechanics. In ES Bennett, BA Weissman (eds), Clinical Contact Lens Practice. Philadelphia: Lippincott, 1993(2);1–17.

6. Moses RA. The Eyelids. In RA Moses (ed), Adler's Physiology of the Eye (7th ed). St. Louis: Mosby, 1981;1–15.

7. Bartlett JD, Melore GG. Diseases of eyelids. In JD Bartlett, SD Jaanus, (eds). Clinical Ocular Pharmacology. Boston: Butterworth–Heinemann, 1995;561–600.

8. Mandell RB. Anatomy and Physiology of the Cornea. In RB Mandell (ed), Contact Lens Practice. Springfield, IL: Thomas, 1988;23–80.

9. Guillon M, Ruben M. Extended or Continuous Wear Lenses. In M Ruben, M Guillon (eds), Contact Lens Practice. London: Chapman & Hall 1994;991–1033.

10. Bergmanson JPG. An expert guide to contact lenses and the corneal epithelium. CL Spectrum 1994;9(7):34–41.

11. Miller D, White P. Infectious and inflammatory contact lens complications. CL Spectrum 1995;10(5):40–46.

12. Thoft RA, Friend J. The x, y, z hypothesis of corneal epithelial maintenance. Invest Ophthalmol Vis Sci 1983;24:1442–1443.

13. Barr JT, Testa LM. Corneal epithelium 3 and 9 o'clock staining studied with the specular microscope. ICLC 1994;21:105–110.

14. Mathers WD, Sachdev MS, Petroll M, et al. Morphological effects of contact lens wear on the corneal surface. CLAO J 1992;18:49–52.

15. Bergmanson JPG. Corneal Epithelium. In ES Bennett, BA Weissman (eds), Clinical Contact Lens Practice. Philadelphia: Lippincott, 1991(4);1–16.

16. Bergmanson JPG. Histopathological analysis of the corneal epithelium after contact lens wear. J Am Optom Assoc 1987;58:812–818.

17. Waltman SR. The Cornea. In RA Moses (ed), Adler's Physiology of the Eye (7th ed). St. Louis: Mosby, 1981;38–62.

18. Huff JW. Corneal Stroma. In ES Bennett, BA Weissman (eds), Clinical Contact Lens Practice. Philadelphia: Lippincott, 1991(41);1–10.

19. Bonnano JA, Polse KA. Hypoxic Changes in the Corneal Epithelium and Stroma. In A Tomlinson (ed), Complications of Contact Lens Wear. St. Louis: Mosby, 1992;21–36.

20. Tomlinson A. Oxygen Requirements of the Cornea. In A Tomlinson (ed), Complications of Contact Lens Wear. St. Louis: Mosby, 1992;3–20.

21. Efron N, Brennan NA. Corneal Oxygen Consumption and Hypoxia. In ES Bennett, BA Weissman (eds), Clinical Contact Lens Practice. Philadelphia: Lippincott, 1991(7);1–14.

22. Efron N. Clinical management of corneal edema. CL Spectrum 1986;1(12):13–23.

23. Ruskell GL. Anatomy and Physiology of the Cornea and Related Structures. In AJ Phillips, J Stone (eds), Contact Lenses (3rd ed). London: Butterworth, 1989;34–71.

24. Grohe RM. A complete guide to detecting and managing limbal complications. CL Spectrum 1994;9(6):26.

25. Efron N. Vascular response of the cornea to contact lens wear. J Am Optom Assoc 1987;58:836–846.

26. Oliver GE, Quinn CJ, Thimons JJ. Diseases of the Conjunctiva. In JD Bartlett, SD Jaanus (eds), Clinical Ocular Pharmacology. Boston: Butterworth–Heinemann, 1995;631–678.

27. Ruskell GL. The Conjunctiva. In ES Bennett, BA Weissman (eds), Clinical Contact Lens Practice. Philadelphia: Lippincott, 1991(3);1–18.

28. Potvin RJ, Doughty MJ, Fonn D. Tarsal conjunctival morphometry of asymptomatic soft contact lens wearers and non–lens wearers. ICLC 1994;21:225–231.

Chapter 2

Anterior Segment Disease and Contact Lenses

Arlene A. Orehek, Joseph P. Shovlin, and Michael D. DePaolis

This chapter discusses numerous anterior segment conditions that can be related to non-contact lens wear problems. The contact lens practitioner should be well versed in lens applications for congenital or acquired conditions when indicated. In addition, he or she should be familiar with the differential diagnosis of anterior segment problems in the contact lens wearer that includes some well-defined non-contact lens–related conditions. Often, non-contact lens–related pathology can mimic contact lens–induced anterior segment conditions.

I. **Congenital abnormalities** are abnormalities in development. New research suggests an arrest in neural crest cell development rather than mesodermal dysgenesis in the third trimester of pregnancy causes congenital abnormalities.[1] The clinician is often called on to fit certain congenital problems such as aniridia, coloboma, etc.

A. **Megalocornea** is a larger than normal cornea. It has a visible horizontal iris diameter of **13 mm or more.** Ninety percent of megalocorneas occur in males and are usually bilateral. Often, there is a high refractive error, especially with astigmatism. Occasionally, there is iridodonesis, a tremulous, unstable iris. The most important clinical management consideration is intraocular pressure (IOP) monitoring. The risk of **elevated IOP** is increased with megalocornea. Increased IOP may occur congenitally or at any age. IOP should be monitored every 3–6 months for patients younger than 5–6 years of age and annually thereafter for a lifetime.[1] **Buphthalmos** may also occur in association with neurofibromatosis or Sturge-Weber syndrome. A large, flat (16 mm) soft lens provides the best centration.

B. **Microcornea** is a smaller than normal cornea. It has a visible horizontal iris diameter of **10 mm or less.** Microcornea is often associated with systemic or ocular syndromes, and the patient should be referred for a pediatric evaluation.[2] There is an association with high refractive errors, and approximately 20% have a risk of **increased IOP** by adulthood.[1] A cornea with microcornea is often very steep. Choose an appropriately steep base curve.

II. **Corneal dystrophies** are primary diseases of the cornea. They are usually inherited as **autosomal dominant** traits but some are recessive, so the sex distribution is a roughly equal.[1-3] They are bilateral, symmetric, and mostly centrally located. Dystrophies are avascular. Onset is early, usually during the first or second decades of life. Most dystrophies develop slowly or are stable so that the visual acuity is not drastically changed throughout a person's life. A few can result in debilitating visual function and can be painful, however. Most dystrophies primarily involve one layer of the cornea, and some may involve more. Diagnosis is based on clinical appearance and careful biomicroscopic examination to assess the corneal layers involved.

   A. **Epithelial layer dystrophies** are dystrophies that affect the most anterior layer of the cornea.

      1. **Epithelial basement membrane dystrophy (EBMD),** also known as **Cogan's dystrophy** or **map-dot-fingerprint dystrophy,** consists of grayish patches (maps), clear or white microcysts (dots), or swirls or refractile lines (fingerprints) within the epithelium.[1] The three types of lesions do not necessarily occur together, but 50% of affected patients have more than one type, generally in the central epithelium.[3,4] Lesions are best seen by retroillumination (Figure 2.1). Although most patients remain asymptomatic, epithelial erosions occur in approximately 10% of all cases and cause great pain.[3,4] Erosions heal in 1–2 weeks but can recur. They become less frequent with time and stop after 1–3 years.[3] Patients are symptomatic in varying degrees on awakening in the morning.[1] Symptoms include severe pain, photophobia, and reduced visual acuity due to irregular astigmatism.[2] Most patients have good vision, but dystrophic changes over the pupil can reduce vision to 20/50 or worse.[3] Negative staining presents early on before any other symptoms.[1] EBMD affects many women older than 30.[2] EBMD may also be acquired as a sequela from an infection or surgery.[3] Management is to treat the erosions with hypertonic drops, ointment, or both every 3–4 hours, to apply a high-water soft bandage contact lens if needed, and to consider photorefractive keratectomy (PTK) in severe cases.[1]

      Pearl: Rigid lenses often help improve acuity and are not contraindicated for EBMD unless there is erosion of the epithelium with or without lenses.

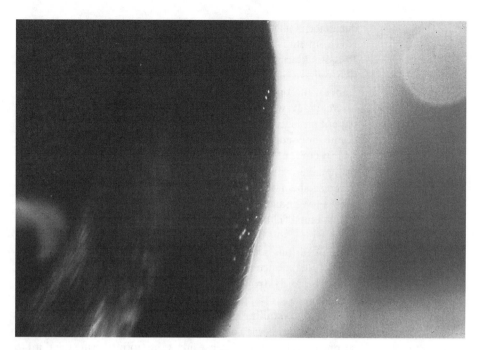

FIGURE 2.1 *Epithelial basement membrane dystrophy. Refractile lines are evident in this patient, with map-dot-fingerprint dystrophy of the epithelium. The retractile lines are often best seen with indirect retroillumination after pupil dilation.*

 2. **Meesmann's juvenile epithelial dystrophy** is bilateral, with symmetric, tiny, cystlike, irregular, clear vesicles in the epithelium that may extend to the limbus. Vesicles are best seen under indirect retroillumination and appear as tiny round or oval bubblelike blebs that form a concentric cluster or focal wedge near the limbus.[2,4] Onset is early, and the patient may be asymptomatic until the third or fourth decade of life. Cysts may cause irregular astigmatism.[2] Generally, visual acuity is quite good. Epithelial erosions may occur, causing transient blur and discomfort.[1,2,4] Management is to treat the erosions if they occur by conventional treatment.[1] Coarse punctate epithelial keratopathy, bleb patterns of EBMD, vapor spray keratitis, and mild corneal edema can mimic Meesmann's vesicles.[3]

B. **Bowman's layer dystrophies** are dystrophies that affect the second most anterior layer of the cornea.

 1. **Anterior mosaic dystrophy (anterior crocodile shagreen)** resembles crocodile skin with central gray polygonal opacities with clear spaces. This dystrophy disappears with limbal pressure and returns when it is removed. This may be a transient finding, similar to a vertical epithelial furrow, associated with **contact lens wear**

due to the ocular surface pressure, and not the result of a dystrophy. No treatment is indicated.[1]

2. **Reis-Bucklers dystrophy** presents with irregular fishnet or thread-like swirls with superficial stromal opacification.[1] In other instances, the opacities take on a more mottled appearance, with discrete gray-white macular spots or linear opacities in a swirling pattern projecting into the epithelium. It is a bilateral, autosomal-dominant condition with early onset. This condition is associated with **recurrent epithelial erosions** and can be painful. Recurrent epithelial erosion usually decreases by the age of 30, possibly due to replacement of Bowman's layer with scar tissue. The cornea becomes rough and irregular and usually affects the visual acuity.[2] Management is to treat the erosions with hypertonic drops and patch with a soft bandage lens. In severe cases, consider keratectomy of fibrous scar tissue to improve vision, PTK, and keratoplasty.[1] Recurrence rates after surgical procedures are high.

C. **Anterior stromal dystrophies** are dystrophies that affect the anterior third of the cornea.

1. In **central crystalline dystrophy,** also known as **Schnyder's dystrophy,** central cornea crystals form an annulus during the first to second decade of life. A dense arcus ring forms during the third to fourth decade. This is the only dystrophy associated with a **systemic hypercholesterolemia.**[3] Visual acuity may be mildly affected. Management is to refer the patient for a systemic workup for cholesterol and lipids. Ocular signs are permanent, but there is a good prognosis systemically with proper controls.[1]

2. **Congenital hereditary stromal dystrophy** is a nonprogressive clouding of the central anterior stroma. Stromal opacities are feathery and fading in intensity as they approach the periphery. This is congenital and bilateral. Visual impairment may lead to **nystagmus** and **esotropia.** Keratoplasty should be performed within the first 2 months of life.[2]

3. **Granular dystrophy (Groenouw's type I)** produces focal white translucent spots resembling cornflakes or bread crumbs.[1,2] The spots have a glassy texture and have a clear stroma in between; they are usually 0.2–0.4 mm in diameter.[2] These spots usually lie in a random distribution but sometimes coalesce into linear or arcuate chains.[2,3] They generally appear by the first decade of life, and over time lesions enlarge and increase in number into the deeper layers of the cornea.[2] Visual acuity can be reduced to 20/200 or worse. The white deposits are composed of noncollagenous, irregularly shaped hyalin.[4] Keratoplasty may be needed, and recurrence is common.[1] Recurrent erosions may occur.[2] **Rigid contact lenses** for increased acuity are often necessary due to anterior surface distortion.

4. **Lattice dystrophy** is divided into three types.[2–4] Lattice type I is characterized by central, anterior stromal refractile lines appearing in the first decade.[1] Lattice type II is associated with **amyloid** deposition throughout the body, resulting in lattice lines.[1,2] Lattice type III develops later in life.[2] Lattice lines thicken, bend, and become more opaque, with a ropy, ground-glass appearance. Characteristics of branching pipe-stemmed lesions are seen at all levels of the stroma with peripheral sparing.[3] There may be a central haze after the third or fourth decade of life.[1] Lattice dystrophy is autosomal-dominant, symmetric, and bilateral.[3,4] Lattice lines are composed of amyloid fibrils 8–10 microns in diameter deposited between the collagen lamellae of the stroma.[2] Lattice dystrophy may become painful, with the thickening of the lines leading to erosion of the overlying epithelium.[2,4] Management is to treat the erosions and consider keratoplasty or PTK with severe acuity loss.[1] Recurrence after these procedures is not uncommon. Contact lenses may be of some value.

5. **Combined granular-lattice dystrophy (Avellino's dystrophy)** is a dystrophy combining common features of granular and lattice dystrophies. The mutation site is located on chromosome 5 for both granular and lattice dystrophies.[2,4]

D. **Full-thickness stromal dystrophies** are dystrophies that affect the entire third layer of the cornea.

1. **Fleck dystrophy** presents with gray to white dandrufflike opacities in wreath-shaped rings with clear centers[2] or comma-shaped spots.[1] Opacities vary in size, shape, and depth. All have distinct margins, which may extend to the periphery.[1,2] This dystrophy is either congenital or has an onset by the age 2. Lesions remain stable. The condition may be associated with a congenital lens opacity, decreased corneal sensation, **keratoconus, limbal dermoid,** and **pseudoxanthoma elasticum.**[1,2] No treatment is indicated.[1]

2. **Macular dystrophy (Groenouw's type II)** presents with diffuse stromal haze, focal gray or white stromal opacities with irregular edges, and irregular Descemet's membrane with corneal guttata.[1,2,4] The dystrophy begins in the central portion of the anterior layers of the stroma, extending to the endothelium and limbus by the second decade of life.[1,2] It resembles ground-glass cloudiness; patches become larger and more confluent with age[3] and can be confused in early stages with a granular dystrophy.[1,4] **Macular dystrophy** is bilateral and symmetric. This is an autosomal-recessive trait.[1] Subepithelial opacities cause elevations, creating an irregular corneal surface.[2] Visual acuity may be reduced by age 30.[1] It is associated with corneal guttata and, superficially, a secondary corneal erosion. Management is to treat the erosions and consider kerato-

plasty with severe visual reduction. Bandage lenses are often an important adjunct.[1]

3. **Congenital hereditary stromal dystrophy** consists of congenital diffuse bilateral flaky-feathery opacities of the stroma, which have been described as distinct entities. This autosomal dominantly inherited dystrophy manifests as a central superficial and deep corneal clouding associated with normal corneal thickness and a relatively clear periphery. It is symmetric and nonprogressive. The early visual deprivation usually results in a searching **nystagmus** accompanied by **esotropia.** Keratoplasty improves acuity, but seldom to better than 20/200 unless performed within the early weeks after birth.[4]

E. **Deep stromal dystrophies** are dystrophies that affect the posterior portion of the third layer of the cornea.

1. **Central cloudy (François) dystrophy** presents with fuzzy gray areas with indistinct margins in a polygonal pattern located in deep central stroma.[1,2] No treatment is indicated, since it rarely affects the vision and is considered nonprogressive. The oval stromal opacity occupies the central third of the cornea and leaves the periphery clear. Corneal thickness and sensation remain normal.[3–5]

2. **Central crystalline dystrophy** appears with fine, needle-shaped crystals forming an oval, discoid, or annular central opacity. Onset is early, within the first decade of life, and becomes stable after the second or third decade of life. Stroma remains clear aside from opacities and a dense corneal arcus and limbal girdle. Visual reduction is usually minor. Central crystalline dystrophy is associated with **hyperlipidemia.** No treatment is indicated, but serum cholesterol and triglyceride levels should be determined because of the importance of the systemic ramifications of lowering serum cholesterol.[2]

3. **Polymorphic stromal dystrophy** presents with a midstromal extension of punctate and filamentous opacities that seem to depress Descemet's membrane toward the anterior chamber. This appears after the age of 50 and progresses very slowly. Corneal sensation and visual acuity are normal. The linear opacities differ from lattice and genu valgum (bend or curved line), and therefore are an exception to the general rule that dystrophies are isolated corneal disorders.[2] This posterior stromal dystrophy appears later in life, does not affect the epithelium, does not progress, and is not familial.

4. In **posterior amorphous corneal dystrophy,** gray irregular sheets of opacities develop across the deep stroma.[2] Onset is early in the first decade of life.[1] This condition may be associated with an occasional endothelial mosaic alteration and corneal thinning of

about 30%.[2-4] Visual acuity is usually only mildly affected (no worse than 20/40). No treatment is indicated.[1]

5. **Pre-Descemet's dystrophy** presents with deep punctate or filamentous gray opacities.[1] It appears between the fourth and seventh decades of life.[2] The opacities may have dendriform, circular, comma, or linear shapes that indent into Descemet's membrane. All shapes may be found in the same cornea in an annular or diffuse pattern.[1] This condition may be associated with posterior polymorphous dystrophy, keratoconus, central cloudy corneal dystrophy, or EBMD.[2]

F. **Endothelial layer dystrophies** are dystrophies that affect the most posterior, or last, layer of the cornea.

1. **Congenital hereditary endothelial dystrophy** has a diffuse **ground-glass** stromal and epithelial edema that involves the entire cornea.[1-3] There is a **"peau d'orange"** (orange peel) effect similar to that found in Descemet's.[2] Focal stromal macular opacities and discrete white dots sometimes appear. Vascularization may be present.[4] The endothelial mosaic may be irregular to absent.[5] Recessive forms are congenital and stationary with an associated **nystagmus** and **esotropia.**[1,2] The dominant form starts in the first to second decade of life; it is slowly progressive with no nystagmus.[1] This dystrophy may cause pain and photophobia due to epithelial effects. Management, begun at an early age, entails referring the patient for keratoplasty to reduce the risk of amblyopia.[1,5,6]

2. **Corneal guttata** is a focal refractile accumulation of collagen posterior to Descemet's membrane[3,5] (Figure 2.2). It starts as a golden hue and progresses to a bronzed, powdered appearance on the endothelium.[4] Primary corneal guttata occurs in three clinical patterns. A few corneal guttata may pepper the posterior cornea as part of the normal endothelium and aging process. Larger numbers of guttata are often accompanied by pigment, forming confluent patches. As the number of guttata increase, the condition is accompanied by corneal edema in endothelial dystrophy.[5,6] Endothelial cells may become decreased in number and irregular in shape. Some endothelial cells may become five times their normal size. Secondary corneal guttata is associated with trauma, inflammation, and degenerations or dystrophies of the cornea. This is a bilateral and symmetric condition with an autosomal-dominant or indeterminable inheritance pattern.[3,4] Patients with no corneal edema are asymptomatic and require no treatment.[5]

Pearl: *If contact lens wear is necessary, a careful selection of high-oxygen-flux materials is important.*

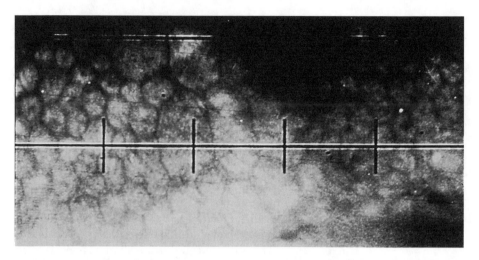

FIGURE 2.2   *Endothelial polymegethism represents significant endothelial morphology in most cases. Polymegethism may be a precursor to reduced cell density. This patient had eight-incision radial keratotomy. The diamond blade, due to its close proximity to the endothelium, has created larger cells with an unusual shape along the incision line. Microperforations are common. (Courtesy of B Weiner, Department of Ophthalmology, University of Maryland, Baltimore.)*

3. **Fuch's endothelial dystrophy,** also known as **late hereditary endothelial dystrophy,** is characterized by **corneal guttata.** It is best seen by retroillumination and is usually asymmetric.[1,5] It is associated with variable stromal and epithelial edema, which may result in microcysts, ground-glass appearance, or bullae.[1] Descemet's membrane may appear thickened and gray.[3] Onset is generally **after 50 years of age,** and the prevalence is higher in females.[1] Visual acuity may be reduced and worsen on awakening because of decreased tear evaporation and increased corneal edema.[1,3] Manage by applying hypertonic drops, ointment, or both; directing warm air from a hair dryer into the eyes in the morning; or using a high-water bandage contact lens. Consider keratoplasty if visual acuity is severely reduced.[1]

   Pearl: It may be prudent to buy time with a bandage lens until a significant cataract develops in order to do a triple procedure. Reducing IOP may lessen edema by allowing less fluid to cross the compromised endothelium into the stroma.[5]

4. **Posterior polymorphous dystrophy** is a dystrophy with grouped vesicles resembling curved linear and geographic lesions of varying shapes producing a "Swiss cheese" pattern with gray thickenings of Descemet's between vesicles. The distribution may be a

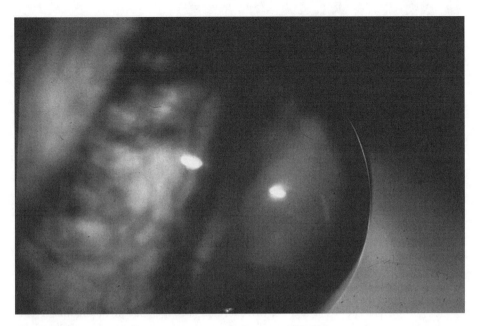

FIGURE 2.3   *Keratoglobus. Keratoglobus represents a significant distortion to a much larger area of the cornea than is typically seen in keratoconus. This patient has rather extensive thinning of the cornea.*

peripheral ring or a focal wedge. Onset is very early (during the first or second decade of life), or may be congenital with a very stable pattern. Visual acuity may be very mildly reduced to 20/30 but can progressively worsen. The condition may be associated with mild stromal or epithelial edema.[1] Generally, edema is less severe than in hereditary endothelial dystrophy.[5] If **iridocorneal adhesions** are present, there is an increased risk of glaucoma.[1,3–5] Manage with hypertonic drops if indicated and annual IOP checks throughout life.[1] Lenses are not contraindicated in this condition.

5. **Keratoconus** is best classified as a **dystrophy** but has some features of degeneration. The central to inferior cornea bulges forward, and thinning is present.[1] It is a bilateral condition, but one eye is usually more involved.[1] The condition may remain stable for a time and begin to progress again later in life.[3,4]

6. **Keratoglobus** is a rare, bilateral condition in which the cornea is of normal diameter and a large area becomes ectatic (Figure 2.3). The stroma becomes thin and sometimes Descemet's membrane ruptures, producing acute **hydrops** and, consequently, irregular myopic astigmatism.[1,3]

III. **Degenerations of the cornea** occur secondary to aging or as a sequela to some other corneal disorder. Sometimes degenerations resemble dystrophies, especially in the rare familial form.[3] Their location can be central or peripheral. Unlike dystrophies, corneal degenerations generally appear **after age 40** and affect mostly the peripheral cornea.[3] These normal changes progress; most are senile changes and are not usually recognized by the patient.[4]

A. **Central degenerations of the cornea** are degenerations that affect the central portion of the cornea. These degenerations will most likely cause a decrease in visual acuity.

   1. **Bullous keratopathy** is an advanced, prolonged epithelial edema with the formation of epithelial **bullae** (bubbling formation) that recurrently break down and reform. It is extremely painful in moderate to severe cases. Eventually, a fibrosis occurs under the bullae, producing a chronically painful and scarred epithelial layer. The most common causes for bullous keratopathy are postoperative complication; **Fuchs' endothelial dystrophy;** and degeneration in which endothelial cells are lost over a lifetime, producing poor corneal dehydration and secondary epithelial edema. Treatment for advanced cases is antiedema therapies, **a soft bandage lens** with **antibiotics,** or PTK in advanced cases.[1]

   2. **Corneal farinata** is a speckling of fine dustlike opacities in the posterior corneal stroma. The deposits may be a degenerative pigment composed of **lipofuscin** that accumulates in cells as a normal aging process.[2,5,6] Visual acuity is usually not affected.[1]

   3. **Mosaic shagreen of Vogt** presents as whitish-gray polygonal opacities separated by clear spaces. It is located centrally in the anterior cornea. Visual acuity may be reduced. Keratoplasty can be considered in severe cases.[2]

   4. **Posterior crocodile shagreen** is a diffuse grayish polygonal degeneration of the posterior corneal surface. Presentation is asymptomatic; no treatment is indicated.[1]

B. **Peripheral degenerations caused by age** are degenerations that affect the peripheral area of the cornea. They are less likely to affect visual acuity.

   1. **Arcus senilis** presents as a broad, whitish, midperipheral ring of lipid substances (Figure 2.4). It is found at the level of Bowman's layer; there is a clear zone between this layer and the limbus. The condition is very common, with 50% of the population affected by age 50 and 100% by age 80.[1] Arcus is asymptomatic, usually bilateral, and more pronounced among blacks. If it appears in those younger than 40 years old, risk factors for **hyperlipidemias** and **atherosclerosis** should be ruled out.[1,2] It is considered a cardiovascular risk factor in patients older than age 40 when it occurs in combination with other classic risk factors, such as a family his-

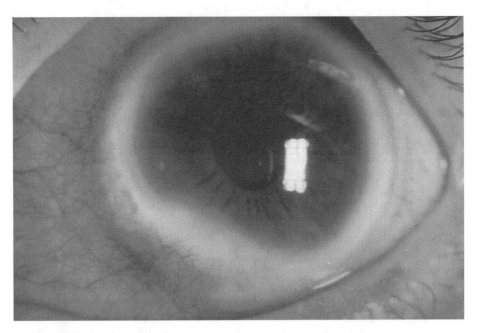

FIGURE 2.4   *Arcus senilis in a young patient with a familial history of lipidemia. The serum levels of this patient should be monitored.*

tory of cardiovascular disease, hypertension, obesity, a diet of polyunsaturated fats, stress, smoking, and lack of exercise.[1] Juvenile arcus occurs in children with **familial lipidemia, megalocornea,** or **blue sclera.**[3]

2. **Cogan's microcystic degeneration** presents as peripheral single or grouped 1- to 2-mm clearish, gray intraepithelial microcysts. It may be unilateral or bilateral and is found in older males. It can be painful if spontaneous **epithelial erosions** occur. Asymptomatic cases should be monitored every 6–12 months; acute erosions can be treated the same as EBMD.[1]

3. **Dellen** are focal, peripheral, saucer-shaped **depressions** approximately half the corneal thickness, producing a "holelike" appearance.[1] Thinning occurs in the epithelium, Bowman's layer, and superficial stroma.[3] Borders are sloped and adjacent to the limbus, frequently in the 3 o'clock and 9 o'clock positions. Size is usually 0.5–1.0 mm in diameter.[1] Dellen are usually transient, lasting only 24–48 hours, but they may last for weeks and lead to scarring.[3] Epithelium remains intact and tissue remains clear or slightly hazy. Dellen are usually associated with an adjacent raised mass such as the thick edge of a **hard contact lens,** or **pterygium.** When possible, the condition should be treated to remove or reduce the cause of

the mass. Protection can be achieved by lubrication, a soft bandage lens, and lid closure. If no treatment is indicated, monitor yearly.[1]

4. **Droplet keratopathy** is the presence of fine, oily-appearing droplets at the limbal areas. This is somewhat common in **agricultural workers** in southern areas of the United States. The cause is controversial and ill-defined but may be related to environmental trauma such as **ultraviolet light, dust,** and **excessive heat.**[3,4,6] PTK may be beneficial for these patients.

5. **Hassall-Henle bodies** are thickenings of Descemet's membrane producing small, round, peripheral endothelial indentations.[1] The thickenings are due to an overproduction of hyaline by the endothelial cells.[2] The condition is identical to **guttata,** which occurs centrally and is associated with edema.[2] **Fuchs' endothelial dystrophy** should not be confused with this condition. No treatment is indicated.[1]

6. **Marginal furrow degeneration** is a bilateral thinning with an associated arcus ring located in the peripheral cornea adjacent to the limbus. Furrow is diagnosed by a depression between arcus ring and limbal border. Sodium fluorescein may pool in the furrow but will not stain because the epithelium remains intact. No treatment is indicated. Remember to rule out Mooren's ulcer, rheumatoid disease, and pellucid and Terrien's marginal degenerations.[1]

7. **Mooren's ulceration** is a chronic progressive marginal ulcer diagnosed by exclusion. It begins as an infiltrate in the anterior stroma and destroys the epithelium. The ulcer then spreads circumlimbally and axially. Some areas of the ulcer are active and inflamed, whereas others seem to be healing.[4] The ulcer runs a course of 3–12 months and can recur. There are two forms, a **unilateral form** that occurs in older people and is less severe, and a **bilateral form** that occurs in younger patients is very severe, and sometimes leads to **perforation.**[1,4] It can greatly reduce visual acuity.[4] Mooren's ulcer responds poorly to therapies, including steroids.[1] The prognosis is poor and the patient should be referred to a corneal specialist.

8. **Pellucid marginal degeneration** presents as inferior corneal thinning near the limbus.[1] This may be an anomaly of connective tissue and has been seen in patients with **skeletal abnormalities.**[3] It is very rare, asymptomatic, and occasionally associated with keratoconus.[1,3] The hallmark sign is an **against-the-rule irregular astigmatism.**[1,3,4]

9. **Pterygium** is a thick, yellowish, triangular mass of tissue growing onto the nasal corneal surface. It is usually rich in surface vascularization and cosmetically unappealing. Subacute symptoms are irritation, foreign body sensation, and reduced vision. Ultraviolet light exposure stimulates pterygia. A ferric (orange-

brown) line called **Stocker's line** may occasionally be seen at the leading corneal edge. The pterygium should be assessed if it is stable or progressive. Recheck the patient every 6–12 months, remembering to measure and diagram the pterygium. Asymptomatic, stable patients require no treatment. If the patient is symptomatic and stable, treatment may include vasoconstrictors, lubrication, and corrective lenses for induced astigmatism and ultraviolet tints. If the condition is progressive or cosmetically unacceptable, recommend surgical intervention. Contact lens wear is not contraindicated.[1,3,4]

10. **Terrien's marginal degeneration** is unilateral or bilateral superior nasal thinning of the peripheral cornea. It has a painful presentation and occurs in males 20–50 years old.[1,4] Bowman's layer and the corneal lamellae may split.[3] **Vascularizing peripheral infiltration** is followed by stromal thinning.[3,4] The thinning may progress circumlimbally and have lipid deposits in the center. Any slight trauma can lead to perforation of this area of marked thinning.[1,4] This condition usually stabilizes with a permanent scar after the initial attack.[1] If thinning becomes extreme, a full-thickness keratoplasty is indicated.[4] Visual deterioration may be due to marked **irregular astigmatism.**[3]

11. **White limbal girdle of Vogt** is a narrow band of fine crystal-like opacities along intrapalpebral regions of nasal or temporal limbal borders of the cornea at the level of Bowman's layer. It is **asymptomatic,** bilateral, and common in women older than age 50. No treatment is indicated.[1,3]

C. **Degenerations not caused by age** are degenerations that may occur at any age.
1. **Band keratopathy** is a whitish-yellow haze of **calcium** accumulation having a Swiss cheese appearance in the intrapalpebral band region of the cornea.[1] The band begins in the corneal periphery and affects the central cornea last.[4] Calcium is deposited in the epithelium, Bowman's layer, and anterior stroma, leaving the remainder of the cornea layers clear.[3] Patients are asymptomatic in early development and progress to symptoms in late stages with painful epithelial erosions. Manage with lubrication for mildly symptomatic presentation and **chelation** with ethylenediaminetetraacetic acid (EDTA), PTK, or penetrating keratoplasty for severe symptoms. Suspicious development should be monitored every 3–4 months. Still's triad, **hyperparathyroidism** (hypercalcemia), and **vitamin D intoxication** should be ruled out.[1,3,4,6]

2. **Coat's white ring** is a ring of iron deposits usually circling related **metallic foreign bodies.** Deposits are found at Bowman's layer or in the superficial stroma.[3]

3. **Corneal amyloidosis** is an amyloid protein defect produced by genetically defective or stressed cells called keratocytes in the stroma. It is deposited in an abnormally thin epithelium. This stains with crystal violet or methyl violet and fluoresces with thioflavine.[3] There is a decrease in visual acuity, and the condition can be painful if corneal erosions develop. Keratoplasty is the preferred treatment. Prognosis is poor for the transplanted cornea, however, because it often develops the same condition.[4]

4. **Climatic droplet keratopathy** appears as fine, oily-appearing droplets at the limbal area. First described in Labrador, it is most often found in **agricultural workers** in the U.S. South.[3] It may be related to environmental trauma or **exposure to ultraviolet light, dust,** and **heat.**[3,4] These factors seem to cause elastic degeneration of the cornea and conjunctiva and deposits of fibroblasts.[4]

5. **Hyaline degeneration** is indicated by yellowish-brown granular opacities appearing in the lower half of the cornea in the shape of a band. This occurs in a geographic pattern and is related to climatic conditions.[3]

6. **Keloid formation** is indicated by white deposits that result in excessive fibrocytic activity originating in the stromal cells. Consider keratoplasty in severe cases when indicated.[3]

7. **Lipid degeneration** is a whitish-yellow degeneration with feathery edges. Lipid deposits are laid down after necrosis; vascularization of the cornea; and in certain diseases, such as **herpes zoster.** Deposits are usually bilateral and central. Consider PTK when necessary, but note that deposits sometimes recur in the donor tissue.[4]

8. **Salzmann's nodular degeneration** consists of bilateral formations of elevated grayish blue nodules peripherally or centrally on the corneal surface.[1] It is a rare degeneration that follows a variety of inflammations, especially **phlyctenular** disease and **trachoma.**[3,4] It occurs in a scarred area or at the edge of a corneal transplant.[1] Epithelium may chronically break down over the nodules, which are composed of hyaline material. Pain occurs in areas of destruction of Bowman's layer and subjacent stroma.[1,4] Vision depends on the location and number of nodules. If asymptomatic, no treatment is indicated. A bandage contact lens is used for symptomatic patients. Consider PTK for severe cases.[1]

IV. **Pigmentations** of the cornea can present in numerous ways. The clinician must be able to recognize when they are due to contact lens wear and when they are not.

A. **Arlt's triangle** is a brownish triangular-shaped pigment deposit at the inferior position on the posterior cornea.[1]

B. **Brawny edema** is a brownish edematous haze in the epithelium that is suggestive of EBMD or recurrent corneal erosions.[1]

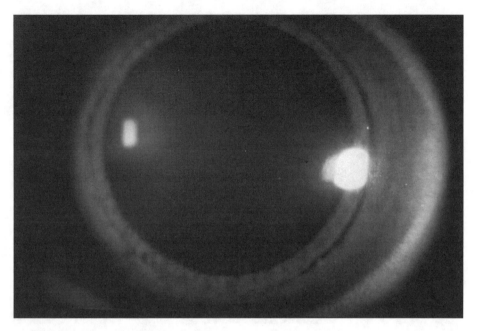

FIGURE 2.5   *Fleischer's line. Iron deposition in keratoconus falls in the basal layer of the epithelium and serves as a guide for the surgeon in penetrating keratoplasty (since it demarcates the base of the cone). Histologically, it is present in most cases of keratoconus and can be detected by slit lamp examination about two-thirds of the time.*

C. **Ferry's line** is a line of orange-brown ferric ions around a surgical filtering bleb.[1]

D. **Fleischer's line** is iron deposition of deep epithelium surrounding the base of the cone found in **keratoconus.** It is frequently incomplete. Blue light makes the ring look darker and more visible[3,4,6] (Figure 2.5).

E. **Goar's line** is pigment granules forming a horizontal line on the inferior posterior cornea; it is suggestive for **pigmentary glaucoma.**[1,6]

F. **Hemosiderosis** is intracorneal or posterior corneal blood staining. It appears after corneal **neovascularization** or **hyphema.**[1,6]

G. A **Hudson-Stähli line** is an orange-brown iron line at the level of the basement membrane of the epithelium in the band region of the normal cornea.[1] It is a roughly horizontal line found in the middle third of the cornea. It is common in older corneas and injured corneas at any age.[3,4,6]

H. A **Kayser-Fleischer ring** is an orange-brown coloration in the posterior cornea ring. It is seen at the level of Descemet's. **Copper** deposits are found in long-standing untreated cases of **Wilson's disease**[1,6] (Figure 2.6).

I. **Keratic precipitates** are white or pigmented deposits on the endothelial surface. They are suggestive for uveitis, trauma, or age.[1]

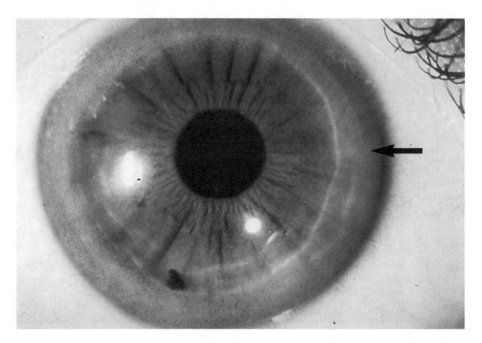

FIGURE 2.6   *Kayser-Fleischer ring (arrow). Wilson's disease is suspected whenever a Kayser-Fleischer ring is found. The ring is annular and is found in the posterior cornea. It signifies copper deposition. Kayser-Fleischer rings are found in Descemet's membrane, whereas Fleischer's line, seen with keratoconus, is in deep epithelium.*

J.   **Keratomelanocystosis** consists of pigmented spokes radiating into the cornea from the limbus. It is seen mostly among blacks and usually appears at the 4 and 8 o'clock positions. Its presence may suggest trauma, infection, or toxic inflammation.[1]

K.   **Krukenberg's spindle** consists of brownish, vertical, spindle-shaped pigment deposits on the posterior cornea. Look for old uveitis or pigment dispersion syndrome and monitor closely for **glaucoma.**[1]

L.   **Melanin** can be deposited in the cornea by patients taking certain systemic drugs. **Phenothiazides** and **chloroquine** can produce fine stippling or whorl-like opacities, respectively, at the layer of Descemet's membrane. Epinephrine can lead to the deposition of adrenochrome in the region of Bowman's layer and the anterior stroma. Trauma can cause pigment deposition in the deeper layers of the epithelium.

M.   **Striate melanokeratosis** occurs when pigment-bearing cells grow from the limbus and remain in the subepithelial peripheral cornea. This is most common in blacks. Melanotic cells can often penetrate far into the deeper cornea in response to stimuli such as trauma, infection, or epithelial breakdown. Pigmentations are permanent and sometimes occur in whorl-like patterns.[3,4]

N.   A **salmon patch** is an orange discoloration of the midstroma in interstitial keratitis. It is pathognomonic for **syphilis.**[1,6]

O.   **Sampaolesi's line** consists of pigment granules deposited at Schwalbe's line. Its presence should make the clinical highly suspicious of **pigmentary glaucoma.**[1]

P.   **Stocker's line** is an orange-brown ferric line at the leading edge of a **pterygium.**[1,4]

Q.   **Tattooing** is variable coloration. It is caused by staining of mucocutaneous membranes by a heavy metallic substance or certain drugs.[1]

R.   **Vortex keratopathy** or **verticillata** is a whorl-like deposition in the epithelium, usually centered in the lower third of the cornea (Figure 2.7). It occurs as a rare congenital disorder unassociated with systemic disease. It is seen much more commonly with **Fabry's disease** or with certain drug treatments, however. These drugs include **phenothiazines, chloroquine, tamoxifen, amiodarone,** and **atovaquone** (used in acquired immune deficiency disease patients; has lipophilic properties). Iodine inclusions are also possible vectors. It is also seen in some contact lens patients using certain solutions.[3]

V.   **Ocular surface disease** usually manifests itself in the contact lens patient as dry eyes (see Chapter 16 for a complete discussion).

A.   **Blepharitis** is a general term for **dermatitis** or **eczema** of the eyelid.[7,8] Inflammation, localized or diffuse, can occur on either the anterior or posterior lid margins and is associated with skin and mucous membrane involvement. Most forms of blepharitis are chronic, but acute forms do exist. Chronic blepharitis is not an isolated problem. Rather, it is one of a group of disorders resulting from disruption of the complex and delicate balance among the eyelids, tear film, and ocular surface. The eyelids are vital to the health of the ocular surface because of their protective function and their role in the production and dispersal of the tear film. Because of the lid's role in producing and distributing the **preocular tear film** (POTF), blepharitis can affect vision by disrupting the surface of the cornea and conjunctiva. There is a strong association between **keratoconjunctivitis sicca (KCS)** and blepharitis. Patients with KCS are more likely to develop blepharitis as a secondary complication.[7] Underlying systemic causes may be associated risk factors for blepharitis. **Seborrheic blepharitis** is associated with seborrheic dermatitis. Atopic dermatitis and psoriasis may also have a blepharitis component. Certain systemic conditions, such as **acne rosacea, chlamydia,** and **viral** infections, may predispose an individual to inflammation of the eyelids. Identifying patients with risk factors for these conditions, offering preventive recommendations, and providing timely intervention help assure high-quality and cost-effective care.[1,7]

1.   **Symptom severity** is related to the degree of inflammation. The milder forms of seborrheic blepharitis may have no associated

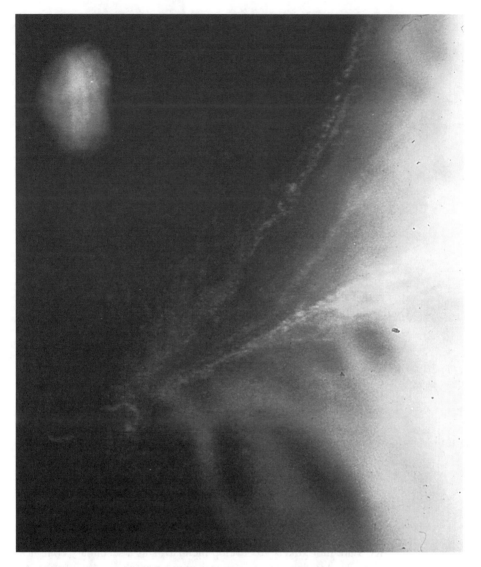

FIGURE 2.7   *Vortex keratopathy in Fabry's disease. Whorl-like depositions occur for several reasons. This patient has lipid inclusions, found in Fabry's disease. The deposition is often in the inferior third of the cornea.*

symptoms. Eyelid margins and dermatologic inflammation can produce various levels of irritation and ocular discomfort. Not only is blepharitis locally painful and cosmetically unappealing, but it causes instability of the POTF, the source of problems related to dry eye. Associated lacrimal disorders, such as lipid deficiency and excessive tear film debris, can disrupt the stability of the POTF to the extent that vision is affected.[7] **Contact lens wear** can become intolerable.[9]

2. **Signs** also vary with degree of inflammation. The milder forms of blepharitis produce **crusting** and **irritation** of the lid margins. Moderate and severe forms are associated with bacterial infections and chronic meibomian gland changes. In severe meibomianitis, the meibomian glands are clogged and the tear film is deficient in normal lipids. **Staphylococcal** infection of the lid margin produces dermatitis, and there is often an aqueous tear deficiency.

3. **Different forms of blepharitis** can generally be identified and categorized by clinical appearance. Each form of blepharitis has its own epidemiologic characteristics. The most common classifications of blepharitis are described below.[7]

   a. **Staphylococcal blepharitis** is usually caused by *Staphylococcus aureus* or *S. epidermidis,* producing a moderately acute inflammation of relatively short duration. It is more prevalent in warmer climates and often occurs in middle-age females who have no other skin abnormalities. In addition to the hallmark signs of lid swelling, erythema of the margins, scaly **collarettes** at the base of the lashes, and possible skin ulceration, an aqueous-deficient (dry) eye frequently results.[10] **Hordeolums** and **chalazions** may also occur. In the early stages, the symptoms are foreign body sensation, irritation, itching, and mild sticking together of the lids. If the condition becomes chronic, thickened lid margins, trichiasis, madarosis, ectropion, or entropion may result. The lower third of the cornea may have staining, erosions, and infiltrates from exotoxins or a disrupted POTF. An associated bacterial conjunctivitis may develop. Treatment includes an antibiotic ointment to control the infection, along with rigorous lid hygiene. Erythromycin, bacitracin, polymyxin-bacitracin, gentamicin, and tobramycin have been shown to be effective. Antibiotic eye drops can be used, but they do not work as well as ointments because drops are not in contact with the microorganisms long enough to be effective. Artificial tears may also be required to alleviate symptoms. For example, if peripheral arcuate corneal infiltrates are present without epithelial defects, topical steroids may be used along with appropriate antibiotics.

   b. **Seborrheic blepharitis** is also known as **squamous blepharitis.** It is part of a dermatologic condition that includes the scalp, face, and eyebrows, all of which culture an abnormal amount of growth of surface organisms. Although skin inflammation is not necessarily evident, the bases of the cilia are surrounded by greasy, foamy scales called **scrufs.** The symptoms include burning, stinging, itching, and ocular irritation or discomfort. The lids may appear hyperemic at the anterior margin, with the hallmark appearance of scales on the lashes. This condition is usually chronic, but there may be periods of exacerbation and remission. Although there is very little inflammation of the lid margin, **KCS** is frequently present and may contribute to meibomianitis and tear film instability. The application of warm, moist compresses to soften and loosen the crusts is followed by washing with a commercial lid scrub or diluted (1:10) baby shampoo on a facial cloth or cotton swab. Care should be taken not to involve the globe. The scalp and eyebrows should be washed with a selenium antidandruff shampoo.[7]

c. **Seborrheic/staphylococcal blepharitis** is also known as **ulcerative** or mixed blepharitis. Associated with seborrheic dermatitis, it is characterized by secondary keratoconjunctivitis, papillary and follicular hypertrophy, conjunctival injection, and mixed crusting and dry eye. The severity waxes and wanes during the course of the disease. Bacterial cultures are usually positive. Histologic examination reveals chronic, moderate, **nongranulomatous** inflammation. There are frequent episodes of mild to moderate inflammatory reaction. The condition is associated with seborrheic dermatitis. Appropriate ophthalmic antibiotic ointments are required. Later, when the lids are more comfortable, warm compresses and lid scrubs can be added. This treatment serves as acceptable control but rarely effects a cure.

d. **Meibomian seborrheic blepharitis** is identified by the presence of increased meibomian and seborrheic secretions without acute inflammation. Tears are sudsy and foamy, producing a burning sensation, especially in the morning. Itching and tearing are common symptoms. The lid glands are dilated, leading to copious meibomian secretions and bulbar injection. Meibomian openings are dilated in this condition, which is associated with **seborrheic dermatitis.** The bulbar conjunctiva is injected, and often there is associated KCS. The treatment includes warm compresses and a shampoo regimen as for seborrheic blepharitis. In addition, the meibomian glands are massaged or expressed to remove the plugs at the openings. Antibiotic ointments or an antibiotic-steroid combination can be helpful.

e. **Seborrheic blepharitis with secondary meibomianitis** is similar to seborrheic blepharitis but produces sporadic episodes of inflammation. The secondary **meibomianitis** causes blocked meibomian glands and anterior seborrhea. Lipid secretions are of toothpaste consistency, producing an unstable POTF. Cultures reveal the presence of normal flora. The treatment includes both lid hygiene and antibiotic or antibiotic-steroid combination therapy. In resistant cases, systemic tetracycline (up to 1 g/day) or doxycycline (100–200 mg/day) for 3–4 weeks may be needed. It is not unusual for patients with this condition to require lower maintenance doses after tapering. **Tetracycline** or its derivatives should not be given to children (ages 7–12) or to pregnant women.

f. **Meibomian keratoconjunctivitis** or **primary meibomianitis blepharitis** is the most severe lid margin inflammation. Typically occurring in individuals older than 50 years, it shows no predilection for gender and is more common in colder climates. It is frequently associated with acne rosacea and is part of a generalized sebaceous-gland dysfunction that clogs the meibomian openings with desquamated epithelial cells. Because lipid secretions have a melting point higher than the ocular surface temperature, stagnation of free fatty acids within the gland and inspissated openings results in lipid-deficient tear film. As part of a generalized sebaceous gland dysfunction, **meibomian keratoconjunctivitis** is frequently associated with acne rosacea.[7,9] The gland openings are obstructed by desquamated epithelial cells, resulting in a poor POTF that can be identified by rose bengal staining. The tear film is very unstable. This condition responds to warm compresses and massage of the lid to express the meibomian contents. When infection is present, topical antibiotic ointments with or without steroids should be used. Oral **tetracycline** may be beneficial by inhibiting lipolytic enzymes, especially when acne rosacea is present. Improvement should be significant within 1–2 weeks, but a lower maintenance dose may be needed for a longer period.

g. **Angular blepharitis** is a localized on the lid at the outer canthus. The staphylococcal form is typically dry and scaly. The *Moraxella* form caused by the ***Morax-Axenfeld diplobacillus*** is wet and macerated with a whitish, frothy discharge. Both forms are treated with antibiotic ointment.

h. **Demodicosis** is an inflammatory reaction to a common mite that inhabits the follicles of lashes in most of those older than age 50. There are two species of mite. ***Demodex folliculorum,*** present in hair and eyelash follicles, consumes epithelial cells, produces follicular distension and hyperplasia, and increases keratinization, which leads to cuffing of the base of the cilia. ***D. brevis,*** present in sebaceous and meibomian glands, may destroy the glandular cells, produce granulomas in the eyelid, and plug the ducts of the meibomian and other sebaceous glands that affect formation of the lipid tear layer. Demodex are present in the lashes of almost all elderly persons. Demodicosis is usually innocuous. When activated, the symptoms are burning and itching. There is lid margin crusting, loss of lashes, and cuffing at the base of the lashes. The diagnosis can be confirmed by **epilating** a lash from the affected area and examining the follicle under a clinical microscope for the presence of a mite. Treatment with a cotton swab saturated with ether may in some cases be supplemented by the application of antibiotic ointment.

    i. **Pediculosis** is an infestation of the lid margin by pubic lice. The organism or its nits (eggs) can often be seen with the slit lamp. Signs and symptoms include redness of the lid margin and conjunctiva, foreign body sensation, and itching. Covering the lice with ointment is acceptable without first removing the live lice or nits.[7] Even bland ointments used for dry eye and lubrication work, and they also avoid toxicity to the ocular surface. Treat for at least 10 days, and re-examine after stopping treatment for 1 week. Retreating is sometimes necessary, since nits may be resistant and may have hatched in the interval.

> ***Pearl:*** *Fluorescein used for retinal angiography has been applied in the office and seems to eradicate the lice easily. Pediculicide shampoo is encouraged.*

  4. **Treatment** is aimed toward controlling the severity of the inflammation and preventing secondary complications. Lid hygiene, consisting of warm compresses and lid scrubs, is the basis for treating all forms of blepharitis. Acute forms of blepharitis are usually the direct sequelae of infection of the lipid-producing glands that open at the lid margin. Most patients have a significant improvement in symptomology when appropriate hygiene is instituted. Although lid hygiene is essential, it alone may not resolve the problem. Based on the clinical findings, an appropriate anti-infective drug can be administered topically, systemically, or in combination. There is no cure for the chronic forms of blepharitis. Aggressive therapy, including **lid hygiene** and appropriate **anti-infectives,** is required for several weeks at the outset to get the condition under control.[10,11] It is followed by variable amounts of continuing treatment to maintain control of chronic blepharitis. Patients must actively participate in steps to control the inflammatory process. Thorough explanation of the disease and the rationale for the therapy help encourage patient compliance and should be reinforced with a follow-up schedule. In addition, associated conditions, such as seborrhea, staphylococcal involvement, and **rosacea,** should be treated. In the event of exacerbation, early diagnosis and treatment can help minimize the degree of inflammation and infection.

    a. **Prognosis** and **follow-up** visits for treatment of blepharitis may be as frequent as every few days at the outset, tapering off to once or twice a year after stabilization. In the absence of other lid or systemic abnormalities, the first acute staphylococcal episode usually can be expected to resolve completely. The chronic forms of blepharitis may be controlled with daily hygiene and topical medication as needed, and when indicated, a course of systemic medication.

    b. **Contact lens wear** may pose a threat to the compromised ocular surface. Additionally, subjective success with contact lenses may be attenuated by complications of tear film deficiency.[7,12] Conversely, contact lenses may play a role in managing selected disorders of the tear film and ocular surface. Identifying and treating conditions before contact lens fitting and managing potential problems aggressively are prerequisites for success. The clinical presence of **rosacea** in almost all cases **contraindicates** contact lens wear. The strategy to help ensure successful contact lens wear by these patients also requires a comprehensive approach to contact lens fitting. First, the lens diameter, thickness, material, and edge designs must be determined to achieve an adequate relationship between lens and cornea and **minimize blink inhibition.** The recommendation of appropriate wearing schedules with rehydration of the soft contact lenses enhances success. Although tear film deficiencies may complicate or contraindicate contact lens wear, they have a role in managing certain types of ocular surface disease. Applying a hydrogel lens to a dry eye may provide a stable, moist environment for desiccated epithelium. There are associated risks, however, including surface deposits, increased inflammation, and potential for infection.

B. A complete discussion of dry eye can be found in Chapter 16.

C. **Ocular surface disease** is a clinical challenge frequently confronting the ophthalmic practitioner. Because dry-eye syndrome and blepharitis constitute the largest component of the ocular surface diseases, the primary care practitioner needs to understand, examine, diagnose, treat, and manage each condition with a careful view toward each treatment's effect on the ocular surface. Educating patients about dry eye and blepharitis is a key element in successful control of these ocular problems. With careful diagnosis and treatment and proper patient education, the long-term comfort of these patients can be maintained.[7]

VI. **Inflammation** is a complex sequence of events that occurs in injured or compromised tissue. Inflammation usually occurs as a sequela of certain anterior segment diseases. The intensity of response depends on the quantity and contact time of an offending stimulus, the degree of prior exposure, and the characteristics of the host tissue.[13] In summary, an **antigen** activates the immune response, leading to vasodilatation, the inflammatory cascade, and elimination of the unwanted stimulus.[1] All types of inflammation are controlled by neurogenic or nonneurogenic factors. Inflammation involves changes in the caliber of the blood vessels, allowing increases in the movement and function of cells. Communication is necessary to trigger these events and occurs mostly by exogenous and endogenous chemical mediators or messengers. An exogenous messenger outside the body, such as a bacterial product, can cause vascular permeability and chemotaxis of leukocytes. Endogenous mediators are located in the plasma and tissues and are interrelated. The plasma contains the complement cascade, the kinin system, and clotting mechanisms. Endogenous mediators in the tissue are histamine and anaphylactic hypersensitivity.[13] **Histamine** is released in the form of granules from mast cells in allergic, traumatic, and inflammatory events. The large number of histamine granules causes vasodilatation, which is initiated by the metabolization of arachidonic acid though the cyclooxygenase and lipo-oxygenase enzymatic pathways.[1] Vasodilatation causes the endothelial pores of vessels to open and increase capillary permeability. This allows plasma, proteins, and white blood cells to leak from the venules.[13] The neutrophils, lymphocytes, and macrophages emigrate and eliminate the antigen at the site of the damaged tissue.[13] The fluids that escape produce swelling and pain. Infiltration is the emigration of white blood cells. There is often an accumulation of edema at the site of the antigen.[1,14] The types of allergic responses[15] are discussed below:

A. **Type I (an immediate, or anaphylactic) reaction,** is the most common ocular response. Allergens attach to two IgE molecules on the surface of mast cells. This causes the cell membrane to **degranulate** and release vasoactive amines and chemotactic factors. Examples are **hay fever, asthma,** and **atopic dermatitis.**

B. **Type II (cytotoxic) reaction,** is produced by exogenous (microbes) or endogenous (drugs) antigens. IgG, IgM, and complement bind to the antigen, which is then **phagocytized** by the macrophages and natural killer cells. Examples are **drug reactions and reactions that occur in response to transfusions, nephritis, organ transplant,** and autoimmune disease.

C. **Type III (immune-complex) reaction** generally occurs when the antigens are diffusible through blood vessels. IgG and IgM activate complement and produce large **antigen-antibody** complexes. Immune-complex reactions are associated with ocular infiltrative and infectious diseases. Examples are **marginal infiltrates, ulcerations, viral infections,** and **contact lens–related infiltrates.**[14,16]

D. **Type IV (cell-mediated immunity or delayed-type hypersensitivity) reaction** occurs when the antigens are numerous, and over time, cell-mediated immunity is acquired by the buildup of sensitized memory T cells to many antigens. **Phlyctenular keratoconjunctivitis** is an example of a **delayed hypersensitivity** reaction to a microbial antigen. Temporal aspects of inflammation can show clinical differences. **Acute inflammation** occurs hours to days after exposure with greater vasodilatation, vascular permeability, pain, ulceration, and loss of tissue function. **Chronic inflammation** occurs weeks to years after exposure and can be with or without noticeable inflammation. The deeper vessels dilate in chronic inflammation, and redness may not be too noticeable. Chronic inflammation produces fibrinization, granulomatous formation, tissue hardening, pannus, neovascularization, and tissue necrosis.[1] A necrotizing inflammatory response can produce considerable tissue damage and can be seen in corneal melting, perforation, and ulcers.[13] The inflammation can be a local reaction without much tissue damage. This is mostly found in reactions to **solution preservatives.**[13] The limbus is rich in mast cells and capillaries. The cornea serves as a site of deposition for circulating immune complexes. Corneal infiltrates are aggregated neutrophils, macrophages, and lymphocytes that migrate from the inflamed host tissue. Corneal infiltrates localize within the epithelium, subepithelium, or stroma. Corneal infiltrates may also be induced by the presence of viruses, contact lens solution preservatives, or bacterial exotoxins and endotoxins.[1,13]

VII. **Contact lens–related inflammation** has many causes.

A. **Preservatives** in contact lens solutions can cause many adverse ocular responses.[13,17,18] Preservatives and disinfectants can cause either allergic or toxic effects on the corneal and conjunctival epithelium.[13,18] Symptoms include redness, tearing, burning, discomfort on insertion, photophobia, decreased lens wearing time, and itching in an allergic response. There are also hyperemia, corneal edema, chemosis, superficial punctate keratitis (SPK), microcysts, perilimbal infiltrates, follicles, papules, and epiphora. Solution characteristics important in adverse ocular responses include the pH, buffering system, preservatives, viscosity, osmolality, and disinfectants used.[13,18] The following is a summary of the most common preservatives and enzymes available on the market today and some of the reported adverse effects (see Chapter 13).

1. **Thimerosal** hypersensitivity was previously very common but it is quickly becoming an event of the past. Almost all solutions are changing to other forms of preservatives that are thimerosal free. Conjunctivitis and keratitis are common consequences of thimerosal hypersensitivity. Thimerosal is still on the market today but is seldom used.
2. **Chlorhexidine** in the past was the most common agent used in hydrogel lens solutions. Patients who are sensitive to chlorhexidine present with adverse ocular responses. Chlorhexidine hypersensitivity presents similarly to thimerosal hypersensitivity, and since these agents are often combined, it is difficult to determine the true culprit.
3. **Benzalkonium chloride** at high concentrations can cause toxicity and produce morphologic disruptions of the epithelium.
4. **Chlorobutanol** is rarely used in contact lens solutions today, occurring in the preservative in one rigid lens lubricating drop.
5. **Benzyl alcohol** causes few adverse responses in patients. It can be used as an alternative for patients who react to the preservatives in other solutions.
6. **Sorbates** are most commonly associated with stinging on insertion of lens. They can discolor and yellow contact lenses. Allergic sensitivities are reported to be low.
7. **EDTA** is used in conjunction with thimerosal, sorbates, and benzalkonium chloride (BAK). There is no indication that this product causes adverse ocular responses except for a rare contact allergy.
8. **Hydrogen peroxide** is a very effective disinfectant. The human body is very efficient in protecting its cells from the effects of hydrogen peroxide. Natural enzymes are available to neutralize any excess hydrogen peroxide on the ocular surface by the tears.
9. **DYMED** is an improved disinfectant due to its larger molecular size. Adverse responses are minor, and it appears that the skin may react more quickly than the conjunctiva due to its molecular size.
10. **Polyquad** is the largest molecule used today. Cytotoxic effects are considered to be very minor.
11. **Papain** was the first enzyme used for hydrogel lenses. Severe discomfort has been reported after papain use with some high-water-content lenses. Patients should be advised to clean and rinse their lenses and if irritation continues change to another enzyme.
12. **Pancreatin** is a naturally occurring enzyme. The adverse effects of ocular irritation to pancreatin are few.
13. With **subtilisin,** adverse reactions depend on exposure dosage and time. If patients have adverse effects the morning after using the enzyme, consider another enzyme or disposable lenses.[13,16]

B. **Acute red eye syndrome,** an acute inflammatory response, is sometimes present in extended and daily wear hydrogel lenses. Anterior stromal infiltrates are often found adjacent to the limbus in this reaction. Symptoms include ocular pain, photophobia, lacrimation, and redness. It can be an inflammatory toxic effect caused by debris and perhaps bacteria trapped under the lens, hypersensitivity to solution preservatives, or dehydration of the tear film during sleep, and hypoxia. **Infectious keratitis** must be ruled out. Acute red eye syndrome is managed by discontinuing contact lenses and applying a topical steroid and a broad-spectrum antibiotic for coverage. Lens wear can be resumed after all signs have resolved. The patient should consider using a preservative-free solution, refitting with a looser lens, and switching to a daily-wear lens with reduced wearing time.[13,18]

C. **Conjunctival hyperemia** is hyperemia of the conjunctiva with or without follicular hypertrophy. It has been reported to be associated with the use of soft contact lenses and preserved solutions. The treatment is to remove the soft contact lens and switch to a preservative-free saline. Inflammatory signs and symptoms should resolve. All other causes for the red eye must be ruled out first, such as bacterial, viral, chlamydial, or amoebic infections; poorly-fitting lenses; and prolonged wearing time in which there is physiologic compromise.[13]

D. **Contact lens–related keratitis** can be secondary to mechanical, physiologic, and immune responses to contact lens wear.[1] Superficial **punctate keratopathy** may also be due to a preservative hypersensitivity or a toxicity reaction. Toxic keratopathy and delayed hypersensitivity reactions to preservatives are both associated with ocular redness, discomfort, photophobia, **epithelial to stromal infiltrates,** and coarse punctate epithelial keratopathy. Treatment is to eliminate the irritating substance and provide an appropriate hiatus from lens wear.[13]

E. **Corneal infiltrates** are a sign of corneal inflammation in a "quiet" eye or a red eye (Figure 2.8). Generally the eyes are "quiet" (without noticeable signs of inflammation), but the condition may be associated with hyperemia follicular hypertrophy and a watery discharge.[13,14] Corneal infiltrates usually occur days to months after wearing contact lenses that were chemically disinfected, soiled, or worn for long periods daily. Contact lens–induced infiltrates are many times observed within 2 mm of the limbus. They may range in appearance from tiny white spherical foci in anterior layers to large, gray-white snowball opacities in corneal stroma.[19] Patients should temporarily discontinue lens wear until the infiltrates resolve.[5]

F. **Giant papillary conjunctivitis (GPC)** is conjunctival hyperemia with small (0.5 mm) to giant (3.0 mm) papillae of the tarsal conjunctiva. The most common causes are soft contact lens wear, hard contact lens wear, protruding sutures postoperatively, use of prosthetic eyes, and mechanical irritants. GPC is 10 times as common with soft lens wear as with hard. Patients may be asymptomatic in response to this nonspecific ocular irritation. There can be an increased lens awareness leading to a

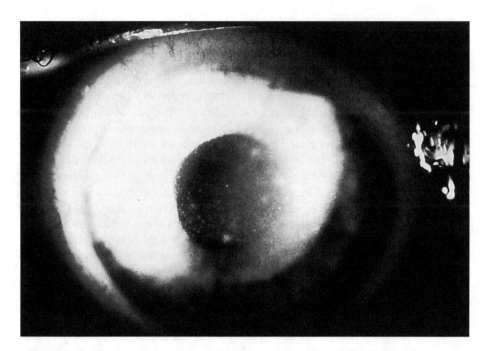

FIGURE 2.8   *Corneal infiltrates in a contact lens wearer. Infiltrates in contact lens wearers are a harbinger of serious tissue damage. Several causes exist, both sterile and infectious. This patient experienced an adverse solution reaction (sterile).*

decreased wearing time or the inability to continue lens wear due to itching and mucus. Mucus discharge may be absent and become a dense and stringy accumulation. Treatment varies with degree of GPC and symptoms. Minor cases can be managed by recleaning lenses or switching to a disposable or a hard contact. More aggressive treatment includes using antihistamines or decongestants, a mast cell stabilizer, nonsteroid and steroid drops, and making significant changes in lenses and care products.[1,16]

G. **Neovascularization** occurs when a small amount of peripheral superficial vascularization is caused by hypoxia, vascular compression from tight-fitting contact lenses, trauma from damaged lenses, or sensitivity to a solution.[13] The microtrauma caused by a contact lens releases enzymes that are chemotactic for inflammatory cells. When the cells reach the area of epithelial damage, they release angiogenic factors that stimulate growth of new vessels toward the site of injury. Normally, small capillaries originating from the episcleral branches of the anterior ciliary artery surround limbal cornea by 1 mm. Under the stimuli mentioned, neovascularization originates from these normal capillaries. If the neovascularization invades the cornea more than 2 mm, it is considered abnormal. The presence of corneal vessels may result in lipid degeneration, **pannus,** scarring, intrastromal hemorrhages, and eventually, reduced visual acuity. Treatment is to remove the causative factor; the vessels may empty and become "ghost vessels."[3] Deeper vessels pose a greater concern.

H. **Pannus** is the extension of the limbal blood vessels into a previously avascular cornea. Pannus always presents by inflammation, whether it is infective, toxic, hypoxic, or of other etiology. Common examples are seen in inclusion conjunctivitis and contact lens–related pathology.[3,4]

I. **Pseudodendritic lesions** are epithelial infiltrates that stain minimally and lack terminal end bulbs (Figure 2.9). They occur in the central or peripheral cornea and are bilateral 70% of the time. Lesions have been reported in soft contact lens wearers who used thimerosal and chlorhexidine preserved solutions. Infiltrates slowly resolve after discontinuation of lens wear.[13,17] This peculiar finding may represent **antigen deposition, hypersensitivity reaction,** or **hypoxic** response. The lesion fortuitously assumes a branching pattern and should not be confused with the dendritic lesions of herpes simplex.[17]

Pearl: The term "pseudodendrite" should be used only when referring to a contact lens–related lesion; otherwise the appropriate term is "dendritiform lesion."

J. **Pseudocysts** are an accumulation of fluid in the intracellular space resulting from ruptured epithelial cell membranes. Microcysts are best viewed on retroillumination. Symptoms include discomfort on lens insertion, photophobia, and epiphora. Intraepithelial microcysts are associated with thimerosal toxicity and chlorhexidine-preserved solutions. Treatment is to discontinue offending agents, at which time all signs and symptoms disappear.[13]

K. **Superior limbic keratoconjunctivitis** induced by contact lenses is an inflammatory reaction that affects hydrogel lens wearers, who often use **thimerosal** or wear a soiled lens with a lot of movement (Figure 2.10). A V-shaped wedge of corneal hyperplasia with the apex directed toward the pupil may be present, creating a sight-threatening situation.[18] Signs include intense laxity and hyperemia of the superior bulbar conjunctiva, fine papillary hypertrophy of superior tarsal conjunctiva, epithelial and subepithelial infiltrates, and superior corneal and limbal punctate staining. The condition is bilateral and can affect the visual acuity if the visual axis is involved.[13] Treatment is a temporary discontinuation of lens for several weeks to months and total abstinence from **thimerosal**-containing lens care products. Old lenses should be discarded, and frequent replacement of lenses is urged.[13] A rigid lens may ultimately prove to be the best option.

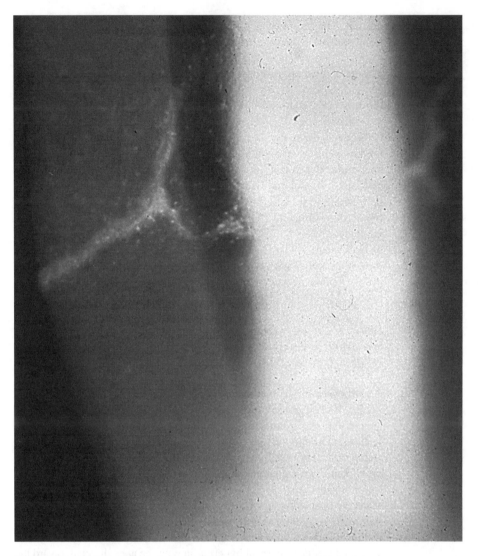

FIGURE 2.9   *Pseudodendritic lesions in a contact lens wearer. Pseudodendrites are not common in a contact lens wearer. When they do occur, however, they can be rather dramatic. They are believed to represent a response to hypersensitivity (antigen deposition), a toxic reaction to solution, or hypoxia. (Courtesy of K Zadnik, The Ohio State University College of Optometry.)*

VIII. **Inflammatory conditions of the conjunctiva** contraindicate lens wear.
   A.   Inflammatory conditions present in many different forms; one type is **allergic inflammatory reactions.**
      1. **Atopic conjunctivitis** appears as red hyperemic bulbar injection with chemosis, a subconjunctival infiltration, and edema. Mucous

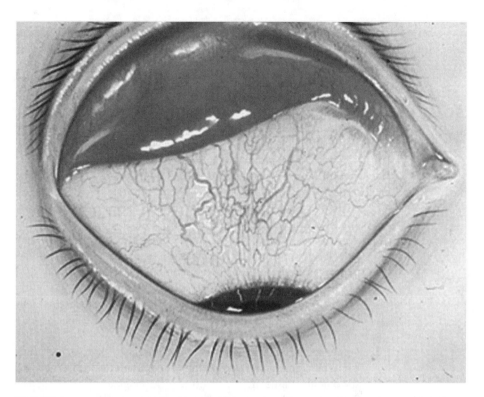

FIGURE 2.10   *Superior limbic keratoconjunctivitis (SLK) in a contact lens wearer. Initially believed to be a solution-related complication (thimerosal reaction), SLK in a contact lens wearer may actually represent a mechanical, deposit-induced change to the superior bulbar conjunctiva, as giant papillary conjunctivitis is to the tarsal conjunctiva. Compared with Theodore's SLK, idiopathic SLK is generally more diffuse about the limbus with more laxity of the superior bulbar conjunctiva.*

membranes may appear glossy. The discharge appears white and stringy, accumulating in the fornices and inner canthus. Atopic reactions may be unilateral or bilateral and vision may fluctuate or remain stable. Reaction can be immediate (type I) or delayed (type IV). It is often seasonal or occurs in response to a nonspecific allergen. Manage by trying to remove the allergen and use cold compresses with a topical decongestant or antihistamine. Delayed reactions (type IV) usually require **steroids.**[1]

2. **Atopic keratoconjunctivitis** presents as a bilateral condition with mild to moderate hyperemia of the bulbar conjunctiva and no chemosis. Papillary changes are found in the inferior palpebral conjunctiva. Corneal findings are concentrated superiorly, with two to five limbal infiltrates approximately 1–2 mm around. A moderate to severe SPK is usually associated. Symptoms, which may persist year-round, always include **itching,** and there may also be a burning sensation,

corneal symptoms, and a nonspecific irritation. The ailment affects primarily men (20–50 years old). Discharge is often thick, white, and stringy. Lids may become edematous, with chronic edema hardening into a leathery texture. Chronic forms show prominent limbal arcades, pannus, and neovascularization. Long-term complications generally produce an anterior stromal haze and scarring. Treatment is with cold packs, oral antihistamines or decongestants, a topical mass cell stabilizer, and topical or systemic steroids.[1] **Plasmapheresis** has been tried in the past in severe cases with some success.

B. **Bacterial inflammatory reactions** are caused by proliferation of bacteria that may be natural flora or other bacteria.

   1. **Acute bacterial conjunctivitis** presents as a meaty red bulbar conjunctiva, with hyperemia greater toward the fornices. The circumcorneal area is clear, and injected vessels are easily movable and blanch with mild vasoconstrictor such as phenylephrine. Papillae may be present in the palpebral conjunctiva. Mucopurulent discharge is greater in the morning, with the lashes matted or eyelids stuck together. There is no associated pain or vision reduction. The history is of 2–3 days of increasingly intense objective signs. Treatment is a **broad-spectrum antibiotic.**[1,13]

   2. **Hyperacute bacterial conjunctivitis** presents with advanced acute bacterial signs, with overflowing **mucopurulent discharge.** The surrounding tissue may be involved to varying degrees. Lid edema, dermatoblepharoconjunctivitis, preseptal cellulitis, conjunctival chemosis, and toxic corneal epithelial staining may be present. Hemorrhagic patterns may change from petechial to gross conjunctival or subconjunctival blood of the bulbar conjunctiva. Pseudomembranes may develop in the fornices. The follicles and preauricular node may be palpable, mimicking a viral presentation. Cultures and Gram's and Giemsa stains are a part of the laboratory workup. Oral antibiotics are usually required in hyperacute forms.[1,13]

Pearl: Cultures in neonatal infections are suggested.

C. **Bacterial corneal ulcer,** or **bacterial keratitis,** presents with polymorphonuclear dense grayish-white opacity associated with epithelial loss and **stromal necrosis.** Any impairment of the corneal epithelium allows bacteria to adhere to the injured epithelium. Different microorganisms produce diverse degrees of infection severity. Corneal ulcers are associated with conjunctival hyperemia and mucopurulent exudate. As the ulcer progresses, it develops neovascularization, increased stromal edema, and hypopyon. Diagnosis cannot be based on clinical features alone—laboratory evaluation is necessary. Initial treatment includes cycloplegic, IOP-lowering medications if needed, and a wide-spectrum an-

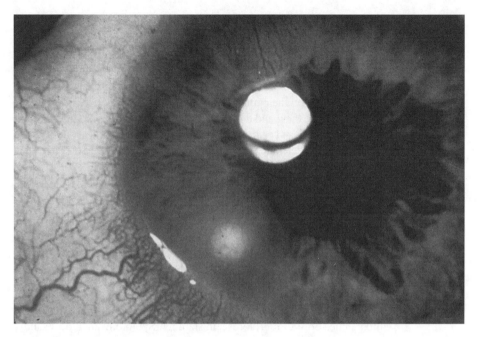

FIGURE 2.11 *Phlyctenular keratoconjunctivitis. Phlyctenular keratoconjunctivitis is a lymphocytic response to any microbial antigen. Corneal lesions are elevated and should not be confused with the stromal necrosis seen in infectious keratitis.*

tibiotic until bacterial morphology is determined[1,20] (see Chapter 15 for a more detailed discussion of bacterial keratitis).

D. Marginal keratitis is an infiltrative immune response to staphylococcal exotoxins. **Exotoxins** produce a sterile response by forming intraepithelial infiltrates in the midperipheral cornea. Lesions are always islands, single or multiple on the peripheral margin, separated by clear cornea. Lesions range from 0.5 to 1.5 mm in size and may be flat or raised. Corneal edema is usually mild to moderate and can produce a haze around the infiltrates. Corneal involvement is most vulnerable at the 4 and 8 o'-clock positions, but lesions may also be superior or circumlimbal. Bulbar conjunctiva is hyperemic. Presentation is usually with a unilateral painful and watery eye. It may be acute or subacute on waking. Corneal symptoms are sandy, gritty sensations. Visual acuity is rarely affected. Rarely do staphylococcal toxins progress and produce anterior stromal necrosis, a sterile ulcer. Treatment depends on the degree of presentation and includes warm compresses, broad-spectrum antibiotics, cycloplegics, and steroids.[1]

E. Phlyctenular keratoconjunctivitis is a raised, circumscribed, pinkish-white limbal nodular reaction to a **microbial antigen** (Figure 2.11). It is a focal superficial infiltrative reaction. The phlyctenulae can progress 1–3 mm into clear cornea and produce thinning, scarring, and vascularization. It is an infiltrate of cells and debris, leading to a fibrin formation. It is caused by an accumulation of superficial epithelial toxins. It is associated with variable degrees of surrounding edema and hyperemia. Lesions may form at any site on the ocular surface. The most common sites for limbal phlyctenules are the 4 and 8 o'clock positions in the inferior circumlimbal areas. Phlyctenules vary from 1 to 4 mm in size. The corneal surface surrounding the phlyctenule demonstrates various degrees of toxic SPK. Presentation is unilateral, with acute onset of symptoms, a sandy, gritty feeling, and foreign body sensation.[1] Healing occurs in 10–15 days.[5] Visual acuity is minimally affected.[1] Corneal involvement can produce severe photophobia.[5] Phlyctenulosis appears to be a local immune type IV **hypersensitivity to *S. aureus* or tuberculin** antigens. Treatment includes **topical steroids** and prophylactic wide-spectrum antibiotics. Cycloplegics may needed in moderate to severe presentations.[1]

F. **Staphylococcal SPK, a form of toxic SPK,** is variable SPK that is concentrated on the inferior corneal surface. It localizes to the 4 and 8 o'clock positions. SPK may become dense, and there may be confluence into patches on sodium fluorescein staining. Symptoms include a sandy, gritty corneal irritation with variable degrees of photophobia or lacrimation. It is associated with corneal edema, inferior bulbar injection, and conjunctival hyperemia. Palpebral conjunctiva produces a mild to moderate degree of papillary conjunctivitis. Staphylococcal lid disease is usually active or residual with crusting and **madarosis.** Marginal anterior stromal scars can be observed on the cornea periphery. Visual acuity may be mildly affected. This condition is most frequent in dry-eye patients and contact lens wearers. Treatment includes ocular lubricants, antibiotic ointment, or antibiotic-steroid combinations.[1]

G. **Trachoma** is a chronic condition caused by *Chlamydia trachomatis.* Moderate to severe superior tarsal follicles with inflammation of the palpebral upper conjunctiva. **Follicles** may be obscured with papillary hypertrophy. Trachoma tends to be endemic in underdeveloped countries and certain ethnic groups. It spreads by direct contact and is associated with genitourinary involvement. Severe forms can be sight-threatening. Treat all cases with **oral tetracycline** and family members and close associates with topical tetracycline ointment. Active corneal response may require topical steroids.[1] Secondary bacterial infection is usually responsible for corneal scarring and blindness.

IX. **Viral and other follicular conjunctivitis** that affect the eye are contraindicated in any type of contact lens wear.

A. **Adenoviral types of conjunctivitis** are the most common form of acute conjunctivitis. The acute phase is mild and short-lived and may be unilateral or bilateral. The condition presents with a purplish-pink bulbar hyperemia. Injection starts at the inner canthus and slowly spreads laterally to involve the entire bulbar conjunctiva. Symptoms include mild to moderate burning irritation and vision fluctuation. Quick tear break-up time can produce secondary SPK with corneal irritation. The discharge is serous, and there are variable degrees of follicular changes, inflammation, and hyperemia. Occasionally there is an ipsilateral **preauricular lymphadenopathy.** Antiviral agents are not effective against adenoviruses. Hot and cold compresses are of some benefit.[1] Steroids should be used judiciously for a severe inflammatory response as in **pseudomembrane formation** or infiltration involving the visual axis.

B. **Axenfeld's conjunctivitis** is found only in children and always follows a low-grade, asymptomatic, chronic course. Palpebral follicles are most abundant on the tarsal conjunctiva with no corneal involvement. The discharge is serous, mild, and chronic. There is no treatment, and the condition is usually self-limiting in months to years. Monitor the patient every 3 months and stress good ocular hygiene.[1]

C. **Chlamydial inclusion conjunctivitis** presents as follicles on the inferior tarsal conjunctiva with superior corneal pannus and tiny white peripheral subepithelial corneal infiltrates. It is usually associated with a stringy mucus discharge and a palpable **preauricular node.** Chlamydia is a **sexually transmitted** disease typically found in young adults. Symptoms include a red eye and ocular irritation of longer than 4 weeks' duration. Treatment includes oral and topical tetracycline.

Pearl: Sexual partners should be treated.

D. **Epidemic keratoconjunctivitis (EKC)** is a follicular adenoviral conjunctivitis producing small **petechial hemorrhages** in the upper and lower eyelids. It is associated at times with **pseudomembranous conjunctivitis,** subepithelial infiltrates, and diffuse or focal keratitis. The presentation of an adenoviral infection is variable. Petechial hemorrhages may coalesce, causing gross subconjunctival or eyelid hemorrhages resembling a black eye. The upper and lower eyelids may be edematous and swollen shut. Preauricular and submandibular lymph nodes are present. Follicular conjunctivitis is highly contagious and bilateral in 75–90% of epidemic outbreak cases. EKC is self-limiting. Patients are made comfortable during the first 2 weeks of ocular involvement with warm or cold compresses. At 2 weeks, if subepithelial infiltrates persist in the central cornea and the patient is symptomatic, topical steroids can be used to eliminate blur or glare. Decongestants and frequent irrigation may help.[6]

E. **Folliculosis** is palpebral conjunctival follicles with no signs of inflammation. Follicles are usually greatest in the inferior cul-de-sac. The condition is found in healthy young children. No treatment is indicated, but the condition should be monitored routinely.[1,3]

F. **Hemorrhagic acute conjunctivitis** is caused by enterovirus 70. It presents hyperacutely with hemorrhages, which can be caused by EKC or any virulent microorganism. It may be unilateral or bilateral. The treatment is to rule out EKC and other infectious syndromes and treat the primary infectious cause.[1,3]

G. **Herpes simplex conjunctivitis** is a unilateral follicular conjunctival reaction associated with **herpetic skin vesicles** along the periocular skin or eyelid margin. Treatment includes trifluorothymidine 1% and cold compresses. The patient should be monitored for corneal involvement until the condition resolves.[3,4]

H. **Herpes zoster conjunctivitis** occurs as a rash of vesicles on an erythematous base that does not cross the midline. It is associated with conjunctivitis, keratitis, uveitis, and secondary glaucoma.[1] Zoster causes hyperesthesia over the affected skin associated with severe burning, pain, and fever.[6] Herpes zoster affects the thoracic area 70% of the time and trigeminal nerve only 25%. There is a 50% chance of ocular involvement when vesicles are located on the tip of nose, called **Hutchinson's sign.**[6] Herpes zoster ophthalmicus may result in corneal scarring, epithelial punctate keratitis, and subepithelial infiltrates, which are usually seen 10–14 days after onset of symptoms.[4] Unfortunately, in severe forms corneal healing is poor with basement membrane damage that results in infection, melting, vascularization, or scarring. It may be accompanied by a total or partial corneal sensation loss and ectropion or other eyelid abnormalities.[3] There may be a postherpetic neuralgia that is painful and usually subsides in 6 months. Herpes zoster is self-limiting but can be fatal. Underlying causes are immunosuppression, chemotherapy, or **malignancy.** Treatment is good hygiene, cold compresses, isolation from immunosuppressed patients, prednisone, antiviral agents such as like famciclovir (Famvir), acyclovir, and sometimes amitriptyline (Elavil).[1]

I. **Molluscum contagiosum** is a viral infection that causes a skin growth (Figure 2.12). It is sometimes confused with **basal cell carcinoma** or papilloma. It can lead to a chronic unilateral conjunctivitis. Diagnosis is made on inspection and confirmed with a biopsy. Treatment is surgical removal.[1] Molluscum contagiosum can cause a low-grade, chronic keratoconjunctivitis with resistance to therapy unless growths are removed. Presumably, keratoconjunctivitis is due to toxic products released from the infection.

J. **Newcastle's disease** is a virus transmitted by infected birds, especially in chicken droppings. Candidates for this disease are poultry workers. If the infectious source is removed, the condition is self-limiting.[1]

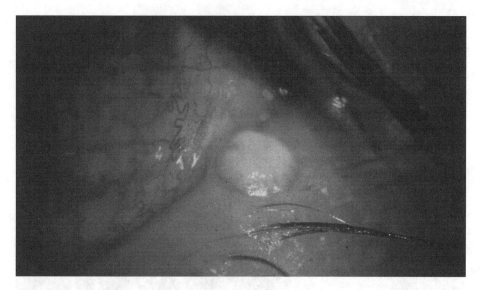

FIGURE 2.12   *Molluscum contagiosum. Molluscum bodies often present with a significant follicular conjunctivitis that results from a toxic reaction to a "pox" virus. This lid lesion must be removed or a persistent conjunctivitis may continue to plague the patient.*

K. **Parinaud's oculoglandular fever** presents as large follicles with yellowish cores associated with diffuse palpebral conjunctival **granulomas.** The presentation is always unilateral and acute, with a dramatic ipsilateral pre-auricular lymphadenopathy. Parinaud's is usually an analogue of "cat scratch fever," and systemic involvement must be considered. Treatment requires systemic antibiotics and nonsteroidal anti-inflammatories. If there is only ocular involvement, it can be treated with a broad-spectrum antibiotic.[1]

L. **Thygeson's SPK** is suspected to have a viral etiology and may follow acute viral keratoconjunctivitis (Figure 2.13). Epithelial infiltrates develop that produce negative staining. Thygeson's is generally a bilateral condition, but it usually affects one eye more seriously. There is a variable degree of SPK, and when it becomes dense it can affect the visual acuity. The eyes remain white and quiet in the presence of a distinct keratitis. There are no associated signs of inflammation or infection. Thygeson's SPK is the only form of keratitis that "keeps no company." It is seen mostly in **females** 15–40 years old. Symptoms range from none to a transient gritty sensation. Symptoms go into remission and exacerbate in 4–6 weeks. Treatment includes lubrication therapy, mild steroids when needed (may prolong the course of the disease), and an antiviral agent

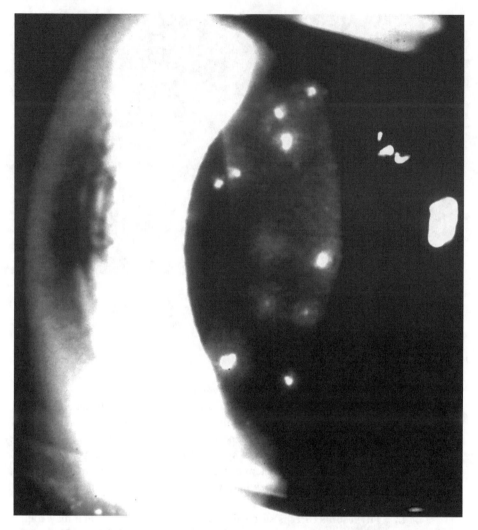

FIGURE 2.13   *Thygeson's superficial punctate keratitis. Intraepithelial infiltrates in Thygeson's may be a response to a viral antigen. As in adenoviral keratoconjunctivitis, steroids may be beneficial but may prolong the course of the disease.*

such as trifluridine (Viroptic). Soft contact lens patients can use their lenses as a bandage with close monitoring.[1]

Pearl: *If a bandage lens is prescribed, treating the most symptomatic eye is generally sufficient, resulting in less reflex tearing and irritation to the fellow eye.*

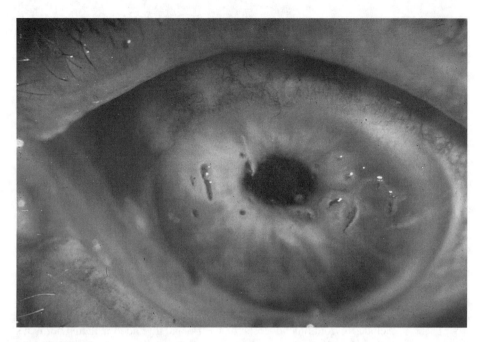

FIGURE 2.14 *Filamentary keratitis in keratitis sicca. Severe keratitis sicca with extra-epithelial threads attached to the cornea is shown. Timely removal is needed to improve patient comfort.*

    M. **Verrucae** are single or multiple consecrating **papillomatous warts.** They are gray-brown to yellow in coloration. Presentations vary, ranging from warts with smooth surfaces to cauliflower-like tissue waves. Lesions that grow at lid margins may cause mild secondary viral keratoconjunctivitis. Verrucae are contagious lesions with an autoinoculation tendency. Patients should be educated about the contagious nature of the warts. Surgical excision can be considered for cosmetic relief.[1]

X. **Other inflammatory reactions** are possible.

    A. **Filamentary keratitis** occurs when dead epithelial cells combine with mucin debris to form chains that accumulate on the cornea (Figure 2.14). Elongated threads can be 1–3 mm or more in length. One end of the filament adheres to a dry spot on the cornea. The unattached end hangs loosely, creating a foreign-body sensation as the lid tugs on filaments with each blink. Symptoms range from annoying in chronic forms to severe in acute presentations. Filaments stain with sodium fluorescein and rose bengal. Primary disease is usually associated with filamentary findings. Manage by treating the primary underlying disease. Filaments can be reduced or removed with lubrication, a pressure patch, jeweler's forceps, acetylcysteine, or a low-water **bandage contact lens.**[1]

    B. **KCS syndromes** present as bands of SPK, with a tear break-up time of less than 10 seconds, mucoid debris, and hyperemia. Symptoms include mid- to late-day corneal irritation. Treatment is eye **lubrications.** Moderate to severe cases need tetracycline or low-dose androgen supplements.[1]

C.   The origins of **physiologic keratitis** are explained in terms of the **"stress immunogen theory."** This theory proposes that the mechanical and physiologic stress factor produced by the inflammatory cascade disrupts normal tissue homeostasis, resulting in dysregulation of control mechanisms in the immune system. The overreaction of the immune system can lead to increasing clinical inflammation and potential tissue changes. An underreaction of the immune system can increase the vulnerability to antigen, as occurs with microbes or nonpathogenic parasites.[1]

D.   **Superior limbic keratoconjunctivitis (SLK)** occurs as an inflammatory thickening and injection of the superior bulbar conjunctiva. Papillary inflammation is found on the upper tarsal conjunctiva.[3,4] It is associated with fine punctate fluorescein staining on the superior cornea, limbus and conjunctiva, and filaments adjacent to the superior corneal limbus. Symptoms include a red, burning eye with possible pain, tearing, mild photophobia, and a foreign body sensation.[20] SLK is usually a bilateral chronic and recurrent external ocular inflammatory disease. Reports have shown that 20–50% of patients with SLK had thyroid dysfunction.[17] Workup includes thyroid function tests for T3, T4, and thyroid-stimulating hormone. Treatment includes artificial tears and ointment, a mild steroid-antibiotic combination if needed, thermal cautery, conjunctival resection, and silver nitrate 0.5–1.0% solution applied for 10–20 seconds to the upper bulbar and tarsal conjunctiva.

*Pearl: If a significant amount of filaments exists, **acetylcysteine 10% drops** are added.[3]*

E.   **Toxic and irritative chronic conjunctivitis** presents as a red eye, but it is difficult to establish the primary cause and effective treatment. Bulbar hyperemia is present, often in an inferior pattern in the 4 and 8 o'-clock positions. There is a mild to moderate mixed papillary or follicular response, which is usually greater in the palpebral conjunctival area. The condition may be unilateral or bilateral. Symptoms may be absent, ranging up to moderate nonspecific irritation. Patients are usually concerned mostly with cosmetic effects. Possible causes are dry air, airborne irritants, allergens, radiation (sun exposure), medications, and contact lens wear. The treatment should be appropriate to the cause and should be modified based on chronicity of response.[1]

XI.   **Fungal infections** are rare but can occur with lens wear.

A.   **Fungi** are primitive nonmotile plantlike organisms. **Yeasts** are unicellular and **molds** are multicellular filamentous structures. Since the mid-1980s, the prevalence of fungal keratitis has definitely increased in certain geographic areas. Forty different genera can cause **keratomycoses;** most are saprophytic. Risk factors include a corneal injury, frequently from a tree branch or vegetative matter in an agricultural setting; **extended or therapeutic soft contact lens wear;** chronic use of topical medication or systemic steroids; diabetes mellitus; and radial keratotomy.[21]

B. The most common organisms can be divided into several classifications.
    1. **Filamentous fungi (molds)** are divided into septate and nonseptate types.
        a. **Septate fungi** are the most common cause of fungal keratitis. Their geographic distribution is variable, but they are found mostly in the southern and southwestern United States. They include the most virulent fungi: *Fusarium, Aspergillus, Curvularia, Paecilomyces,* and *Phialophora.*
        b. **Nonseptate fungi** are rare corneal pathogens. Mucoraceae are included in this category.
    2. **Yeasts** have a worldwide distribution in the genus *Candida: C. albicans, C. parapsilosis,* and *C. tropicalis.* Risk factors for yeast infection include protracted ulceration of the epithelium, topical steroid therapy, penetrating keratoplasty, and bandage soft contact lenses.[22] The clinical features of a typical yeast infection are an ulcerated epithelium with suppurative stromal inflammation. The site of corneal infection can be focal or diffuse. Rare, atypical yeast infections may have an intact epithelium, a nonsuppurative stomal inflammation, and a multifocal inflammation site. A ring infiltrate or abscess is possible with an intact epithelium.

C. The **clinical features** of a typical fungal infection include an intact or ulcerated epithelium, nonsuppurative stromal involvement, and feathery infiltrates with a focal or multifocal site of inflammation with satellite infiltrates (Figure 2.15). An atypical or severe fungal infection shows an ulcerated epithelium, a suppurative stroma, and diffuse sites of inflammation. Fungal infections may also be associated with a mild iritis, endothelial plaque, and a hypopyon in severe infections. Confocal microscopy is beneficial in making a diagnosis.

D. **Keratomycosis** is diagnosed by clinical suspicion, corneal scrapings, or superficial keratectomy (paracentesis). Diagnosis is confirmed with such stains as Gram's, Giemsa, GMS, periodic acid–Schiff, potassium hydroxide, and calcofluor white. **Sabouraud's dextrose agar** with gentamicin and without cycloheximide, blood agar, and brain-heart infusion agar with gentamicin are diagnostic culture media. Seventy-five percent of keratomycosis cases can be detected by stains. Prevention should be to minimize use of extended-wear and therapeutic contact lenses and avoid indiscriminate use of topical steroids.[21]

E. The **initial therapy** is drugs, which are generally not introduced until definitive diagnosis is made by culture.[21]

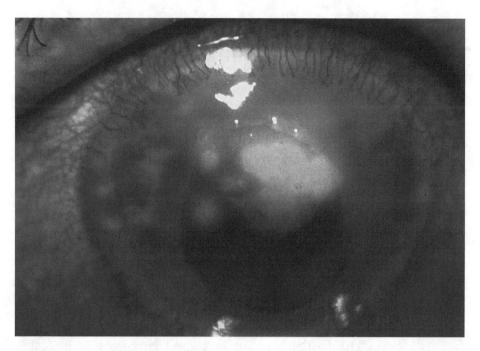

FIGURE 2.15   *Fungal keratitis in a contact lens wearer. Feathery infiltrates without epithelial disruption may be present. Hypopyon are not diagnostic for this infection.*

1. **Topical drugs** are often continued for 6 weeks or longer, and the patient must be watched for signs of toxicity. Natamycin 5% suspension every hour for 24 to 48 hours is used for hyphae. Amphotericin B should be used every 15–20 minutes for 24–48 hours for yeast. Miconazole, 10 mg/ml, can used every hour but can become very toxic.
2. **Oral drugs** are generally used for hyphae because *Candida* generally respond to topicals alone. The oral drugs used are ketoconazole (200–600 mg/ml) or fluconazole (100–200 mg/ml).
3. **Other agents** are atropine 1% or isopto-hyoscine 0.25% qid. Glaucoma medication is used as needed; the role of collagen shields as a delivery device is not well defined. Excimer laser ablation may be of some value unless there is deep penetration.

XII. **Protozoan infections** can be a result of contact lens wear.
    A. In the past, *Acanthamoeba* **keratitis** was regarded as a curiosity, but recently this pathogen is being recognized with increased frequency. It affects primarily the cornea and sclera. Early detection alters the course of therapy and ultimately affects the outcome, so early diagnosis is critical. Five or six species can be ocular parasites. *Acanthamoeba* can take two forms: a sessile **cyst** and a motile **trophozoite.** The cyst form is more dif-

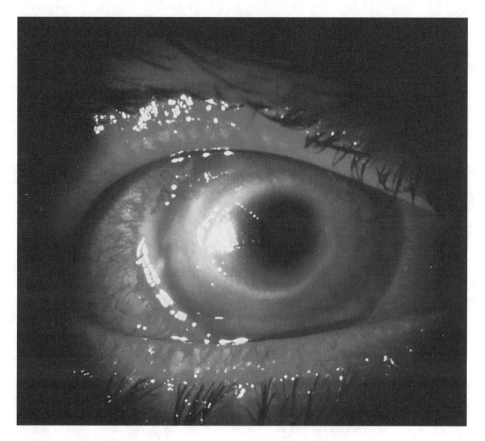

FIGURE 2.16   Acanthamoeba *keratitis in a contact lens wearer. Protozoan infection of the cornea can be ravaging due to the organism's ability to resist treatment. Ulcerative keratitis in a contact lens wearer must include a differential diagnosis that excludes ameba.*

ficult because it is resistant to freezing, desiccation, standard chlorination, and a variety of antimicrobial agents. The organism is a "free living" motile protozoan with worldwide distribution. *Acanthamoeba* can be isolated from fresh water, well water, sea and brackish water, sewage, hot tubs, air, soil, wheat, and barley. The incidence of infection may be high in an area after a disaster such as a flood or hurricane.[21]

B.   The **clinical features** are initially nonspecific signs, such as patchy epithelial involvement resembling an irregular or pleomorphic focal or stellate epitheliopathy, mild nonsuppurative stromal keratitis, iritis, and pseudoguttata. More advanced signs include **radial keratoneuritis, ring infiltrate, scleritis,** and hypopyon or hyphema (Figure 2.16). A pseudomembrane or adenopathy may be present. A remarkable lack of vascularization is often the only feature to help differentiate this infection from **herpes simplex.**[23,24]

C. **Symptoms** are usually a unilateral **pain** despite ocular findings, and often there is a history of trauma, **contact lens wear,** or both. Symptoms generally wax and wane over time with chronicity.[21,25]

D. **Laboratory confirmation** is by corneal scrapings, which are examined with Giemsa or trichrome stains. Also, the ameba can be cultured by plating on **non-nutrient agar** with heat-killed *E. coli.* Other valuable tests include immunofluorescent techniques, including **calcofluor white** and indirect immunofluorescent antibody testing. Standard cultures for bacteria, fungi, and virus are expected to be negative. Cysts can sometimes be seen on soft lenses with high magnification.[26] **Confocal microscopy** is invaluable in making a diagnosis and monitoring for an appropriate response to treatment.[26]

E. **Treatment** should include one agent from at least two of the following four categories, as a topical every 30–60 minutes. Oral ketoconazole or fluconazole should be administered as well.[21]

   1. **Antibiotics**–paromomycin (Humatin), neomycin
   2. **Antifungals**–clotrimazole, ketoconazole, itraconazole, miconazole, fluconazole
   3. **Antiparasitics**–propamidine isethionate (Brolene), hydroxystil-bamidine, hexamidine di-isethionate (Desomedine)
   4. **Biocides**–polyhexamethylene biguanide (PHBG, Baquacil)

   Supportive and adjunct therapy is frequent **debridement,** conjunctival flaps, bandage lenses, debulking procedures, cryotherapy, and, with caution, steroids. Grafts show a high rate of recrudescence.[21] Some authorities suggest with recalcitrant disease alternating applications of Brolene or hexamidine on day 1, paromomycin on day 2, and chlorhexidine digluconate or a biocide on day 3, since most of these topicals are quite toxic with prolonged usage. Repeated drug therapy may select out cells that can encyst rapidly. **Tandem scanning confocal microscopy** has been helpful in distinguishing drug epithelial toxicity from recurrent disease.[27]

F. The **risks factors** described here are contact lens–related risk factors that have been identified by epidemiologic studies,[21,23] including use of **distilled water,** saliva, and **tap water** to rinse lenses. Tap water has recently become a concern, especially with rigid lens wear. Bacterial contamination of the lens case and care system is a common factor. There is some risk of amebic resistance to chemical disinfection. Other risks associated with lens wear are corneal insult from hypoxia and mechanical trauma. Contact lenses should be avoided during swimming and during the use of hot tubs.[21]

G. **Additional protozoan infections** may be caused by other ameba besides *Acanthamoeba,* such as infection with *Naegleria, Hartmannella,* or *Vahlkampfia.*[21,27] *Microsporida,* a protozoan, has been recently found on corneal scrapings of patients infected with human immunodeficiency virus **(HIV).** It generally presents as superficial punctate, multifocal keratitis and may be confined to the superficial cornea for months. A slight improvement in one patient was noted with trimethoprim/sulfisoxazole.[28] Itraconazole and fumigillin have recently been used with some success in treatment of *Microsporida*.[27]

REFERENCES

1. Catania LJ. Diagnoses of the Cornea. In LJ Catania (ed), Primary Care of the Anterior Segment. Norwalk, CT: Appleton & Lange, 1995;241–341.

2. Waring GO, Rodrigues MM, Laibson PR. Corneal dystrophies. I. Dystrophies of the epithelium, Bowman's layer and stroma. Surv Ophthalmol 1978;23:71–113.

3. Smolin G. Dystrophies and Degenerations. In G Smolin and RA Thoft (eds), The Cornea: Scientific Foundations and Clinical Practice. Boston: Little, Brown, 1983;329–354.

4. Waring GO, Rodrigues MM, Laibson PR. Corneal Dystrophies. In HM Leibowitz (ed), Corneal Disorders: Clinical Diagnosis and Management. Philadelphia: Saunders, 1984;57–99.

5. Waring GO, Rodrigues MM, Laibson PR. Corneal dystrophies. II. Endothelial dystrophies. Surv Ophthalmol 1978;23:147–166.

6. Buckley RJ. The Cornea. In DJ Spalton, RA Hitchings, PA Hunter (eds), Atlas of Clinical Ophthalmology. Philadelphia: Lippincott, 1984;1–16.

7. Scott CA, Catania LJ, Larkin KM, et al. Care of the Patient with Ocular Disease, Clinical Guidelines. St. Louis: American Optometric Association, 1995;1–48.

8. Kantor GR, Spielvogel RL, Yanoff M. Skin and Lacrimal Drainage System. In TL Duane (ed), Biomedical Foundations of Ophthalmology. Philadelphia: Lippincott, 1993;1–45.

9. Henriques AS, Korb DR. Inadequate or deficient meibomian gland secretion can adversely affect the success of contact lens wear. Br J Ophthalmol 1981;65:108–111.

10. Shine WE, Silvany R, McCulley JP. Relation of cholesterol-stimulated *Staphylococcus aureus* growth to chronic blepharitis. Invest Ophthalmol Vis Sci 1993;34:2291–2296.

11. English FP, Nutting WB. Demodicosis of ophthalmic concern. Am J Ophthalmol 1981;91:362–372.

12. Serrander AM, Peek KE. Changes in contact lens comfort related to menstrual cycle and menopause. A review of articles. J Am Optom Assoc 1993;64:162–166.

13. Silbert JA. The Role of Inflammation in Contact Lens Wear. In JA Silbert (ed), Anterior Segment Complications of Contact Lens Wear. New York: Churchill Livingstone, 1994;123–142.

14. Snyder C. Infiltrative keratitis with contact lens wear—a review. J Am Optom Assoc 1995;66:160–177.

15. Weissman BA, Mondino BJ. Ulcerative Bacterial Keratitis. In JA Silbert (ed), Anterior Segment Complications of Contact Lens Wear. New York: Churchill Livingstone 1994;247–270.

16. Allansmith MR. Immunology of the external ocular tissues. J Am Optom Assoc 1990;61:16–22.

17. Shovlin JP, DePaolis MD, DeSando MA. The great masqueraders—and how to unmask them. Rev Optom 1991;128:33–37.
18. Udell IJ, Mannus MJ, Meisler DM. Pseudodendrites in soft contact lens wear. CLAO J 1985;11:51–55.
19. Matoba AY. Infectious Keratitis. In Focal Points: Clinical Modules for Ophthalmologists. San Francisco: American Academy for Ophthamology, 1992;1–10.
20. Shovlin JP. What to expect the morning after. Optom Management 1992;24:73.
21. Aquavella JA, Shovlin JP, DePaolis MD. Protozoan and Fungal Keratitis in Contact Lens Wear. In JA Silbert (ed), Anterior Segment Complications of Contact Lens Wear. New York: Churchill Livingstone 1994;271–288.
22. Wilhelmus KR, Robinson NM, Font RA. Fungal keratitis in contact lens wearers. Am J Ophthalmol 1988;106:708–713.
23. Berger ST, Mondino BJ, Hoft RH. Successful management of *Acanthamoeba* keratitis. Am J Ophthalmol 1990;110:335–340.
24. Hirst LS, Green WR, Mertz W. Management of *Acanthamoeba* keratitis—a case report and review of the literature. Ophthalmology 1984;91:1105–1109.
25. John KJ, Head WS, Parrich CM. Examination of hydrophilic contact lenses with light microscopy to aid in the diagnosis of *Acanthamoeba* keratitis. Am J Ophthalmol 1989;108:329–332.
26. Pfister DR, Cameron JD, Krachmer JH, et al. Confocal microscopy findings of *Acanthamoeba* keratitis. Am J Ophthalmol 1996;121:119–128.
27. Mathers WD, Sutphin JE, Folberg R, et al. Outbreak of keratitis presumed to be caused by *Acanthamoeba*. Am J Ophthalmol 1996;121:129–142.
28. Davis RM, Font RL, Keisler MS, et al. Corneal microsporidiosis—a case report including ultrastructural observations. Ophthalmology 1990;97:953–957.

Chapter 3

Examination and Instrumentation

Milton M. Hom

I. **Patient history** is important in establishing the viability of contact lens wear. A case history to which several questions pertaining to contact lenses have been added should be taken.
   A. A **general history** concerning allergy, hay fever, and systemic drugs is indicative of potential dry-eye problems (see Chapter 16). Knowledge of past conditions concerning **ocular health,** such as surgery or infection, is helpful.
   B. A **past contact lens history** is extremely helpful in avoiding future problems. It is important to know about past successes or failures, reasons for lens wear, and previous care regimens.[1]
   C. **Patient motivation** is a necessary ingredient. The patient needs sufficient motivation to overcome the fear, discomfort, and possible visual compromise commonly seen with contact lenses. The patient needs to be responsible and compliant with regard to lens care[2] (see Chapter 13).
   D. **Indications** for contact lenses are anisometropia, high myopia, irregular cornea, eye color change, bandage or therapeutic needs, cosmesis, and inability to wear spectacles (due to skin allergies, nasal problems, epidermolysis bullosa); they are also used in sports and by theater and film performers.[1,3]
   E. **Contraindications** may include low refractive errors, horizontal prism, ocular infections and inflammations, recurrent corneal erosions, diabetes, sinus and allergy problems, sensitive eyes, dry eyes, poor blinking, acne rosacea, seborrheic conditions, and a dusty environment.[1]
II. **Contrast sensitivity function** is an evaluation of visual perception across a range of object sizes and contrast levels. The test consists of five rows of sinewave grating targets, or patches, in a nine-by-five matrix. The targets decrease in contrast from left to right. The test is scored and a "signature" plotted. Contrast sensitivity function can be used to demonstrate to the patient differences in vision between old and new soft lenses. High-frequency defects may indi-

cate corneal edema and early retinal pathology. Middle- and low-frequency defects appear with optic nerve and cerebellum lesions.[4]

III. **Binocularity** can be affected by contact lenses.

    A. **Myopes** must converge and accommodate more with contact lenses than with spectacles. Insufficient accommodation can be a problem, as can esophoria. Myopes with intermittent or occasional **exotropia** may benefit more from contact lenses.[5,6]

    B. **Hyperopes** accommodate less and converge less with contact lenses. A beginning **hyperopic presbyope** will do better with contact lenses than myopic patients. **Hyperopic esophores** and **hyperopic accommodative esotropes** can also benefit from contact lenses.[5,6]

    C. **Vertical phorias** can be corrected with up to two prism diopters in contact lenses. Lateral phoria, however, is corrected with lateral prism and is better corrected with scleral lenses.[5]

IV. A **biomicroscope**, or **slit lamp**, offers a detailed, stereoscopic, noninvasive view of the anterior segment. The transparent ocular tissues allow the use of several different types of illumination. Types of illumination vary with the positioning, size, shape, focus, and filtration of the beam. Mastery of the biomicroscope is essential for the competent contact lens practitioner.

    A. **Diffuse illumination** gives a large, uniform view of the living eye. A ground-glass filter is placed in front of the beam to diffuse the focused light. The recommended angle is 45 degrees with low magnification.

    B. **Direct illumination** is used when the oculars are viewing where the beam is focused. The type of direct illumination varies with the size of the beam. The beam can be a small, thin optic section; a larger, thicker parallelepiped; or an even larger broad beam. When an optic section is shortened, it becomes a conical beam.[7,8]

        1. An **optic section** is a very thin beam designed to give a cross-section of the cornea. It is used primarily to give the location of a structure within the corneal layers. The front part of the section (closest to the light source) is the epithelium or tears; the back part is the endothelium[7] (Figure 3.1).

            a. The **angle** is set between 30 and 60 degrees to the oculars, on the same side as the corneal section being viewed. A beam narrowed as much as possible is required. More of the stroma can be revealed by increasing the angle between the oculars and light source.[7,8]

            b. **Corneal layers** and depth can be distinguished with an optic section. Depth can be localized with an optic section and a simple knowledge of the corneal layers. Apparent depth, however, is approximately two-thirds of the actual depth. One use of the optic section is determination of the depth of an embedded **foreign body.**[7,8] **Corneal dystrophies** are also more easily identified with an optic section because the layer can be localized.

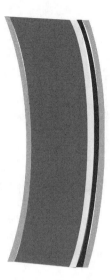

FIGURE 3.1 *Optic section. An optic section reveals a cross-section of the cornea. The light source is positioned to the right of the optic section. Closest to the light source is the bright tear layer. The epithelium appears as the dark layer adjacent to the tear layer. Next to the epithelium on the right is another bright layer, which represents Bowman's membrane. The wide area is the stroma. The bright layer on the left of the optic section is the posterior cornea.*

    c. **Flare** and **cells** in the anterior chamber can be detected by positioning the upper part of the optic section against the dark background of the pupil.[8] Some practitioners prefer an optic section over a conical beam (see the discussion of conical beam, section IV.B.4).

2. A **parallelepiped** is the most commonly used illumination. It is essentially a wider optic section. The beam is widened to approximate the corneal depth, anywhere from 0.1 to 0.7 mm. A wide block of **stroma** with broad views of the anterior and posterior surfaces is easily seen[7,8] (Figure 3.2). The width, height, and depth of an object can be determined at the same time. Most objects in the cornea can be assessed with a parallelepiped. The slit width and focus need continual adjustment during an examination.

3. **Broad-beam illumination** is similar to the optic section and parallelepiped, except that the beam is widened to more than corneal thickness. **Larger objects** and structures are more easily assessed with the broad beam. These include pterygia, corneal nerves, and large scars and opacities.[7] Remember to turn down the light inten-

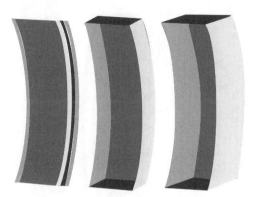

FIGURE 3.2   *Parallelepiped. On the left, a narrowed parallelepiped is an optic section. In the center is a thinner parallelepiped. On the right, a wide parallelepiped is shown. The stroma and anterior and posterior surfaces are easily seen. The light source is positioned on the right.*

sity with broad-beam illumination. The widened beam is usually too bright if the intensity is kept the same as with a parallelepiped.

4. **Conical beam illumination** is primarily used for viewing **cells** and **flare** in the anterior chamber. Its use is based on **Tyndall's phenomenon.**[9] The optic section is shortened to 1–2 mm in height. There should be no illumination in the room because of the low intensity of the small conical beam. Cells appear as whitish reflections passing by the conical beam. Flare appears as yellowish particles. Red blood cells appear as reddish-yellow dots. White blood cells appear grayish-white. Pigment granules are brown. Cells and flare show best against the dark pupil.[7,8]

5. **Specular reflection** is commonly used to view the endothelium. The angle of the light source must be set to equal the angle of the oculars. The light and objective are moved until a bright, glaring reflection off of the anterior corneal surface is seen. Oculars are first moved 20 degrees away from the light source. The light source is then moved in the opposite direction until the bright, glaring reflection is seen in one ocular. There should be three reflexes: a bright reflection off the tear layer, a dimmer reflex off the endothelium, and the blurred image of the light source filament.[10] The endothelium appears in the dimmer reflection between the two reflexes as a patch of beaten gold[11] (Figures 3.3 and 3.4). Focus on the endothelium patch and increase magnification to observe the endothelial cells.[7]

   Pearl: *A considerable area of endothelium can be examined by having the patient change fixation.*[9]

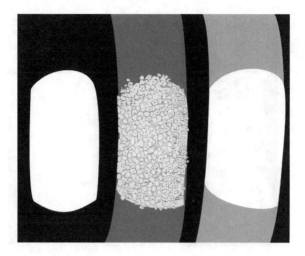

FIGURE 3.3   *Specular reflection of endothelium. In the center is specular reflection off the endothelium. The endothelial mosaic is visible and in focus. On the left is the reflection of the light filament. On the right is the specular reflection off the anterior corneal surface. Both the anterior cornea surface and the light filament are out of focus.*

a. The **lipid layer** of the tears can also be observed with specular reflection. The oculars are focused on the tear film around the bright reflection off the lipid layer.[7,12] Increasing the angle between the light source and oculars makes the endothelial reflex easier to view. The anterior reflection becomes less distracting. The Tearscope (Keeler Instruments, Broomall, Pennsylvania) uses specular reflection to view the lipid layer (see the discussion of the Tearscope, section VII).

b. **Endothelial cell features** are seen with specular reflection. The clarity of specular reflection depends on the smoothness of the reflecting surface. An example is the sun's reflection on the surface of a lake: Undisturbed water reflects an almost mirror image of the sun, but any surface disruption, such as rippling of water, makes the reflection uneven and breaks it with dark areas. Elevations and depressions in the endothelium, such as **guttata** or **folds,** disturb the evenness of the surface. They appear as dark defects within the specular reflection. With good optics, the borders of the endothelial cells are visible. The flat surface of the endothelial cell itself is highly reflective. The junctional borders are uneven and appear as a dark mosaic, however. These characteristics are used in detecting **polymegethism** and **pleomorphism** with specular reflection.[7-9]

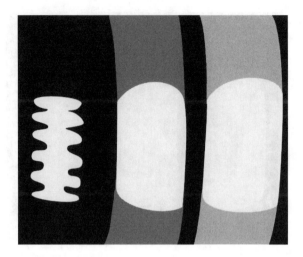

FIGURE 3.4   *Specular reflection and light filament. On the left is the light filament reflection in focus. When the filament is in focus, both the posterior and anterior cornea to the right are blurred.*

6. Oblique, or **tangential, illumination** is used to view elevations in the iris surface. The angle between the oculars and light source is increased to almost 90 degrees. The beam is positioned tangential to the eye, creating long shadows for any elevations.[7,8]

C. **Indirect illumination** entails viewing what is not in the focused light beam. It is the secondary illumination of the reflected light from the direct beam. Normally, the oculars and beam are linked together. Offsetting the beam or taking the beam out of **click stop** disengages the linkage and creates indirect illumination. Taking the beam out of click stop is not necessary to allow indirect illumination. Indirect illumination is used whenever structures not within the focused light beam are viewed. Direct illumination is used when the structures are within the focused light.[7,9]

  1. **Proximal illumination** entails viewing the area adjacent to the focused light beam. Objects are observed with scattered light. The scattering increases contrast and produces a silhouette of the area of interest against a light background. Many **changes in transparency** can be seen only with proximal illumination, but this form of illumination does not reveal the texture of the object. Proximal illumination, for example, can be used to see changes in transparency in front of the leading edge of a **pterygium**.[7,9] **Infiltrates** can be viewed with direct or indirect illumination. The center of the infiltrate is made of densely packed cells that thin out toward

the periphery. Infiltrates are either epithelial or stromal and can be differentiated with an optic section.

    a. **Epithelial infiltrates** are small grayish-white clusters. They reflect light with direct illumination. With marginal retroillumination, small refractile bodies, or gray bodies, appear within the infiltrate. The refractile bodies differ from **microcysts** in that they appear in patches within the infiltrate. Microcysts are usually spread out over the cornea and not densely clustered in a specific area. **Vacuoles** also differ from infiltrates by not reflecting light and almost disappearing with direct illumination.[13]

    b. **Stromal infiltrates,** or **subepithelial infiltrates,** appear snowball-like with a white or buff center.[13] They may have an "orange peel" appearance with indirect illumination. Medium magnification, bright illumination, and a parallelepiped are needed to see the hazy, diffuse, whitish infiltrate.[14]

  2. **Sclerotic scatter** is used to detect **central corneal clouding.** Polymethyl methacrylate lenses, as well as steeply fitted, low oxygen permeable (Dk) silicone acrylates, can display central corneal clouding. A parallelepiped is focused at the limbus and positioned at an angle between 45 and 60 degrees, creating a circumcorneal glow. The cornea is viewed against the dark background of the pupil with the naked eye, outside the oculars. The whitish haze of **edema** within the pupil can be detected.[7]

D. **Retroillumination** makes use of the reflection of the focused beam to view the cornea. Refractile bodies appear best with retroillumination. When direct focal illumination is applied, it sometimes overpowers and washes out an abnormality. Retroillumination deliberately avoids the use of direct light.[9] Anterior corneal objects are backlighted with light reflected from the deeper iris or retina.[7]

  1. **Direct retroillumination** entails viewing the object entirely illuminated with reflected light against an **illuminated background.** A parallelepiped normally hits the eye in two places, the focused bright area of light on the cornea and the associated reflected area on the iris or retina. The reflected light is directed behind the object being viewed. Objects that normally appear light will appear dark with direct retroillumination. Direct retroillumination can also use the light reflected off the **retina.** An object in the more anterior lenticular lens or cornea becomes illuminated against the red glow of the retina.[7]

  2. **Indirect retroillumination** occurs when the object is illuminated indirectly against a dark background.[7] Indirect retroillumination is similar to direct retroillumination, but in indirect retroillumination, the object is viewed against a **dark** rather than a light background. The beam is positioned such that the dark background is behind

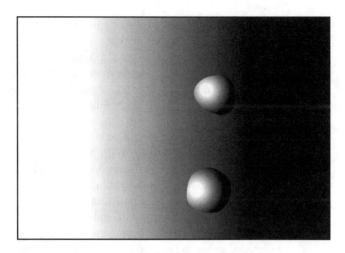

FIGURE 3.5   *Unreversed illumination and vacuoles. Unreversed or reversed illumination refers to the side the shadow is cast on. With the light coming from the left, vacuoles display unreversed illumination.*

the object. The object is not within the pathway of the reflected light. Light-colored and almost transparent objects appear best against a dark background.[8]

3. **Marginal retroillumination** is used for viewing refractile bodies such as **microcysts** and **vacuoles.** The junction between the light and dark iris-reflected background areas is placed alongside the refractile body. Lesions with a lower index, such as vacuoles, will appear as **unreversed illumination.** The lower-index vacuole acts like a converging lens. A higher-index material, such as that contained by microcysts, shows **reversed illumination** (Figures 3.5 and 3.6). Sometimes, however, microcysts show both reversed and unreversed illumination because the contents may vary.[13]

E. A **cobalt filter** is used to view fluorescein dye. Abrasions, ulcers, edema, epithelial defects, and foreign bodies appear vivid green with a cobalt filter or blue light.[7,15] The cause of any staining in the cornea should be ascertained.[3] Remember, however, that areas of staining can indicate places where epithelial cells are not tightly attached to each other.[6] The natural fluorescence of the cornea tends to obscure staining. Affixing a yellow Kodak Wratten 12 or 15 or Tiffen 2 filter (Bausch & Lomb [B&L], Rochester, New York) to the observation system greatly enhances contrast of contact lens fluorescein studies[11,15] (see Chapter 6).

1. **Sequential staining** involves instilling fluorescein up to six times, 5 minutes apart. Staining that may otherwise go undetected will appear with the sequential application of fluores-

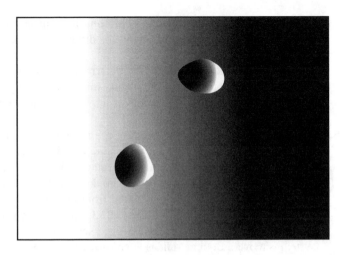

FIGURE 3.6 *Reversed illumination and microcysts. Microcysts display reversed illumination, the illumination coming from the left.*

cein.[15] Possible contact lens intolerance can be predicted with
sequential staining.[3]

2. **Negative staining** indicates **elevations** or **irregularities** in the epithelial surface. The staining appears as a dark blue area similar to
that seen in tear break-up testing. The break-up area appears in-
stantaneously, however, and the area does not move with blinking.
Epithelial basement membrane disorders and emerging microcysts
can cause negative staining.[16,17]

F. **Red-free filters** block all red wavelengths. Use of a red-free filter allows
the hemoglobin-rich vessels to appear as dark branching against a green
background. Another method, indirect retroillumination with white light,
is not as effective due to shadowing and cloaking effects.[18]

G. A **routine slit lamp examination** is best accomplished by following a system. Some practitioners prefer an **"inside out"** system (starting with the
lenticular lens and moving out to the lids); others prefer an **"outside in"**
system (starting with the lids and working inward to the lenticular lens).

V. The **keratometer** is the most commonly used instrument for cornea curvature measurements. It not only measures radius of curvature, but it can also
verify base curves of rigid lenses and detect corneal distortion. Although it is
the standard, keratometry (K) has many drawbacks. The measurement encompasses the central 2.8–4 mm cornea, depending on the corneal power. The
small size of the area measured may lead to errors in determining the exact
toricity of the cornea. For contact lens fitting, K readings are good approximations of toricity. For larger surface area procedures such as excimer or radial keratotomy, however, K readings are not as useful. The same cornea can

also produce a variety of readings with different instruments. This may be due to the use of different mire separations and different indices of refraction for calibration.[11,19]

A.　The **principle of keratometry** is to determine the difference between the object or target size and the virtual image formed by the cornea. Since the cornea is considered a convex mirror, the radius of curvature is calculated with mirror formulas.[20]

B.　**Doubling** greatly reduces the effect of eye movement when a measurement is being taken. A prism splits the mire into two images. The prism or doubling system is moved until the images touch. At that point, the separation between the images is equal to the virtual image size. The actual image size can then be calculated from magnification formulas.[8] Keratometers use **variable doubling** (B&L) and **fixed doubling.** With variable doubling, the mires have a fixed separation and the doubling system is moved. Both meridians are measured at the same time, as with the B&L keratometer. With fixed doubling, the doubling system is fixed and the mire separation is varied. These are two-position keratometers that require rotation to measure both meridians.[11,21]

C.　The **measurement procedure** entails focusing the eyepiece and lining up the patient's eye. A penlight directed through the eyepiece is a helpful guide for proper alignment. The instrument is then moved forward with the focusing knob. With the B&L keratometer, there should be four images. Although the mires are not in focus, they still can be seen because of **Scheiner's principle.** The two mires in the lower right are made to overlap as perfectly as possible with the focusing knob.[11] To determine the axis of the principle meridians, the keratometer barrel is rotated so that the pluses are in direct line with each other. The pluses and minuses are superimposed over each other with the dioptric wheels to determine the corneal curvature.[8]

D.　**Irregular corneas** distort the mires. Distorted mires do not appear smooth or equal in size. Sometimes, **doubled mires** appear. These are mires that cannot be made to overlap properly despite the best focusing efforts. At other times, the mires may appear not round but oval or shaped like a **racetrack.** All of these can indicate an irregular cornea or keratoconus (see Chapter 17).

E.　**Front surface keratometry,** or overkeratometry, is a variation of standard keratometry.[22] Keratometry is performed over rigid lenses while the lenses are being worn, which gives an idea as to the amount of lens flexure.

F.　The **range** of the keratometer can be extended by adding a +1.25 D lens to the front end of the instrument. This enables measurement of the excessively steep corneas seen in **keratoconus.** Adding a –1.00 D lens helps in measuring excessively flat corneas.[11] There are tables showing the equivalent curvature measurement after the keratometer has been extended with trial lenses (see Appendix A).

G. **Autokeratometry** is faster and more convenient than regular manual keratometry. The corneal radius reading is similar to manual keratometry. Mires or infrared beams are reflected off the cornea and measured by photosensors.[21] Some autokeratometers are combined with autorefractors.

VI. **Videokeratography** has been a significantly powerful advance in the assessment of corneal topography. It works on the same general principle as keratometry. Several concentric target rings are projected onto the cornea, creating a virtual image.[20] That image is compared with the target size, and the curvature is calculated by computer. **Color-coded maps** that encompass a large area of the cornea are produced. Usually, redder colors are the steeper areas and the bluer colors are the flatter areas. The location of the corneal apex is easily found with videokeratography. For some bifocals, such as the **Lifestyle Hi-Rider** (Lifestyle Company, Morganville, New Jersey), this may be invaluable (see Chapter 18). Use of the **subtractive analysis** feature can dramatically demonstrate any changes in corneal topography. For changing topographies such as those found in keratoconus, periodic assessments can be useful to determine the course of the condition.[23] Drawbacks of videokeratography include errors in alignment, focusing, calibration, software, and hardware.[19]

VII. The **Tearscope** is a hand-held instrument used with a biomicroscope to view the lipid layer of the tear film using specular reflection. It is a hemispheric illumination system with a central hole for viewing. The Tearscope is placed over the eye and the hole aligned with the biomicroscope objective. Different patterns are formed according to the thickness of the layer (see Chapter 16). Normal layers lack interference patterns and appear as varying shades of gray.[12,24]

REFERENCES

1. Gasson A, Morris J. Preliminary Considerations and Examination. In A Gasson, J Morris (eds), The Contact Lens Manual. Oxford, England: Butterworth–Heinemann, 1992;20–37.

2. White PF, Gilman EL. Preliminary Evaluation. In ES Bennett, BA Weissman (eds), Clinical Contact Lens Practice. Philadelphia: Lippincott, 1991(17);1–18.

3. Stone J. Assessment of Patient Suitability for Contact Lenses. In AJ Phillips, J Stone (eds). Contact Lenses (3rd ed). London: Butterworth,1989;270–298.

4. Baldwin JS, Lawner R, Keep GF. Could contrast sensitivity help your contact lens practice? CL Spectrum 1993;8(10):61–66.

5. Harris MG, Gilman E. Consultation, Examination and Prognosis. In RB Mandell (ed), Contact Lens Practice. Springfield, IL: Thomas, 1988;136–170.

6. Caffrey B. A better way to do sodium fluorescein staining. CL Spectrum 1994;9(2):56.

7. Zantos S, Cox I. Anterior Ocular Microscopy. In M Ruben, M Guillon (eds), Contact Lens Practice. London: Chapman & Hall, 1994;360–388.

8. Mandell RB. Contact Lens Instruments. In RB Mandell (ed), Contact Lens Practice. Springfield, IL: Thomas, 1988;913–953.

9.   Martonyi CL, Bahn CF, Meyer RF. Clinical Slit Lamp Biomicroscopy and Photo Slit Lamp Biomicrography. Ann Arbor, MI: Time One Ink, 1985;12–46.
10. Berliner ML (ed). Biomicroscopy of the Eye, Vol. 1. New York: Paul B. Hoeber, 1949;64–123.
11. Gasson A, Morris J. Instrumentation. In A Gasson, J Morris (eds), The Contact Lens Manual. Oxford, England: Butterworth–Heinemann, 1992;12–19.
12. Guillon JP, Guillon M. The Role of Tears in Contact Lens Performance and Its Measurement. In M Ruben, M Guillon (eds), Contact Lens Practice. London: Chapman & Hall, 1994;453–483.
13. Josephson JE, Caffrey BE, Rosenthal P, et al. Symptomatology and Aftercare. In M Ruben, M Guillon (eds), Contact Lens Practice. London: Chapman & Hall, 1994;559–580.
14. Grant T, Terry R, Holden BA. Extended Wear of Hydrogel Lenses. In MG Harris (ed), Problems in Optometry. Philadelphia: Lippincott 1990;599–622.
15. Schnider CM. Dyes. In JD Bartlett, SD Jaanus (eds), Clinical Ocular Pharmacology. Boston: Butterworth–Heinemann, 1995;389–407.
16. Silbert JA. Complications of extended wear. Optom Clin 1991;1(3):95–122.
17. Catania LJ. Diagnoses of the Cornea. In LJ Catania (ed), Primary Care of the Anterior Segment (2nd ed). Norwalk, CT: Appleton & Lange, 1995;203–351.
18. Grohe RM. A complete guide to detecting and managing limbal complications. CL Spectrum 1994;9(6):26.
19. Binder PS. Videokeratography. CLAO J 1995;21(2):133–144.
20. Mandell RB. Corneal topography. In RB Mandell (ed), Contact Lens Practice. Springfield, IL: Thomas, 1988;107–135.
21. Stone J, Rabbetts R. Keratometry and Specialist Optical Instrumentation. In M Ruben, M Guillon (eds), Contact Lens Practice. London: Chapman & Hall, 1994;283–311.
22. Schnider CM, Ames KS. Rigid Gas-Permeable Lens Design, Fitting, and Problem Solving. In ES Bennett (ed), Contact Lens Problem Solving. St. Louis: Mosby 1994;1–17.
23. Szczotka L, Lebow KA, Caroline P, et al. Mapping the future of contact lenses. CL Spectrum 1996;11(3):28–33.
24. Tomlinson A. Tear Film Changes with Contact Lens Wear. In A Tomlinson (ed), Complications of Contact Lens Wear. St. Louis: Mosby, 1992;159–194.

PART II

Rigid Lenses

Chapter 4

Rigid Lens Design and Fitting

Milton M. Hom

I. **Rigid gas-permeable (RGP) lenses** offer superior vision, long-term comfort, durability, and ease of care when compared with soft lenses.[1,2] RGP lenses are safe and effective.

A. **Comfort** is a major factor in choosing between RGP lenses and soft lenses. Patients with sensitive eyes may not have the adaptability to overcome the initial discomfort. Diagnostic fitting is an excellent method of detecting these patients before ordering lenses.

*Pearl: A patient who continues to tear and does not want to gaze straight ahead after the initial 15–20 minutes of rigid lens wear is a **high reactor**. **High reactors** usually have better success with soft lenses.[1]*

B. **Use of positive terms** when presenting rigid lenses to patients is advised by RGP experts. Negative terms such as "pain" should be avoided. For example, the clinician can refer to a lens as "having a tickling sensation" rather than being irritating. Positive terms are preferred to encourage the patient (Table 4.1).[3]

C. **Vision** is usually better with RGP lenses than with soft lenses. Rigid materials produce superior vision because they do not conform to the eye as soft lenses do. Greater amounts of spectacle cylinder are masked with rigid lenses.

II. **Determining which patients should wear lenses** is based on several factors, including age of the patient, motivation, and lifestyle.

A. **Myopia control** is a worthwhile benefit of RGP lenses for younger patients. RGP lenses have been shown to stabilize a child's myopic refraction.[4] When discontinued, the effect of lenses on myopic progression is diminished, but the increase in myopia is significantly less than would have occurred if spectacles were worn.[5]

Table 4.1   Terms to Avoid and Positive Terms to Use When Presenting Rigid Lenses to Patients

Terms to Avoid	Terms to Use
Hurt	Initial sensation
Pain	Edge awareness
Discomfort	Lid sensation
Irritation	"Tickling" sensation
Uncomfortable	Lid awareness
Painful	"Itchy" sensation

Source: Adapted from ES Bennett. How to present rigid lenses more effectively. Rev Optom 1994;131(Suppl):8A–10A.

Pearl: For advancing myopia, RGP lenses should be your first choice for contact lens patients younger than 18 years old.

B. **Polymethyl methacrylate (PMMA) rehabilitation** is an excellent reason to fit RGP lenses. PMMA lenses are not oxygen permeable, and 98% of patients have edema.[6] Refitting with RGP lenses is recommended whether or not there are any symptoms.[7,8] Lower-Dk fluorosilicone acrylates (FSAs) are an excellent choice, largely because high-Dk lenses are vulnerable to warpage.[9] There is no distinct advantage of higher Dk lenses for daily wear, unless there are signs of RGP-induced edema developing later.[6,10,11]

   1. **Signs and symptoms** of patients needing rehabilitation are **spectacle blur** of 30 minutes or longer, **mire distortion,** 20/25 visual acuity with lenses, decreased wearing time, **corneal changes** of 0.75 D or more, and **poor endpoint refraction** without lenses.[7,12] Biomicroscopic signs are increasing or persistent **staining, microcystic edema, neovascularization,** and **central corneal clouding**[12,13] (see Chapter 3).

   2. **Corneal topography** shows relative flattening in the superior cornea accompanied by inferior steepening for high-riding PMMA lenses. This change in topography resembles a keratoconic topography.[14]

   3. The **Rengstorff curve** describes the changes in cornea curvature after PMMA lenses have been removed.[7,15] Myopia decreases during the first 3 days after cessation of lens wear, then increases over several weeks until it stabilizes (Figure 4.1).

   4. **Immediate refitting** with rigid lenses is advised for long-term PMMA wearers.[10,12] Rengstorff found that the curvature measured immediately after removal closely matches the cornea after stabilization has taken place.[7] Refitted RGP lenses can continue to be worn on a full-time basis after dispensing. Immediate refitting with soft lenses is not advisable, however.

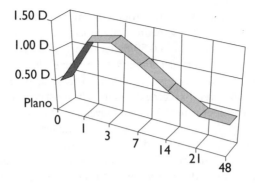

FIGURE 4.1 *Rengstorff curve. Rengstorff found that myopia decreases over the first 3 days after stopping polymethyl methacrylate (PMMA) wear and then increases over several weeks until it stabilizes. Refitting the cornea immediately after lens removal is advised. The horizontal axis indicates the number of days. The vertical axis indicates the mean amount of myopic change. (Adapted from ES Bennett. Treatment Options for PMMA-Induced Problems. In ES Bennett, RM Grohe [eds], Rigid Gas-Permeable Contact Lenses. New York: Professional Press, 1986;283.)*

> ***Pearl:*** *That PMMA lens wear should be discontinued for 3 days before examination is a common myth. After 3 days without wear is probably the worst time to perform a refraction.*[12]

5. **PMMA parameters** can be used for the RGP lenses. Some authors, however, advise modifying the design to a larger, flatter, thicker lens with lower edge lift.[6,10,16,17]

6. **Foreign body sensitivity** may be experienced by former PMMA patients.[18] Corneal sensitivity returns to a more normal state with RGP lenses. Foreign bodies that were once undetected by the patient become noticeable.

7. **Corneal warpage syndrome (CWS)** is usually due to extreme hypoxia related to PMMA lenses.[15,19] Large amounts of astigmatism appear after long-term PMMA wear. Sometimes it takes up to 5 months after lens cessation before stabilization occurs.[15] Patients with CWS rarely have K readings of more than 50 D. It needs to be diagnostically differentiated from keratoconus because both conditions display corneal distortion. CWS does not display the classic biomicroscopic signs such as Fleischer's ring or Vogt's striae. Immediately refitting RGP lenses is advised but with reduced wearing time until stabilization is reached.

III. **Rigid lens fitting and management** require more skill than fitting soft lenses. Instead of the "one size fits all" approach used with soft lenses, additional expertise is necessary.

A. **Lens selection** is usually around 9.0-mm diameter ± 0.3 mm, although larger diameters are sometimes suggested.[20] If diagnostic fitting, the initial base curve ranges from 0.50 flatter than K (9.2-mm diameter) to "on K" (9.0-mm diameter), depending on the fitting philosophy.[20-25] K is designated as the flat keratometer reading. The initial base curve can be steepened with increasing corneal toricity. The most common RGP fit is usually **lid attachment** with 1–2 mm of movement. If the lens can be centered better with the help of the upper lid, a larger, flatter lens is used.[26] If the lens is centered better without lid influence, a smaller lens is used.[27] Presently, **FSAs** are the material of choice for most cases[22,28] (see Chapter 5).

B. **Fluorescein pattern and centration** require interpretation with a biomicroscope or Burton lamp. Ideally, the lens should have an alignment-fitting relationship (see Chapter 6). Centration should be within the corneal diameter and completely cover the pupil.[26] The base curve should be adjusted to achieve alignment fit and proper centration.

C. **Vision** needs to be checked with a spherical cylindrical over-refraction. If the cylinder power in the over-refraction is necessary for adequate vision, a toric lens should be considered[16] (see Chapter 8).

Pearl: For residual astigmatism of 0.75 D or higher, consider a lens designed for astigmatism.[16]

D. The **lens surface** should be examined while on the eye for deposits and poor wetting. The surface should be clean without hazing or dry patches.[26] If deposits are present, the patient may be predisposed to soilage in the future. Lens care procedures may need to be customized (see Chapter 9). Poor wetting is often associated with deposits, and poor wetting and deposits are warning signs of a possible dry eye (see Chapter 16).

E. The **follow-up schedule** after dispensing is usually appointments at 1 week, 2 weeks, 1 month, 2 months, 3 months, and 6 months. Subsequent follow-up is every 6 months.[26] **Procedures** during every follow-up include history (comfort, vision, and wearing times), visual acuity, over-refraction, fluorescein pattern, biomicroscopy (with and without lenses), and lens inspection. Keratometry and refraction are also advisable. Other helpful tests are retinoscopy and overkeratometry (also called front surface keratometry) (see Chapter 3).

IV. **Spherical rigid lens design** is important to understand when fitting rigid lenses.

A. **Physical parameters** are covered in Figures 4.2 and 4.3.

B. **Fitting philosophies** can be divided into two categories: **empirical** or **diagnostic.** Empirical fitting is a simple method that generates a design based on patient data. No lenses are placed on the eye until the ordered lenses are dispensed. With diagnostic fitting, lenses are actually trial-fitted on the patient's eye and tested. Although more time-consuming,

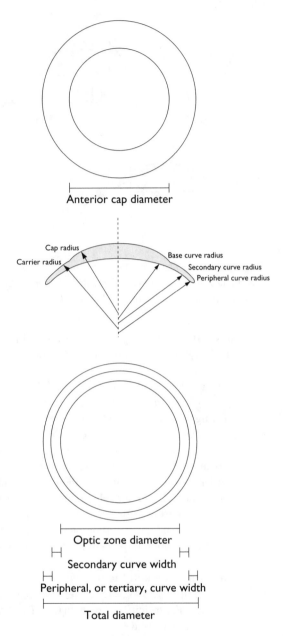

FIGURE 4.2   *Physical parameters. The top diagram shows the front surface of a tricurve lenticular rigid lens. The different lens radii are shown in the middle diagram. At the bottom is the back surface of the lens. (Adapted from AJ Phillips. Rigid Gas-Permeable and Hard Corneal Lens Fitting. In AJ Phillips, J Stone [eds], Contact Lenses [3rd ed]. London: Butterworth, 1989;337.)*

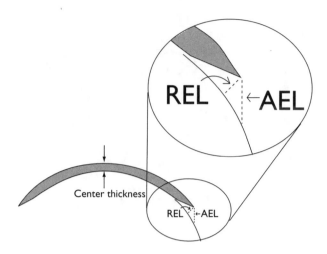

FIGURE 4.3   *Edge parameters. The center thickness, relative edge lift (REL), and axial edge lift (AEL). (Adapted from AJ Phillips. Rigid Gas-Permeable and Hard Corneal Lens Fitting. In AJ Phillips, J Stone [eds], Contact Lenses [3rd ed]. London: Butterworth, 1989;367.)*

diagnostic fitting has a higher success rate.[22] In 1937, the first trial-fitting sets made by Zeiss cost a prohibitive $1,000–3,500.

1. **Empirical fitting methods,** or **direct ordering,** ensures that a new, unworn lens is placed on the eye.[24] The fitting visit is eliminated, making this method easy to perform. Compared with diagnostic fitting, however it produces lower success rates and less patient confidence in the practitioner.[29] Performance factors such as residual astigmatism and centration cannot be evaluated and corrected in advance.[22,24] Despite the disadvantages, the majority of rigid lens orders are empirically prescribed by laboratories.[30]

   a. **Mandell's** empirical method is referred to as **custom.** The custom lens is defined by factors such as corneal diameter, lid position, lid tension, scotopic pupil size, and K readings. Custom lenses are interpalpebral—that is, they are primarily fit within the palpebral aperture.[31]

   b. **Harrison and Stein** use a nomogram for a 90% success rate in fitting FSAs.[32] Diameters are increased as base curves flatten. For toricity of less than 0.75 D, a base curve 0.75 D flatter than K is used.[32]

   c. **Computer programs** are available for lens design.[33,34] Corneal topographers can come equipped with fluorescein pattern simulators and lens design programs. Some programs will not only empirically design lenses, but also can process "what if" changes in lens parameters. Other information such as axial edge lift, flexure, and Dk/L or Dk/t are also calculated.[33]

Table 4.2   Interpalpebral Base Curve Selection

Corneal Cylinder (D)	Base Curve
0–0.75	0.25 D steeper than flat K
1.00–1.50	0.50 D steeper than flat K
1.75–2.50	0.75 D steeper than flat K
2.75–3.25	1.00 D steeper than flat K

Note: The base curve selection for an interpalpebral fit is steeper than K for an apical clearance fit. Twenty-five to 33% of the toricity is added to the flat K.
Source: Adapted from ES Bennett. Lens Design, Fitting, and Troubleshooting. In ES Bennett, RM Grohe (eds), Rigid Gas Permeable Contact Lenses. New York: Professional Press 1986;189–224.

    d. **Sag heights** are assumed to be alike for most eyes under empirical methods. When steep K readings are presented, it is assumed that the cornea is small (small and steep). If the cornea is large (large sag height), however, an improper lens is designed. The same applies to flat lenses. Flat lenses are designed with large corneas in mind. Again, if the flat cornea is small (small sag height), another improper lens is designed. Unfortunately, patients who have corneas with larger or smaller than usual sag heights can end up with unexpectedly flat or steep lenses.

  2. **Diagnostic fitting** is the preferred method by most authorities.[22,24]

    Pearl: Storing trial lenses dry avoids the problems of dried encrusted solute and base curve changes associated with wet storage.[35]

    Success with trial fitting can be assured when four factors are taken into account: spectacle astigmatism, lens itching, lens awareness (comfort), and spherical refractive error.[36] According to one study, high success rates are obtained with low astigmatism, no itching, good comfort, and low spherical error. For high astigmats, those with more than 0.75 D, the presence of itching is pivotal. When there is no itching, the success rate is 90%. When there is high astigmatism with itching, the success rate is 62%.

    Pearl: Some experts recommend an anesthetic to enhance the trial lens fitting. It can be used with no significant physiologic problems.[37]

C. **Interpalpebral,** or **"small and steep,"** fitting is originally a PMMA fitting philosophy. The smaller-diameter lens is typically 8.0–8.6 mm and centers primarily between the lids. Sometimes there is upper lid contact. The lens has an apical clearance fluorescein pattern with 1–2 mm of lens movement. The initial base curve is determined by adding 25–33% of the corneal toricity to the flat K (Table 4.2). Lid attachment philosophies

Table 4.3   Bennett's Diameter Selection

Diameter (mm)	Pupil Size in Dim Illumination (mm)	Corneal Curvature (D)	Palpebral Fissure Size (mm)
8.8–9.0	≤6	≥45	≤9.0
9.2–9.4	6–8	42	9.0–10.5
9.6–9.8	≥8	≤42	≥10.5

Source: Adapted from ES Bennett. Master the art of rigid lens design. Rev Optom 1994;131(Suppl):15A.

call for an interpalpebral type of fit for corneas greater than 45.00 D.[24] For large palpebral apertures when lid attachment is not feasible, interpalpebral fitting is the philosophy of choice. Another use of a small apical clearance interpalpebral lens is to help raise lens positioning.[23]

D. **Bennett** uses a tricurve or tetracurve design for spherical RGP lenses.[22]

   1. **Diameter** ranges between 9.2 and 9.4 mm; optic zones (OZs) range between 7.6 and 8.2 mm. A 9.2-mm diameter with a 7.8-mm OZ is most often prescribed. If a larger lens is needed, a 9.6-mm with an 8.2-mm OZ is used. When a smaller lens is indicated, an 8.8-mm with a 7.4-mm OZ is used. Bennett does not recommend small, 0.1-mm to 0.2-mm base curve changes when fitting because they have little effect on lens performance.[22] Diameter selection depends on pupil size, curvature, and palpebral fissure[38] (Table 4.3).

   2. **Base curve** radius (BCR) selection depends on corneal toricity. Bennett likes to use lenses that are basically **0.50 D flatter than K**.[24] The base curve needs to be adjusted if the OZ is changed. For every 0.25 D change in BCR, there needs to be a corresponding adjustment of 0.50 mm in OZ. For instance, if the OZ is increased 0.50 mm, the base curve must be flattened by 0.25 D. If the OZ is decreased 0.50 mm, the BCR must be steepened 0.25 D (Table 4.4).

   3. A **peripheral system** consists of a tricurve for an 8.8-mm diameter or a tetracurve for larger lenses. Tricurve design has a secondary and peripheral curve. The secondary curve has 1.0–1.5 mm added to the BCR. The peripheral curve has 1.5–2.0 mm added to the BCR. The widths are 0.3–0.4 mm.[38] The tetracurve has a secondary curve, intermediate curve, and peripheral curve, with 0.8 mm, 1.0 mm, and 1.4 mm added to the base curve radii, respectively. The widths are 0.3 mm for the secondary curve and 0.2 mm for both the intermediate and peripheral curves. A minimum of a medium blend is recommended.[24]

   4. **Center thickness** varies with power and Dk. Higher Dk materials (Dk 45–70) need an additional 0.02 mm. For every diopter toricity, another 0.02 mm of thickness should also be added.

Table 4.4   Bennett's Base Curve Selection

Corneal Cylinder (D)	Base Curve
0–0.50	0.50–0.75 D flatter than K
0.75–1.25	0.25–0.50 D flatter than K
1.50	On K
1.75–2.00	0.25 D steeper than K
2.25–2.75	0.50 D steeper than K
3.00–3.50	0.75 D steeper than K

Note: Based on corneal toricity measured by keratometry, base curves are selected with relationship to the K (flat keratometry reading). Lens diameter is 9.2 mm.
Source: Adapted from ES Bennett. Basic Fitting. In ES Bennett, BA Weissman (eds), Clinical Contact Lens Practice Philadelphia: Lippincott, 1991(23);1–22.

5. **Edge design** is important in Bennett's system. The edge should be thin, tapered, and rolled. Thickness is approximately 0.08–0.10 mm. With a tetracurve design, the edge lift (0.10–0.12 mm) is designed to be lower compared with PMMA. **Plus lenticular design** is indicated at powers of more than –5.00 D. **Minus lenticular design** is recommended for powers of less than –1.50 D and all plus lenses.[22,24]

6. **Hyperopic lenses** need some adjustment in lens parameters to optimize performance. BCR selection is steeper than K; diameter and OZ are larger than in other lenses.[22] Plus lenses have a higher mass, causing them to drop inferiorly. Minus lenticulation is advised.[24] The most common changes for hyperopic lenses are usually those made to enhance centering.

E. **Korb** design, otherwise known as **lid attachment** or **Polycon** (Wesley-Jessen, Des Plaines, Illinois) design, optimizes interaction with the upper lid.[22] Korb defines the optimum contact lens as an additional thin layer attached to the tear film. Since the tear film moves with the lid, the lens must move as if it was a part of the upper lid. Attachment to the upper lid enhances wetting, decreases staining, and facilitates blinking.[39]

1. **Correct blinking** is required. Proper blinking must be complete, relaxed, and frequent. Poor blinking contributes significantly to staining. If blinking is poor, it must be corrected with training[35] (see Chapter 16).

2. A **diameter** of 9.5 mm is suggested. Based on a study of 105 patients, 9.5 mm was the most accepted diameter (86%), offering optimal visual and fitting performance.[40] Diameters of 8.5 mm and 9.0 mm were later released in thicker parameters.[20]

3. An **OZ** of 8.4 mm allowed movement from superior to inferior limbus and back without causing visual fluctuation or a physical sensation.[40] Horizontal centration has been shown to be better with an 8.4 mm OZ.[41] Smaller OZs resulted in flare and distortion on

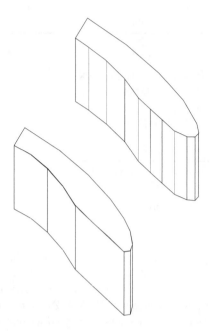

FIGURE 4.4   *Korb edge contour in computer-generated three-dimensional edge cross-sections. The Korb edge (top) slopes toward the upper lid. The edge is designed to attach to the lid. Conventional designs (bottom) slope away from the upper lid. (Adapted from ES Bennett. Lens Design, Fitting, and Troubleshooting. In ES Bennett, RM Grohe [eds], Rigid Gas-Permeable Contact Lenses. New York: Professional Press, 1986;206.)*

movement. Larger OZs resulted in loss of maximum comfort.[40] Another consideration was flexure. The larger 8.4-mm OZs have significantly higher flexure compared with smaller OZs.[42]

4.   The **base curve** is 0.25 mm flatter than flat K for a 9.0 mm diameter.[31]

5.   An **edge lift** of 0.12 mm was chosen over a 0.06-mm design because there was less peripheral corneal desiccation.[40]

6.   **Lenticular construction** was used to give an **edge profile** of a −3.00 lens, the profile that offered the best comfort.[40] For high powers, lenticular design was used to make an edge as optimal as possible. If the edge is too thick, too much of a lid effect takes place, causing superior decentration. A thin, 0.08-mm edge is optimal.[39] The edge contour was designed to slope toward the lid to enhance contact. Other edge designs slope away from the lid (Figure 4.4). **Peripheral corneal desiccation** is greatly reduced with a thin-edge, lid-attachment design.[3,24] Superiorly

Table 4.5 Inside-Out Philosophy and Lens Diameter

Visible Iris Diameter	Lens Diameter (mm)
Small (11.0 mm)	8.7
Medium (11.5 mm)	9.2
Large (12.0 mm)	9.7

Note: A guideline for lens diameter is the visible iris diameter. The lens should be 2.3 mm less than the iris diameter.

centered lenses have the lowest incidence of 3 o'clock and 9 o'clock staining.[37,43]

7. **Center thickness** is as thin as 0.07 mm to decrease lens mass and increase oxygen permeability.[40]

8. **Movement** of the lens is with the upper lid. Lens lag, or a dropping movement after the blink, must be eliminated.[44] This is achieved by corrective blinking, flattening the lens (often 0.40–0.50 mm flatter than flat K), or using a lenticular design.

F. **Inside-out design** begins with the base curve (inside) and adds the OZ and secondary and peripheral curves outwardly to establish the overall diameter.[22,23]

1. The **base curve** selected is **0.50 mm flatter than K,** regardless of corneal toricity, for an OZ of 7.0–7.5 mm.[23,45] A true alignment fit can only be achieved with a flatter radius of curvature than the cornea.[23]

2. **OZ diameter** is unique to give alignment for any given corneal curvature.[45] The OZ should equal, not exceed, the BCR. For every 0.5 mm increase in OZ, the base curve must be flattened by 0.25 D to maintain the same lens-to-cornea relationship.

3. The **peripheral system** has a **secondary curve radius** 1 mm flatter than the base curve. The secondary curve width is considered an **"accordion curve"** that adjusts depending on the OZ, peripheral curve, and overall diameter. **Peripheral curve** or **limbal clearance curve** has a radius of 12.25 mm and a standard width of 0.4 mm for peripheral clearance. The blend is heavy and between the two peripheral curve radii.[23,45]

4. The **diameter** is based on visible iris diameter. The lens should be 2.3 mm less than the visible iris diameter (Table 4.5).

5. **Lid position** is an important factor in size determination. If the upper lid covers a portion of the cornea, the lens can be designed to take advantage of its stabilizing effect. A larger-diameter lens (greater than 9.0 mm) is used to attach to the upper lid. A smaller diameter would be needed if the lower lid covers part of the cornea. If the upper lid is located above the cornea, a lid attachment fit may

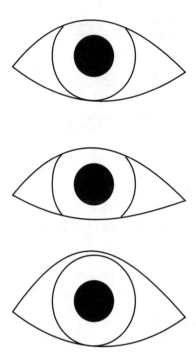

FIGURE 4.5   *Lid positioning and diameter. Top. This eye is ideal for lid attachment because the upper lid covers a portion of the cornea. Middle. Another lid-attachment eye, but the lens must be made smaller to gain the same effect. The lower lid covers a portion of the cornea. Bottom. The upper lid has no corneal coverage, which would make lid attachment difficult. A smaller and steeper interpalpebral lens would be better. (Adapted from GE Lowther. Review of rigid contact lens design and effects of design on lens fit. ICLC 1988;15[12]:379.)*

not be practical. A smaller, steeper lens fitted interpalpebrally may be better[44] (Figure 4.5) (CD-ROM: RGP lens fitting and eyelid geometry).

6. **Edge design** is usually lenticular for low minus and all plus lenses.[16] Thickening of the edge **(myoflange)** is needed for –2.00 D and below and for all plus lenses. Thinning of the edge **(hyperflange)** is for higher minus lenses.
7. **Center thickness** is 0.18 mm for a plano and decreases 0.01 mm for every diopter to –5.00. Above –5.00, edge thickness is 0.13 mm.
8. **Positioning** of the lens is under the upper lid for comfort and support. If the upper lid is at or above the superior limbus, the lens will lose support and drop. An **interpalpebral fit** is then needed.[23,45]
9. **Lens movement** along the vertical meridian should be smooth.[21] For with-the-rule corneas, the horizontal meridian acts as a fulcrum and limits lateral decentration. Lens movement on against-the-rule

Table 4.6 Mandell's Base Curve Selection

Corneal Toricity (D)	Base Curve
Spherical	On K or 0.25 D flatter than K
0.25–1.00	On K or 0.25 D steeper than K
1.00–2.00	0.50 D steeper than K
More than 2.00	Add ⅓ the difference in K to flat K

Note: Base curve in relationship to flat K for a 9.2 mm diameter lens is chosen according to amounts of corneal toricity.
Source: Adapted from RB Mandell. Fitting Methods and Philosophies. In RB Mandell (ed), Contact Lens Practice. Springfield, IL: Thomas, 1988;203–242.

    corneas tends to decenter laterally. The lens needs to be kept in place with the upper lid.[27]

G. **Mandell** defines his trial lens-fitting method as **standard.**[31]

1. **Standard lenses** are diagnostically fitted with a trial lens set of 8.8-mm diameter and 7.5-mm OZ; 9.2-mm diameter and 7.8-mm OZ; and 9.6-mm diameter and 8.0-mm OZ.

2. The **diameter** of 9.2 mm with a 7.8-mm OZ is the most often used. For corneas flatter than 42.00, a 9.6-mm diameter can be used. For corneas steeper than 44.00, a 8.8-mm diameter can be used.

3. The **base curve** is chosen to achieve minimal apical clearance (Table 4.6).

4. Regarding the **peripheral system,** the steepest system is sought that allows tear exchange (Table 4.7).

5. The **center thickness** is a minimum of 0.13 mm in the low minus lens for flexure considerations. This yields a 0.11-mm edge thickness.

H. **Bayshore** uses smaller lenses of around 8.0-mm diameter and an apical clearance relationship.[21] The lens is fitted interpalpebrally and centers without lid interaction. The edge lift is average to high, with a well-blended periphery and rapid but limited movement.[21]

V. **Power** can be determined empirically or with over-refraction.

A. The **spherical power** of the spectacle refraction (vertexed) should equal the power of an lens fitted "on K" (flat keratometry reading). Tear layer power must be accounted for if the base curve is different from the flat keratometry reading.

B. **Vertex distance** must be taken into consideration for powers of 4.00 and higher. The power at the spectacle is different than at the corneal plane. Any spectacle power must be "vertexed" to the corneal plane for higher powers. Usually, the vertex power can be looked up in tables (see Appendix B) or calculated. The formula is as follows:

Table 4.7   Mandell's Peripheral System

Base Curve (D)	SCR/Width (mm)	PCR/Width (mm)
41.00–41.50	9.5/0.4	11.1/0.3
42.00–43.00	9.0/0.4	10.8/0.3
43.50–44.50	9.0/0.4	10.5/0.3

SCR = secondary curve radius; PCR = peripheral curve radius.
Source: Adapted from RB Mandell. Fitting Methods and Philosophies. In RB Mandell (ed), Contact Lens Practice. Springfield, IL: Thomas, 1988;203–242.

$$F \text{ vertexed} = \frac{F(\text{spectacle sphere power})}{1 - d(\text{vertex distance})\, F(\text{spectacle sphere power})}$$

1. For **example,** for a spectacle power of +14.50 –3.00 × 010, the meridian powers are +14.50 and +11.50.[22] Each meridian is vertexed separately (for a 12-mm vertex distance):

$$\frac{+14.50}{1 - (0.012)(+14.50)} = +17.55 \text{ D}$$

$$\frac{+11.50}{1 - (0.012)(+11.50)} = +13.34 \text{ D}$$

The vertexed prescription is +17.55 –4.21 × 010 or, rounded off, +17.50 –4.25 × 010.

2. **MJK effectivity charts** are easy-to-use tables for determining vertex power at a standard 13 mm.[46] The need for meridional powers is eliminated (Table 4.8).

3. **Tear layer power** must be taken into account in determining rigid lens power. A steeper lens induces a plus tear lens. The plus tear lens needs to be compensated for in the lens power by adding minus. Flatter lenses create a negative tear lens and plus must be added.[22]

   a. The **SAMFAP rule** is useful for remembering how to compensate for tear lens power. "SAMFAP" stands for "Steeper Add Minus, Flatter Add Plus."[23,47] If the lens is steeper, then add the minus dioptric equivalent of base curve change. For a flatter lens, add the corresponding amount of plus power compensation.

   b. **For example,** for Ks of 45.00/46.50 (7.50 mm/7.25 mm), a BCR of 44.50 D (7.58 mm), and a spectacle Rx of –3.50 –1.00 × 180, the tear layer power must be accounted for.[23] Since the lens is flatter by 0.50 D, according to Flatter Add Plus (FAP), 0.50 would be added to the lens power, yielding a –3.00 D (–3.50 +0.50 = –3.00).

Table 4.8 MJK Effectivity Charts

Minus Sphere	Sphere Vertexed	-0.25	-0.50	-0.75	-1.00	-1.25	-1.50	-1.75	-2.00	-2.25	-2.50	-2.75	-3.00
Minus Sphere													
-3.00	-2.87	-0.25	-0.50	-0.75	-1.00	-1.25	-1.25	-1.50	-1.75	-2.00	-2.25	-2.50	-2.75
-3.25	-3.12	-0.25	-0.50	-0.75	-1.00	-1.25	-1.25	-1.50	-1.75	-2.00	-2.25	-2.50	-2.75
-3.50	-3.37	-0.25	-0.50	-0.75	-1.00	-1.25	-1.25	-1.50	-1.75	-2.00	-2.25	-2.50	-2.75
-3.75	-3.62	-0.25	-0.50	-0.75	-1.00	-1.00	-1.25	-1.50	-1.75	-2.00	-2.25	-2.50	-2.75
-4.00	-3.75	-0.25	-0.50	-0.75	-1.00	-1.00	-1.25	-1.50	-1.75	-2.00	-2.25	-2.50	-2.50
-4.25	-4.00	-0.25	-0.50	-0.75	-1.00	-1.00	-1.25	-1.50	-1.75	-2.00	-2.25	-2.50	-2.50
-4.50	-4.25	-0.25	-0.50	-0.75	-1.00	-1.00	-1.25	-1.50	-1.75	-2.00	-2.25	-2.25	-2.50
-4.75	-4.50	-0.25	-0.50	-0.75	-0.75	-1.00	-1.25	-1.50	-1.75	-2.00	-2.25	-2.25	-2.50
-5.00	-4.75	-0.25	-0.50	-0.75	-0.75	-1.00	-1.25	-1.50	-1.75	-2.00	-2.25	-2.25	-2.50
-5.25	-4.87	-0.25	-0.50	-0.75	-0.75	-1.00	-1.25	-1.50	-1.75	-2.00	-2.25	-2.25	-2.50
-5.50	-5.12	-0.25	-0.50	-0.75	-0.75	-1.00	-1.25	-1.50	-1.75	-2.00	-2.00	-2.25	-2.50
-5.75	-5.37	-0.25	-0.50	-0.75	-0.75	-1.00	-1.25	-1.50	-1.75	-2.00	-2.00	-2.25	-2.50
-6.00	-5.62	-0.25	-0.50	-0.75	-0.75	-1.00	-1.25	-1.50	-1.75	-2.00	-2.00	-2.25	-2.50
-6.25	-5.75	-0.25	-0.50	-0.75	-0.75	-1.00	-1.25	-1.50	-1.75	-1.75	-2.00	-2.25	-2.50
-6.50	-6.00	-0.25	-0.50	-0.75	-0.75	-1.00	-1.25	-1.50	-1.75	-1.75	-2.00	-2.25	-2.50
-6.75	-6.25	-0.25	-0.50	-0.75	-0.75	-1.00	-1.25	-1.50	-1.75	-1.75	-2.00	-2.25	-2.50
-7.00	-6.37	-0.25	-0.50	-0.50	-0.75	-1.00	-1.25	-1.50	-1.75	-1.75	-2.00	-2.25	-2.50
-7.25	-6.62	-0.25	-0.50	-0.50	-0.75	-1.00	-1.25	-1.50	-1.75	-1.75	-2.00	-2.25	-2.50
-7.50	-6.87	-0.25	-0.50	-0.50	-0.75	-1.00	-1.25	-1.50	-1.50	-1.75	-2.00	-2.25	-2.50
-7.75	-7.00	-0.25	-0.50	-0.50	-0.75	-1.00	-1.25	-1.50	-1.50	-1.75	-2.00	-2.25	-2.50
-8.00	-7.25	-0.25	-0.50	-0.50	-0.75	-1.00	-1.25	-1.50	-1.50	-1.75	-2.00	-2.25	-2.50
-8.25	-7.50	-0.25	-0.50	-0.50	-0.75	-1.00	-1.25	-1.50	-1.50	-1.75	-2.00	-2.25	-2.50
-8.50	-7.62	-0.25	-0.50	-0.50	-0.75	-1.00	-1.25	-1.50	-1.50	-1.75	-2.00	-2.25	-2.25
-8.75	-7.87	-0.25	-0.50	-0.50	-0.75	-1.00	-1.25	-1.50	-1.50	-1.75	-2.00	-2.25	-2.25
-9.00	-8.00	-0.25	-0.50	-0.50	-0.75	-1.00	-1.25	-1.50	-1.50	-1.75	-2.00	-2.25	-2.25

Table 4.8   *(continued)*

Minus Sphere	Sphere Vertexed	−0.25	−0.50	−0.75	−1.00	−1.25	−1.50	−1.75	−2.00	−2.25	−2.50	−2.75	−3.00
−9.25	−8.25	−0.25	−0.50	−0.50	−0.75	−1.00	−1.25	−1.25	−1.50	−1.75	−2.00	−2.00	−2.25
−9.50	−8.50	−0.25	−0.50	−0.50	−0.75	−1.00	−1.25	−1.25	−1.50	−1.75	−2.00	−2.00	−2.25
−9.75	−8.62	−0.25	−0.50	−0.50	−0.75	−1.00	−1.25	−1.25	−1.50	−1.75	−2.00	−2.00	−2.25
−10.00	−8.87	−0.25	−0.50	−0.50	−0.75	−1.00	−1.25	−1.25	−1.50	−1.75	−2.00	−2.00	−2.25
−10.25	−9.00	−0.25	−0.50	−0.50	−0.75	−1.00	−1.25	−1.25	−1.50	−1.75	−2.00	−2.00	−2.25
−10.50	−9.25	−0.25	−0.50	−0.50	−0.75	−1.00	−1.25	−1.25	−1.50	−1.75	−2.00	−2.00	−2.25
−10.75	−9.37	−0.25	−0.50	−0.50	−0.75	−1.00	−1.25	−1.25	−1.50	−1.75	−1.75	−2.00	−2.25
Plus sphere													
+4.00	+4.25	−0.25	−0.50	−0.75	−1.00	−1.25	−1.75	−2.00	−2.25	−2.50	−2.75	−3.00	−3.25
+4.25	+4.50	−0.25	−0.50	−0.75	−1.00	−1.50	−1.75	−2.00	−2.25	−2.50	−2.75	−3.00	−3.25
+4.50	+4.75	−0.25	−0.50	−0.75	−1.00	−1.50	−1.75	−2.00	−2.25	−2.50	−2.75	−3.00	−3.25
+4.75	+5.12	−0.25	−0.50	−0.75	−1.00	−1.50	−1.75	−2.00	−2.25	−2.50	−2.75	−3.00	−3.25
+5.00	+5.37	−0.25	−0.50	−0.75	−1.25	−1.50	−1.75	−2.00	−2.25	−2.50	−2.75	−3.00	−3.25
+5.25	+5.62	−0.25	−0.50	−0.75	−1.25	−1.50	−1.75	−2.00	−2.25	−2.50	−2.75	−3.00	−3.25
+5.50	+5.87	−0.25	−0.50	−0.75	−1.25	−1.50	−1.75	−2.00	−2.25	−2.50	−2.75	−3.00	−3.25
+5.75	+6.25	−0.25	−0.50	−0.75	−1.25	−1.50	−1.75	−2.00	−2.25	−2.50	−2.75	−3.00	−3.25
+6.00	+6.50	−0.25	−0.50	−1.00	−1.25	−1.50	−1.75	−2.00	−2.25	−2.50	−2.75	−3.00	−3.50
+6.25	+6.75	−0.25	−0.50	−1.00	−1.25	−1.50	−1.75	−2.00	−2.25	−2.50	−2.75	−3.00	−3.50
+6.50	***+7.12***	−0.25	−0.50	−1.00	−1.25	−1.50	−1.75	−2.00	−2.25	−2.50	***−3.00***	−3.25	−3.50
+6.75	+7.37	−0.25	−0.50	−1.00	−1.25	−1.50	−1.75	−2.00	−2.25	−2.50	−3.00	−3.25	−3.50
+7.00	+7.75	−0.25	−0.50	−1.00	−1.25	−1.50	−1.75	−2.00	−2.25	−2.50	−3.00	−3.25	−3.50
+7.25	+8.00	−0.25	−0.50	−1.00	−1.25	−1.50	−1.75	−2.00	−2.25	−2.75	−3.00	−3.25	−3.50
+7.50	+8.25	−0.25	−0.50	−1.00	−1.25	−1.50	−1.75	−2.00	−2.50	−2.75	−3.00	−3.25	−3.50
+7.75	+8.62	−0.25	−0.50	−1.00	−1.25	−1.50	−1.75	−2.00	−2.50	−2.75	−3.00	−3.25	−3.50
+8.00	+8.87	−0.25	−0.50	−1.00	−1.25	−1.50	−1.75	−2.25	−2.50	−2.75	−3.00	−3.25	−3.50
+8.25	+9.25	−0.25	−0.50	−1.00	−1.25	−1.50	−1.75	−2.25	−2.50	−2.75	−3.00	−3.25	−3.50

		−0.25	−0.75	−1.00	−1.25	−1.50	−1.75	−2.25	−2.50	−2.75	−3.00	−3.25	−3.75
+8.50	+9.50	−0.25	−0.75	−1.00	−1.25	−1.50	−1.75	−2.25	−2.50	−2.75	−3.00	−3.25	−3.75
+8.75	+9.87	−0.25	−0.75	−1.00	−1.25	−1.50	−1.75	−2.25	−2.50	−2.75	−3.00	−3.25	−3.75
+9.00	+10.25	−0.25	−0.75	−1.00	−1.25	−1.50	−2.00	−2.25	−2.50	−2.75	−3.00	−3.50	−3.75
+9.25	+10.50	−0.25	−0.75	−1.00	−1.25	−1.50	−2.00	−2.25	−2.50	−2.75	−3.00	−3.50	−3.75
+9.50	+10.87	−0.25	−0.75	−1.00	−1.25	−1.50	−2.00	−2.25	−2.50	−2.75	−3.25	−3.50	−3.75
+9.75	+11.12	−0.25	−0.75	−1.00	−1.25	−1.50	−2.00	−2.25	−2.50	−2.75	−3.25	−3.50	−3.75
+10.00	+11.50	−0.25	−0.75	−1.00	−1.25	−1.50	−2.00	−2.25	−2.50	−3.00	−3.25	−3.50	−3.75
+10.25	+11.87	−0.25	−0.75	−1.00	−1.25	−1.75	−2.00	−2.25	−2.50	−3.00	−3.25	−3.50	−3.75
+10.50	+12.12	−0.25	−0.75	−1.00	−1.25	−1.75	−2.00	−2.25	−2.50	−3.00	−3.25	−3.50	−3.75
+10.75	+12.50	−0.25	−0.75	−1.00	−1.25	−1.75	−2.00	−2.25	−2.50	−3.00	−3.25	−3.50	−4.00
+11.00	+12.87	−0.25	−0.75	−1.00	−1.25	−1.75	−2.00	−2.25	−2.75	−3.00	−3.25	−3.50	−4.00
+11.25	+13.12	−0.25	−0.75	−1.00	−1.25	−1.75	−2.00	−2.25	−2.75	−3.00	−3.25	−3.50	−4.00
+11.50	+13.50	−0.25	−0.75	−1.00	−1.25	−1.75	−2.00	−2.25	−2.75	−3.00	−3.25	−3.75	−4.00
+11.75	+13.87	−0.25	−0.75	−1.00	−1.25	−1.75	−2.00	−2.25	−2.75	−3.00	−3.25	−3.75	−4.00

Note: At a vertex distance of 13 mm, MJK effectivity charts easily determine the vertexed powers for prescriptions in the spherocylindrical format. The first two columns refer to the spherical power. The spherical component is located in the first column. The second column indicates the corresponding vertexed spherical power. The rest of the columns refer to the cylindrical power. The cylindrical component is located on the top row. Following the column down to the corresponding spherical power indicates the vertexed cylindrical component. An example is +6.50 −2.50 × 180. This corresponds to +7.12 −3.00 × 180, shown in bold italics. The axis remains the same.

Source: Adapted from JC Krohn, M Jensen. Determining the effective power of a sphero-cylinder refraction at the corneal plane. CL Spectrum 1989;4(9):56–62.

4. **Over-refraction** is used with diagnostic fitting. Refraction is performed over the trial lens with the desired base curve. The final power is calculated by simply adding the over-refraction. If there are large amounts of astigmatism in the over-refraction (**residual astigmatism**), a toric lens may be necessary for better vision (see Chapter 8).

5. **Dioptric conversions** are necessary to convert between diopters (D) and millimeters (mm). Base curves are presented in either format. The formula for converting to millimeters[31] is as follows:

$$\text{Radius (in mm)} = \frac{\text{Index of refraction} - 1}{\text{Power (in diopters)}} \times 1000$$

The index of refraction normally used is 1.3375. This value is used to convert keratometer readings into millimeters.

VI. **Lenticular design** adds a carrier or flange to the front surface of the lens to increase or decrease edge thickness. A peripheral curvature is cut onto the front surface of the lens at a particular radius and size to create the lenticular carrier. This peripheral radius is referred to as **anterior carrier** or **flange radius.** The anterior surface of the lenticular lens is left with two curves.[48] The remaining size of the central area is the **anterior cap size, or front OZ.**[44,49]

A. The **indication** is usually the use of higher-power lenses where thickening or thinning of the lens edge is needed. Lens performance and comfort improve with lenticular designs.[44,49,50] Most agree that thick minus lenses of more than –4.00 to –5.00 D need the thinning offered by a lenticular design.[44,49] Some authors say that all plus and low minus lenses of –2.00 D and less need an edge-thickening lenticular design.[22–24,50]

B. The **anterior cap size** is typically smaller than the posterior OZ to decrease **junction angle.** It is usually 1.6–1.8 mm smaller than the overall diameter (for 9.2-mm or greater diameter).[49] A larger cap size is not recommended. It will make the lens heavier and make it ride lower on the eye.[51]

C. **Peripheral flange radius,** or **anterior peripheral radius,** is the curvature of the front surface lenticular carrier. It is specified relative to the base curve.[51] The flatter the radius, the thicker the edge. The steeper the radius, the thinner the edge.[23]

D. **Junction thickness** is determined where the anterior cap meets the peripheral flange. It is usually the thinnest point of the lens and is prone to breakage. Minimum thickness required for safety is 0.15–0.18 mm. The lens can break apart if it is too thin.[52]

E. A **minus carrier design,** or **myoflange,** thickens the edge of the lens.[23] The anterior peripheral radius is made 1.0–3.0 mm flatter than the base curve.[48,51] The flatter the carrier, the higher it will position on the eye.[51] Lenses with unwanted thin edges benefit from a minus lenticular. This includes low minus lenses of –2.00 D and lower, as well as all plus lenses.[22]

F. **Plus carrier, hyperflange, myodisk,** and **myolenticular** designs thin the lens edge.[23,49,51] Higher minus lenses of more than –5.00 benefit from this design.[2] The carrier radius is made steeper by at least 1.0 mm.[51]

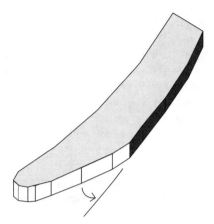

FIGURE 4.6   *Junction angle. A lenticular lens is shown. The junction angle is formed by the cap and flange. The dark surface represents the anterior cap. The light surface represents the flange or carrier. The angle between the cap radius and the flange radius is the junction angle. (Adapted from CF Moore, RB Mandell. The design of high-minus contact lenses. CL Spectrum 1989;4[11]:44.)*

    G. **Junction angle** affects comfort. A high junction angle creates a greater lid sensation. High junction angles can be lowered by decreasing anterior cap size or by increasing diameter[49] (Figure 4.6).

VII. An **aspheric rigid lens design** is desired by many practitioners because it more closely follows the contour of the cornea. The lenses progressively flatten toward the periphery. The cornea itself is aspheric, and a much closer fit is achieved. Many times, centration and comfort improves. Disadvantages include the difficult in-office verification of lens parameters and the usually higher expense.

    A. Regarding **selection,** aspheric lenses allow better centration and comfort for patients with spherical lenses who have inferior or superior decentration.[53–55] Patients with 3 o'clock and 9 o'clock staining should also be considered. Postradial keratotomy corneas may also benefit.[53]

    B. **Maximum gradient bearing theory** may help to explain the benefits of aspheric lenses. Aspheric lenses spread the lens weight over a wider corneal surface.[56,57] The localized pressure areas seen in the junctional blends of a spherical lens are eliminated. This allows for better peripheral alignment and less peripheral staining.[56] A wider bearing area makes the lens easier to fit because base curve selection is more forgiving. More than one specific aspheric base curve works for a particular eye.[57,58]

    C. **Fluorescein patterns** appear with apical pooling, midperipheral bearing, and approximately 0.3 mm of edge pooling. Lenses should be fitted from the steep side because flat lenses can deceptively appear as alignment lenses.[59]

D. **Basic designs** are divided into four categories: **conic section** (ellipse, parabola, or hyperbola), **nonconic** (an aspheric curve with continuous curves with no transition zones), **angled cones** (the peripheral zone of the contact lens is a section of the cone surface), and **combination designs.** The combination designs include toric base curves with aspheric peripheral curves, aspheric base curves with spherical peripheral curves, front-surface spherical with an aspheric periphery, and **bi-aspherics** (central and peripheral aspheric base curves).[53,56,60] From a clinical standpoint, the difference among designs is the degree of flattening from the lens center (or midcenter) to the periphery.[61] Lenses with **low to moderate flattening** (e values [eccentricity] of less than 1.0) are used to enhance fitting characteristics such as centration. Lenses with **moderate to high flattening** (e values of more than 1.0) are used for presbyopic patients. The higher amounts of flattening induce plus power in the periphery.[62]

Pearl: If the lenses initially recommended by the manufacturer were 0.1 mm steeper than K, it usually indicates that the lenses have low to moderate flattening. If the lenses were 0.2–0.3 mm steeper than K, it indicates a lens with moderate to a high degree of flattening.[62]

E. **Z values** roughly describe the actual stand-off from the cornea.[63] Smaller Z values indicate a steeper periphery. Larger Z values indicate a flatter periphery and larger edge lifts.

F. **E values** are used to describe corneal asphericity for conic sections. Not all types of aspheric lenses can be described accurately with e values, however. Spheres have a value of zero. Ellipsoidal shapes have an e value of less than 1.0. Paraboloidal shapes have an e value of 1.0. E values of more than 1.0 are hyperboloidal shapes[60,62] (Figure 4.7). Corneas typically have a e value of 0.4. A proper fit for a 0.4 e is 0.5 to allow adequate tear exchange. Larger e values are steeper than K. Smaller e values are flatter than K. A 0.4 e value is 0.50 flatter than K.

G. **Inferior decentration** can be corrected by reordering in a minus carrier lenticular design or making the lens larger, steeper, or both. **Superior decentration** can be corrected by reducing lens diameter, steepening the base curve, or both.[64]

VIII. **Troubleshooting spherical rigid gas-permeable lens performance** is sometimes necessary.

A. **Lens decentration** is a common problem for RGP lenses. Flare during night driving is a common symptom.[12,65] In many cases, the natural inclination is to try a larger lens in the hope that increasing corneal coverage will solve the problem. Unfortunately, increasing diameter can sometimes make the problem worse.

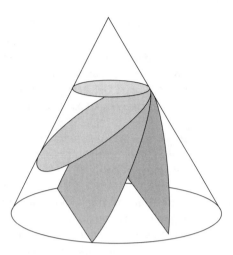

FIGURE 4.7   *Conic sections. Conic sections are shown from top to bottom. At the top, circles or spheres have a value of zero. Below the circle are ellipses with e values of less than 1.0. Below the ellipse are paraboloidal shapes with an e value of 1.0. Hyperbolas, shown at the bottom, have e values greater than 1.0. (Adapted from AJ Phillips. Rigid Gas-Permeable and Hard Corneal Lens Fitting. In AJ Phillips, J Stone [eds], Contact Lenses [3rd ed]. London: Butterworth, 1989;336.)*

1. **Inferior decentration** is largely influenced by upper lid positioning.[9] If the upper lid covers the superior limbus, then it can be used to raise the lens position. A larger diameter and flatter base curve should be tried. If the upper lid has a high position and does not cover the superior limbus, the influence of the lid must be decreased as much as possible. A smaller diameter and steeper base curve are indicated.

   a. **Thinning the lens** can be helpful. Thick lenses have unnecessary mass and cause the lens to drop. The recommended thickness for a given power and diameter should be adhered to and must be verified.[9] A **lenticular design** for reducing overall mass can be effective.[10,55]

   b. A **superior flat cornea** may be obstructing lens excursion. A simple test can determine if this is the case. While lifting the upper lid out of the way, the lens can be digitally moved over the superior cornea. If there are **dark areas** in the peripheral fluorescein pattern, the peripheral system of the lens may be too steep. The steepness will inhibit the lens from moving smoothly over the superior cornea, resulting in inferior decentration. A flatter peripheral system may be necessary.[27,45]

    c. A **specific gravity** change is helpful for low-riding lenses and much more effective than reducing lens thickness.[66] **Low-specific-gravity** materials are effective for improving inferior centration. Low-Dk materials have lower specific gravities and can be cut thinner. Use of **high-specific-gravity** materials for high-riding lenses is not as effective.[66,67]

        Pearl: Changing to a lighter, lower-specific-gravity material is the most effective means of improving the centration of a low-riding lens.[68]

    d. **Edge lift** of a lens that is too great will cause the lens to be easily pushed downward, forcing inferior decentration. A flat and wide peripheral curve can be the cause. An aspheric, quasi-aspheric or multiperipheral curve design can decrease the edge lift, help centration, and at the same time increase comfort.[57] On the same note, increasing edge lift can help centration by acting like a hook for the upper lid.[68]

2. **Superior decentration** can be corrected by keeping in mind lens mass and upper lid forces when designing the lens. **Increasing the center thickness** of the lens will increase mass and help to drop the lens position.

    Pearl: Thickening improves centration for high-riding lenses.[66]

    a. **Upper lid influence** may be the cause of the decentration. The upper lid may be picking up the lens because the edge is too thick. The edge needs to be thinned with a **lenticular design.** Upper lid influence can also be minimized by **reducing the diameter.**[10,55] The effectiveness of a reduced diameter depends on lid positioning. Smaller diameters will work for upper lids with no corneal coverage.

    b. **Steepening** the lens or using aspheric designs is useful.[55] Both strategies are effective if a displaced corneal apex is causing the decentration. Aspheric lenses have the added advantage of producing less upper lid interaction[57] (CD-ROM: RGP Cases: Case 1).

    c. **With-the-rule** corneal toricity of a large degree can cause superior decentration. A toric lens may be necessary to allow proper centration[10] (see Chapter 8).

3. **Lateral decentration** is usually caused by an against-the-rule cornea. A toric lens may be necessary to enhance centration for higher toricities. Another strategy is to use the upper lid to stabilize the lens. Lens diameter is increased to enhance a lid attachment fit.[23] Aspheric lenses are also useful.[69]

B. **Discomfort** for an already adapted patient can be differentially diagnosed by manually moving the lens while holding away the lids. If the sensation remains, then lens quality or poor lens-to-cornea relationship may be the cause. If the sensation goes away, the edge profile or high edge lift should be suspected. This can be confirmed if the sensation returns upon blinking (after releasing the lids and lens).[45]

    1. **Poor edges** definitely cause discomfort. Polishing the edges is very effective (see Chapter 7).

    2. **High edge lift** causes discomfort. Narrow peripheral curves are more comfortable than wide peripheral curves.[70] **Aspheric designs** have good initial comfort because of the uniform edge clearance.[53–55]

    3. **Decentration** can cause discomfort. The sensation of the upper lid is mainly at the margin.[23] Whenever the lens is not in constant contact with the upper lid, lens awareness results.[27] The design should be changed to enhance centration and lid attachment.

C. **Peripheral corneal desiccation,** or **3 o'clock and 9 o'clock staining,** usually stems from inferior centration, poor tear film, or inadequate peripheral lens design. Improving centration, blink exercises, and decreasing excessive edge lift are effective.[10,71]

D. **Flexure** can be a problem with the modern RGP materials in thin designs.[72,73] Normally, rigid lenses do not conform to the cornea. Astigmatism caused by corneal toricity is masked by the lens. Unfortunately, for higher toricities, some conforming does take place and flexure is created. When the lens flexes, a portion of the corneal astigmatism is not masked and becomes apparent in over-refraction. Usually, visual acuity suffers from flexure. Lenses typically flex about 30% of the corneal toricity.[16]

    1. **Corneal topography, lens thickness,** and **cornea-to-lens relationship** determine the amount of flexure. Higher toricities and thinner and steeper lenses result in greater amounts of flexure.

    2. **Flexure effects** are indicated by the cylinder in the over-refraction. **Overkeratometry** readings can actually measure flexure amounts.

    3. **Increasing lens thickness** is effective in reducing flexure, but may change the fitting relationship. A flatter lens (by a minimum of 0.50 D) may be more desirable. Reducing OZ by at least 0.3 mm or changing to a lower Dk material will also work.[1]

E. **Warpage** can develop through use of excessive force when rubbing the lens.[8,9,25] Sometimes the lens warps from trying to remove an upside-down lens adhered to the bottom of a smooth-welled case. The BCR will verify as a toric, but the power in the lensometer is spherical. Increasing the lens thickness by 0.02 mm can help if it does not change lens performance.[55]

F. A **power change** can also occur when a patient uses overly aggressive cleaning techniques with an abrasive cleaner.[9] For patients prone to warping lenses or changing powers, a hands-off cleaning regimen may be the best option.

G. **Reduced wettability** can be thought of as initial or acquired.
1. **Poor initial wettability** is usually due to the manufacturing process. Cleaning and conditioning the lens during the 24 hours prior to inserting the lenses often prevents this problem. Use of a laboratory cleaner or a light surface polish is sometimes necessary. In some cases, the lens needs to be replaced.
2. **Acquired wettability** usually results from a dirty lens. Lenses should be cleaned immediately after removal, and a more aggressive abrasive cleaner can be prescribed. Sometimes residue from the patient's hands can adhere to the lens and cause problems. A careful cleaning regimen is the best option. An FSA material can be used because of its inherent deposit resistance.[9]

H. **Cracking and crazing** of the lens surface may provide harbors for bacteria and viruses.[74] There are two reported cases of corneal ulcers caused by crazed lenses.[75] Crazing appears as a translucent hazy film with filmy deposits. Cracking has a transparent stained-glass pattern on a clean lens.[6]

I. **Lid geometry effects** are important areas for troubleshooting. Comfort and lens positioning are heavily influenced by upper and lower lids. Lid geometry can be classified as **narrow, ideal, unusual,** and **wide aperture** depending on the configuration (CD-ROM: RGP lens fitting and eyelid geometry). Adjusting the lens parameters to the characteristics of the lid geometry can be extremely helpful in optimizing the fit.

J. **Changing optic zone diameters (OZD)** can be helpful for enhancing lens performance (CD-ROM: RGP Cases: Case 4). Smaller OZDs fit flatter due to smaller sagittal heights. Changing to a larger OZD can minimize excessive movement and help center the lens better.

REFERENCES

1. Bennett ES. Lens Design, Fitting, and Evaluation. In ES Bennett, VA Henry (eds), Clinical Manual of Contact Lenses. Philadelphia: Lippincott, 1994;41–88.
2. Gasson A, Morris J. Preliminary Considerations and Examination. In A Gasson, J Morris (eds), The Contact Lens Manual. Oxford, England: Butterworth–Heinemann, 1992;20–37.
3. Bennett ES. How to present rigid lenses more effectively. Rev Optom 1994;131(suppl):8A–10A.
4. Hansen DW. Getting a head start on myopia control. CL Spectrum 1994;9(4):27.
5. Grosvenor T, Perrigin D, Perrigin J, et al. Rigid gas-permeable contact lenses for myopia control: effects of discontinuance of lens wear. Optom Vis Sci 1991;68(5):385–389.
6. Grohe RM, Bennett ES. Problem Solving. In ES Bennett, BA Weissman (eds), Clinical Contact Lens Practice. Philadelphia: Lippincott, 1991(29);1–16.
7. Bennett ES. Treatment Options for PMMA-Induced Problems. In ES Bennett, RM Grohe (eds), Rigid Gas-Permeable Contact Lenses. New York: Professional Press, 1986;275–295.
8. Superpermeables as fitting alternative. CL Forum 1988;13(2):59–61.
9. Bennett ES. A practical guide to troubleshooting rigid gas-permeable lenses. CL Spectrum 1994;9(10):22.
10. Schwartz CA. 10 worst fitting problems and how to solve them. CL Forum 1988;13(8):32–37.

11. Pole JJ, Lowther GE. Clinical comparison of low, moderate, and high rigid gas-permeable lenses. CL Forum 1987;12(7):47–51.
12. Moore CF. Eliminating persistent refitting problems. CL Forum 1986;11(2):21–26.
13. Lowther GE. Microcystic edema versus microcysts. ICLC 1992;19:5.
14. Wilson SE, Lin DTC, Klyce SD, et al. Rigid contact lens decentration: a risk factor for corneal warpage. CLAO J 1990;16(3):177–182.
15. Rengstorff RH. Corneal rehabilitation. In ES Bennett, BA Weissman (eds), Clinical Contact Lens Practice. Philadelphia: Lippincott, 1991(48);1–10.
16. Silbert JA. Conquering residual astigmatism and RGP flexure. CL Forum 1990;15(11): 15–28.
17. Fontana FD. RGP fitting and refitting made easy. CL Forum 1990;15(9):56–61.
18. Moore JW. Researchers turn to RGP materials, complications. CL Forum 1987;12(12):60–62.
19. Shovlin JP, DePaolis MD, Kame RT. Contact lens–induced corneal warpage syndrome vs. keratoconus. CL Forum 1986;11(8):32–36.
20. Rouault CE, Sagan W. Effects of base curve and diameter changes on the cornea with RGP lenses. CL Spectrum 1988;3(11):87–90.
21. Schnider C. The RGP highway. CL Spectrum 1995;10(2):17.
22. Bennett ES. Basic Fitting. In ES Bennett, BA Weissman (eds), Clinical Contact Lens Practice. Philadelphia: Lippincott, 1991(23);1–22.
23. Caroline PJ, Norman CW. A blueprint for rigid lens design: part 1. CL Spectrum 1988;3(11):39–49.
24. Bennett ES. Lens Design, Fitting, and Troubleshooting. In ES Bennett, RM Grohe (eds), Rigid Gas-Permeable Contact Lenses. New York: Professional Press, 1986;189–224.
25. Rakow PL. Clinical impressions of the Boston RXD material. CL Forum 1989;14(12):21–26.
26. Fonn D. Progress Evaluation Procedures. In ES Bennett, BA Weissman (eds), Clinical Contact Lens Practice. Philadelphia: Lippincott, 1991(28);1–10.
27. Caroline PJ, Norman CW. A blueprint for RGP design. CL Spectrum 1991;6(11):15–19.
28. Legerton JA. Problem solving with mid-Dk fluorinated siloxane acrylate RGPs. CL Forum 1989;14(5):25–27.
29. Bennett ES. Henry VA, Davis LJ, et al. Comparing empirical diagnostic fitting of daily wear fluoro-silicone/acrylate CLs. CL Forum 1989;14(11):38–44.
30. Bennett ES. How important are diagnostic lenses in RGP fitting? CL Spectrum 1993;8(12):19.
31. Mandell RB. Fitting Methods and Philosophies. In RB Mandell (ed), Contact Lens Practice. Springfield, IL: Thomas, 1988;203–242.
32. Harrison K, Stein HA. A nomogram for fitting fluorosilicone acrylate contact lenses. CLAO J 1988;14(3):136–138.
33. Computer-aided RGP design: a roundtable discussion. CL Spectrum 1989;4(9):29–34.
34. El Hage SG, Bacigalupi M, King KB. RGP design based upon computerized corneal topography. CL Spectrum 1992;7(2):47–50.
35. Snyder C, Campbell JB. Considerations in the maintenance of large RGP fitting sets. CL Spectrum 1990;5(7):37–39.
36. Andrasko G, Billings R. A simple nomogram for RGP fitting success. CL Spectrum 1993;8(12):28–31.
37. Bennett ES, Schnider C. 6 ways to improve initial comfort. CL Spectrum 1993;8(12):33–36.
38. Bennett ES. Master the art of rigid lens design. Rev Optom 1994(suppl);131:11A–14A.
39. Korb DR, Korb JE. A new concept in contact lens design—parts I and II. J Am Optom Assoc 1970;41(12):1023–1032.

40. Williams E. New design concepts for permeable rigid contact lenses. J Am Optom Assoc 1979;50(3):331–336.
41. Theodoroff CD, Lowther GE. Quantitative effect of optic zone diameter changes on rigid gas-permeable lens movement and centration. ICLC 1990;17:92–95.
42. Brown S, Baldwin M, Pole J. Effect of optic zone diameter on lens flexure and residual astigmatism. ICLC 1984;11(11):759–763.
43. Businger U, Treiber A, Flury C. The etiology and management of three and nine o'clock staining. ICLC 1989;16(5):136–140.
44. Lowther GE. Review of rigid contact lens design and effects of design on lens fit. ICLC 1988;15(12):378–389.
45. Caroline PJ, Norman CW. A blueprint for RGP design. Diagnostic lens fitting and fluorescein pattern interpretation: part III. CL Spectrum 1992;7(1):35–39.
46. Krohn JC, Jensen M. Determining the effective power of a sphero-cylinder refraction at the corneal plane. CL Spectrum 1989;4(9):56–62.
47. Schnider C. Simplify (not nullify) your job with corneal topography. CL Spectrum 1995;10(4):14.
48. Weissman BA, Bennett ES. Contact Lens Design. In ES Bennett, BA Weissman (eds), Clinical Contact Lens Practice. Philadelphia: Lippincott, 1991(15);1–6.
49. Moore CF, Mandell RB. The design of high-minus contact lenses. CL Spectrum 1989;4(11):43–47.
50. Pole JJ, Dominguez A, McNamara N. Lenticular vs. single cut for low plus RGPs—the better design for your patient. CL Spectrum 1994;9(10):31–32.
51. Mandell RB. Optional Lens Features. In RB Mandell (ed), Contact Lens Practice. Springfield, IL: Thomas, 1988;440–471.
52. Bennett ES. What you should know about RGP edge design. CL Spectrum 1993;8(10):17.
53. Bennett ES. Aspheric lens designs: what you need to know (part 2). CL Spectrum 1994;9(7):21.
54. Feldman G, Bennett ES. Aspheric Lens Designs. In ES Bennett, BA Weissman (eds), Clinical Contact Lens Practice. Philadelphia: Lippincott, 1991(16);1–10.
55. Ames KS, Schnider CM. Rigid Gas-Permeable Lens Design, Fitting, and Problem Solving. In ES Bennett (ed), Contact Lens Problem Solving. St. Louis: Mosby, 1995;1–17.
56. Bennett ES. Aspheric lens designs: what you need to know. CL Spectrum 1994;9(6):21.
57. Ames KS, Jones WF. Spherical vs. aspheric designs: a clinical difference? CL Forum 1988;13(5):18–22.
58. Ames KS, Andrasko G. More efficient RGP fitting by design. CL Spectrum 1991;6(1):55–59.
59. Koetting RA. Are you ready to try aspherics again? CL Spectrum 1989;4(1):71–73.
60. Goldberg JB. Basic principles of aspheric corneal lenses. CL Forum 1988;13(5):35–38.
61. Caroline PJ, Garbus C, Garbus JJ, et al. Comparison of aspheric RGP lens contours. CL Spectrum 1992;7(7):43–45.
62. Ames K. Aspheric Rigid Gas-Permeable Lenses. In CA Schwartz (ed), Specialty Contact Lenses: A Fitter's Guide. Philadelphia: Saunders, 1996;49–57.
63. Goldberg JB. The "Z" values of aspheric contact lenses. CL Spectrum 1992;7(2):16.
64. Goldberg JB. Modification procedures for aspheric corneal lenses. ICLC 1991;18:110–112.
65. Hodur NR, Gandolfi B, Wojciechowski S. Flare with rigid contact lenses. CL Forum 1986;11(3):48–49.
66. Carney LG, Mainstone JC, Quinn TG, et al. Rigid lens centration: effects of lens design and material density. ICLC 1996;23:6–12.
67. Quinn TG, Carney LG. Controlling rigid lens centration through specific gravity. ICLC 1992;19:84–88.

68. Sobara L, Fonn D, Holden BA, et al. Centrally fitted versus upper lid attachment rigid gas-permeable lenses. Part 1. Design parameters affecting vertical decentration. ICLC 1996;23:99–103.
69. Gruber E. Material vs. design: expand your fitting philosophy. CL Spectrum 1994;9(9):32–34.
70. Picciano S, Andrasko G. Which factors influence RGP lens comfort? CL Spectrum 1989;4(5):31–33.
71. Cotie B. How to manage three and nine o'clock staining. CL Forum 1990;15(5):42–43.
72. Lebow KA. Does RGP thinness adversely affect lens performance? CL Spectrum 1993;8(9):31–34.
73. Miller WL, Andrasko G. An analysis of flexure characteristics of the Boston Rx material. CL Forum 1989;14(8):57–59.
74. Moody KJ, Tanner JB, Mannarino A. Bacterial adherence to gas-permeable contact lenses. CL Spectrum 1991;6(10):49–50.
75. Moody K, Mannarino A, Tanner J, et al. Staphylococcal ulceration with RGP contact lens wear. CL Spectrum 1989;4(3):61–64.

Chapter 5

Rigid Lens Materials

Milton M. Hom

I. **Polymethyl methacrylate (PMMA)** has excellent optic clarity, good machinability, and outstanding wettability, stability, and durability.[1] It is the same material that older toothbrush handles are made from. PMMA would be the first choice among contact lens materials if not for its inability to transmit oxygen (see Chapter 4). For some practitioners, an ideal material is PMMA with high oxygen flux.[2]

II. The **oxygen permeability** of contact lens materials is commonly measured in two ways: Dk and equivalent oxygen percentage (EOP).

   A. **Dk** is the industry standard for measurement of contact lens oxygen permeability. **D** represents **diffusion** and **k** represents **solubility**. For rigid lenses, the permeability is from diffusion of oxygen through the spaces in the polymer. The higher the Dk, the more permeable the material. The total oxygen transmissibility of the lens is denoted by **Dk/t** or **Dk/L**, where **t** (or **L**) is the thickness. **Dk/t** is the current term under ISO contact lens terminology (see Table 10.2 in Chapter 10). When the lens is thicker (higher t value), the oxygen transmissibility is reduced. When the lens is thinner (lower t value), the transmissibility is increased.[3]

   B. The **boundary layer effect** reduces the effective Dk/t of a contact lens while on the eye. Gas and oxygen molecules travel at different rates through water than through polymers. A boundary layer is formed when oxygen molecules arrive at the front surface of the lens faster than they can penetrate. At the back surface of the lens, depending on the interfacing surfaces, a boundary layer can form if the oxygen arrives faster than it can be carried away. This overcrowding forms the boundary layers that entrap oxygen at the interfacing surfaces. The interface with fluid on the front or back surface of the lens slows down the transmission of oxygen. A correction procedure in oxygen transmissibility measurement can be used to compensate for boundary layer effects.[4]

   C. **EOP** is a clinical measurement that quantifies oxygen permeability. EOP measures the amount of oxygen delivered to the cornea while the total barrier effect of the lens in the eye is taken in account. The EOP with no lens on the eye is 21%. EOPs of 17.9% and 9.9% are recommended for extended and daily wear, respectively.[5]

III.   Rigid gas-permeable (RGP) monomers are the ingredients that make up rigid lenses. Each monomer is polymerized into the material to give the lenses certain properties.[6] Polymer chemists use different percentages of monomers to develop recipes for RGP materials.[3] There are three basic ingredients: oxygen, rigidity and stability components, and wetting components.

   A.   Oxygen components make the material gas-permeable.

      1.   Silicone gives the polymer oxygen permeability as a result of the silicone-to-oxygen bond in the polymer side chains.[7] The bond angles are larger and more flexible than in the carbon-to-carbon bonds found in PMMA. The bonds freely rotate and allow more space for the oxygen to pass through.[3] Oxygen relies on **diffusion** to move through the voids in the material.[8] Silicone is also hydrophobic and soft.[6] The hydrophobicity gives the material poor wetting qualities and a propensity toward attracting deposits. The softness reduces dimensional stability and makes the lenses prone to warpage and flexure.[9] Reduction of dimensional stability is clinically seen as a change in base curve radius.[10] A related monomer is silicate, found in Fluorex lenses (G.T. Laboratories, Glenview, Illinois).[11]

      2.   Fluorine adds oxygen permeability and deposit resistance to the polymer. **Solubility** is the additional mechanism by which oxygen permeates through fluorinated polymers. Whereas silicone depends on diffusion, fluorinated polymers also rely on solubility.[8] Although fluorine is not as permeable as silicone, oxygen dissolves into the material containing fluorine. Fluorine literally soaks up the oxygen molecules like a sponge.[7,8]

      3.   The low coefficient of friction and **low surface tension** of fluorine prevent deposits from sticking and permit removal with blinking.[2,7,12] Another commonly known fluoropolymer is **Teflon.** Fluorine alone is acutely hydrophobic and has the same affinity for deposits as silicone.[9] The proper combination of monomers can take advantage of fluorine's deposit resistance, however, and counteract the deposit affinity of silicone.[6]

   B.   Rigidity and stability components are necessary to make the lens rigid. Without these components, the lens would be soft like a soft lens.

      1.   Methyl methacrylate (MMA) adds stability, strength, optic clarity, and machinability to the polymer. Many of these attributes are found in the related material, **PMMA.** Another monomer that adds rigidity is **dimethyl itaconate.**[3]

      2.   Cross-linkers bind the polymer chains to prevent them from sliding past one another. Stability is increased by locking these chains into position. A commonly used cross-linker is **ethylene glycol dimethacrylate.**[7]

   C.   Wetting components make the lens more wettable and help to overcome the hydrophobic properties of fluorine and silicone.[3] Tears are bound to the lens surfaces via surface interactions. These interactions are **hydrogen bonding, electrostatic interaction,** and **hydrophobic interaction.**[6] Of the three, electrostatic interactions are the strongest. With RGP materials, a positively charged molecule (e.g., water) is electrostatically attracted to the negative sites on the lens surface. A critical balance must be maintained with the wetting agents. Insufficient hydrophilic monomers do not produce sufficient wetting, and excessive hydrophilic monomers allow too much softness.[3]

    1. **Methacrylate acid** is an organic acid also found in soft lens polymers. A negative charge is added to the surface to attract water via electrostatic interaction.[3,6,13]

    2. **N-vinyl pyrrolidone** is a wetting agent that helps to produce wettability by adding an electrostatic charge to the polymer. This monomer is also used in soft lens polymers.

    3. **Polyvinyl alcohol** and **hydroxyethylmethacrylate (HEMA)** are two other components added for better wetting.[3]

  D. **Additives** such as an ultraviolet light absorber can add desirable features to the lens. **Boston Equalens** (Polymer Technology, Wilmington, Massachusetts) is one lens that uses such additives.

IV. **Wetting angles** indicate a polymer's affinity for water. The lower the angle, the better the wettability. Sessile drop, captive bubble, and Wilhelmy plate are different in vitro methods for measuring wetting angle. Some authors believe that wetting angles have little clinical importance because the lens is rapidly wetted and coated when placed into the eye.[10,13] The surface coating, or pellicle, acts as "camouflage," giving materials essentially the same wetting angles while on the eye.[14] Wetting usually improves when material soaks in solution. The hydrophilic groups in the polymer chain are attracted to the surrounding water and migrate to the surface. It is advisable to soak the lenses in solution 24–48 hours before dispensing to avoid "first day nonwetting syndrome" (see Chapter 9).

  A. The **sessile drop** approach is the traditional method for measuring wetting angles. A drop of water is placed on the test material, and the angle of contact between the liquid and solid is measured. An angle of less than 90 degrees indicates hydrophilicity; an angle of greater than 90 degrees indicates hydrophobicity. Unfortunately, this method of measurement does not specify exacting controls, and numerous factors can cause variability. These factors include liquid drop material, drop size and purity, time of measurement after drop placement, and surface preparation.[1,15]

  B. The **captive bubble** method was developed by Maurice Poster in 1978. In this technique, the angle is measured in a bubble chamber under controlled conditions. The material surface is immersed in saline or water, and an air bubble is formed. This method takes into account the polymer's improved wetting after soaking in liquid. Wetting angles are usually one-third to one-half those of angles measured by sessile drop methods.[1,15]

    C. With a **Wilhelmy plate,** the angle is deduced from force measurements as a function of the immersion depth of the material in water. Two angles are measured, an **advancing angle** and a **receding angle.** The advancing angle relates to the tendency of the liquid to be spread over the lens surface (i.e., as the lid pushes tears on blink closure). The receding angle relates to the tendency to withdraw from the surface (i.e., when the lid pulls tears on blink opening). The advancing angle is larger than the receding angle because of a phenomenon called **hysteresis.**[1,15]

    D. **In vivo wetting angle** measurements are more helpful than in vivo methods in predicting the consequences of poor wetting. Lenses with high wetting angles usually experience more deposits and irritation. Even more predicative of wetting is a wetting angle measurement **after lens wear.**[16,17]

V. **Geometries** can be used to describe the linkages of the polymers. The different geometries are linear, branched, and cross-linked. The silicone-to-oxygen side chains inhibit close packing of the polymer chains. Permeability by way of diffusion requires the chains to be loosely packed and flexible. Unfortunately, this makes the polymer softer. To counteract flexibility and flexure, cross-linkage density is increased. Cross-linkers are added for stability. Adding too much cross-linkage, however, can make the material brittle and easy to break.[3,7]

VI. **Silicone acrylates (SAs)** are copolymers of MMA and alkylsiloxanyl-methacrylate. In the latter part of the 1980s, there was a **"great Dk race."**[10] Formulating new polymers to increase Dk was the primary goal of manufacturers. Some of the polymers developed were **Paraperm** (Paragon Vision Sciences, Mesa, Arizona), **Boston** (Bausch & Lomb, Rochester, New York) and **Optacryl** materials.

    A. In the 1980s, **high-Dk** RGP lenses were manufactured by increasing silicone content. Lenses were more permeable, but there were clinical tradeoffs. More deposit accumulation, surface scratching, and instability were seen with high-Dk SA lenses.[18] Because of the silicone content, dimensional stability may be a problem with **minus lenses flattening** and **plus lenses steepening.** Crazing and cracking after about a year of use have also been reported.[10]

    B. **Hydrophilic components** such as methacrylic acid are added for better wetting. The surface of an SA can be thought of as primarily hydrophobic with highly hydrophilic methacrylic acid zones. A small proportion of these zones have a negative charge.[19] More silicone content requires more wetting agents and often increases deposits.[20]

    C. **Polycon** (Wesley-Jessen, Des Plaines, Illinois) was the first well-known SA lens, seen first in the late 1970s.[10] The lens had a Dk of 8, extremely low by today's standards. The lens was cut very thin and displayed great flexibility. It was fitted in a flat, lid-attachment manner (see Chapter 4).

    D. A **suction cup effect** of high-Dk SA lenses can be induced if the lens is fitted too steep. The tendency to trap itself on the eye may be related to the hydrophobicity of the material. Negative pressure is created under the lens, causing it to adhere. There is an associated loss of vision and central staining.[18,21]

VII. **Fluorosilicone acrylates (FSAs)** are the first-choice materials for many practitioners. FSAs differ from SAs in the addition of fluorine. FSA lenses typically have better deposit resistance, higher oxygen permeability, and more stability than SA lenses. The addition of fluorine allows the silicone content to be decreased, resulting in better resistance to protein.[20] FSA lenses include Boston **Equalens** (Bausch & Lomb), **Fluoroperm** (Paragon Vision Science), **SF-P** (Menicon, Clovis, California), and **SGP 3** (Permeable Technologies, Morganville, New Jersey).

A. The **Boston RXD** (Bausch & Lomb) has a large amount of fluorine and very little silicone. The lens can be cut thin without the typical flexure seen in RGP lenses. It is resistant to deposits.[12] Compared with SA lenses, which are cut thicker, the RXD showed greater resistance to flexure.[22]

B. The **Boston 7** lens has a very low (5–7%) silicone content. A backbone is added to the material to give the polymer more durability. **Boston ES** (Bausch & Lomb) material uses the same technological principles as Boston 7 (Bausch & Lomb) but with more stiffness added.[23]

C. **Silicone sicca** is the lens binding seen with SA lenses. FSA lenses have less binding because of their ability to repel rather than attract debris from beneath the contact lens.[2]

D. The **surface haze** seen on SA lenses is much less common with FSA lenses. Because of their hardness, FSA lenses have better surface quality than SA lenses. The surface of an FSA lens can be polished better, and the more polished surface gives the lens better deposit resistance and subsequently less surface haze. Comfort is also enhanced when surfaces are cleaner.[2,20]

E. **Enzyme cleaning** is needed less with FSA lenses because they have enhanced protein resistance.[10] Weekly enzyme cleaning is recommended for SA lenses.[9]

F. **Lipid-based deposits** are more likely with FSA lenses. Lipids on lens surfaces appear oily and greasy. Cleaners such as **Boston Advance** (Bausch & Lomb) have been optimized for lipid deposits related to FSA lenses[20] (see Chapter 9).

G. **Glycocalyx** formation enhances the comfort of FSA lenses. The fluorine component has an inherent affinity for mucus. This mucus affinity forms a glycocalyx around the lens and increases comfort. The lens glycocalyx is a layer of tear film mucin adhering to the lens.[9] Clinically, the time before dehydration and tear breakup time are lengthened.[12] As a result, the adaptation times of FSA lenses are shorter than those of SA lenses.[2]

VIII. **Fluorocarbon** materials are composed of fluorine and MMA to create a **polyperfluoroether.** N-vinyl pyrrolidone is added for better wetting.[9,12] The much larger amounts of fluorine produce a rather high Dk/t of around 100. The high fluorine content (40–50%) makes the lens flexible like a soft lens.[10,12] The **Advent** lens (Ocular Sciences/American Hydron, South San Francisco), originally brought to market by 3M, was the first commercially available fluorocarbon lens.[12,24] The lens has good wettability and protein resistance.[10]

IX.   **Novalens** by Nova Vision (Morrisville, North Carolina) has a neutral surface charge, making it more deposit-resistant.[12] The lens is made of strylsilicone.[25] The specially treated surface is unlike that of other rigid lenses because it is hydrophilic, which produces better comfort. Because of the surface treatment, however, the lens cannot be modified without special procedures.

X.   **Silicone elastomers** are available in two forms: elastomeric or resin.[9] Both forms have excellent permeability once they have received surface treatment for their inherently intense hydrophobicity. A treated polar elastomeric surface is said to be passivated.[26] Elastomeric lenses handle like soft lenses but feel like rigid lenses on the eye. These lenses suffered from poor long-term wettability, deposits, and high cost. They are currently in use as a pediatric Bausch & Lomb **Silsoft** lens. Silicone resin lenses, such as Dow Corning's **Silcon** lens, are rigid and no longer available.[10]

XI.   Cellulose acetate butyrate **(CAB)** was the first commercially available gas-permeable material. Originally developed in 1938 by Kodak, it was first used for contact lenses in 1974.[5] CAB is less rigid and less brittle than PMMA.[27] The disadvantages are poor wettability, dimensional instability, and low Dk compared with today's materials.[5,10] The wettability comes from the free **hydroxyl groups** located on the cellulose rings. The permeability and flexibility are a result of the **butyrl groups.** Some hydroxyl groups are replaced with acetyl and butyrl groups when the material is polymerized. One problem is that the material does not have a fixed composition. There could be a large number of hydroxyl groups, making the material more wettable, or there could be more butyrl groups, making it more permeable and flexible. Supplies from different sources can have different properties.[27] Some practitioners still use CAB for applications such as keratoconus because it is nonsensitizing.

XII. **Polystyrene** first appeared in the mid-1980s. This material has greater resistance to flexure and lower specific gravity than SAs. Problems with styrene are surface stability, brittleness, and low Dk. Styrene is currently in use in Wessley-Jessen's **Softperm** lens. It is the rigid center in the styrene-HEMA combination lens[5,10] (see Chapter 17).

REFERENCES

1. Zhang J, Herskowitz R. Is there more than one angle to the wetting characteristics of contact lenses? CL Spectrum 1992;7(10):26–32.
2. Advantages of fluoropolymers. CL Forum 1988;13(2):50–55.
3. White P. RGP material and immaterial clichés. CL Spectrum 1988;3(11):63–65.
4. Benjamin WJ. Oxygen Transport Through Contact Lenses. In M Ruben, M Guillon (eds), Contact Lens Practice. London: Chapman & Hall, 1994;43–70.
5. Lembach RG. Rigid gas-permeable contact lenses. CLAO J 1990;16(2):129–134.

6. Grohe RM, Caroline PJ. Surface Deposits on Contact Lenses. In ES Bennett, BA Weissman (eds), Clinical Contact Lens Practice. Philadelphia: Lippincott, 1992(24);1–12.

7. Weinschenk JI. A look at the components in fluorosilicone-acrylates. CL Spectrum 1989;4(10):61–64.

8. Caroline PJ, Ellis EJ. Review of the mechanisms of oxygen transport through rigid gas-permeable lenses. Int Eyecare 1986;2(4):210–213.

9. Lippman JI. Clinical surface characteristics of high-Dk hydrogel and gas-permeable CLs. CL Forum 1989;14(8):45–48.

10. Tomlinson A. Choice of materials—a material issue. CL Spectrum 1990;5(9):27–35.

11. Burke WJ. Polymer Chemistry. In ES Bennett, BA Weissman (eds), Clinical Contact Lens Practice. Philadelphia: Lippincott, 1992(20);1–13.

12. Lippman JI. Contact lens materials: a critical review. CLAO J 1990;16:287–291.

13. Terry R, Schnider C, Holden BA. Rigid gas-permeable lenses and patient management. CLAO J 1989;15(4):305–309.

14. Benjamin WJ. Pellicle, biofilm, mucin layer, surface coating, or contact lens camouflage. ICLC 1989;16:183–184.

15. Benjamin WJ. Wettability. In ES Bennett, RM Grohe (eds), Rigid Gas-Permeable Contact Lenses. New York: Professional Press, 1986;117–136.

16. Benjamin WJ, Yeager MD, Desai NN, et al. In vivo analysis of contact angles. Int Eyecare 1986;2(3):163–170.

17. Madigan M, Holden BA. Preliminary report: lens wear and its effect on wetting angle. Int Eyecare 1986;2(1):36–44.

18. Benjamin WJ. "Super-perm" or "Normo-perm": what risks accompany high oxygen permeability? ICLC 1989;16:94–96.

19. Hoffman WC. Ending the BAK-RGP controversy. ICLC 1987;14:31–35.

20. Ames KS. The surface characteristics of RGP lenses. CL Spectrum 1991;6(6):45–48.

21. Olson A. Polymer Chemistry. In ES Bennett, RM Grohe (eds), Rigid Gas-Permeable Contact Lenses. New York: Professional Press, 1986;77–92.

22. Blehl E, Lowther GE, Benjamin WJ. Flexural characteristics of SoftPerm, Boston IV, and RXD contact lenses on toric corneas. ICLC 1991;18:59–62.

23. O'Connor D. Great expectations. Optom Manage 1995;30(9):37–40.

24. Issacson WB, Rodrigues OP. Flexible fluoropolymer: a new category of contact lenses. CL Spectrum 1989;4(1):60–62.

25. White P, Scott C. Contact lenses and solutions summary. CL Spectrum 1994(suppl); 9(12):1–24.

26. Rae ST, Huff JW. Studies on initiation of silicone elastomer lens adhesion in vitro: binding before the indentation ring. CLAO J 1991;17(3):181–186.

27. Tighe BJ. Contact Lens Materials. In AJ Phillips, J Stone (eds), Contact Lenses (3rd ed). London: Butterworth, 1989;72–124.

Chapter 6

Fluorescein Patterns

Milton M. Hom

I. **Fluorescein** instillation is the best way to determine the relationship between a rigid contact lens and the cornea. **Straub** first used fluorescein for investigating corneal lesions in 1888. Fluorescein was used only with white light[1] until 1938, when **Obrig** discovered that a cobalt-blue filter greatly enhanced viewing of fluorescein patterns. With such a filter, almost 100% of the absorbed light is converted to fluorescent light.[2]

A. The **intensity** of fluorescence varies with the relative thickness of the tears. It is because of this property that fluorescein patterns are useful to rigid lens fitters. Thicker areas of tears appear as bright yellow; thinner areas and areas of touch appear as dark blue. Varying thicknesses of tear film appear as varying intensities of green. Below a critical thickness, there is no visible fluorescence. For example, the tear film needs to be at least 60 μm in thickness to fluoresce with a fluorescein concentration of 0.025%, the normal concentration used when doing the test. There is greater intensity of fluorescence with a higher concentration of fluorescein and increased thickness of solution. Intensity diminishes as the tears dilute the concentration over time.[2]

Pearl: Dark areas are not necessarily areas of touch. The tear film may be too thin to fluoresce.[2]

B. **Fluorescein pH** has a significant effect on fluorescent properties. A pH below 6.0 has half the fluorescence of a neutral pH of 7.0. Great variations in pattern reading can result if unbuffered saline is used to dissolve the strip. Buffered saline is a much better choice.[2]

C. **Fluorescein** is available in impregnated-strip or sterile liquid form.

1. **Fluorescein-impregnated paper strips** were developed by Kimura. The strips are dry and require wetting with a liquid, preferably a buffered solution.[2] The problem with liquid fluorescein is its susceptibility to bacterial contamination. *Pseudomonas* grows easily in fluorescein.[3] The strip circumvents this risk and greatly reduces the risk of contamination.

2. **Sterile fluorescein** is available in a liquid form. As mentioned previously, fluorescein is an excellent medium for culturing *Pseudomonas*. The sterile liquid is available in single doses to help prevent contamination.[3]

3. **Fluorexon** (Fluoresoft, Holles Laboratories, Kohasset, Massachussets) is high-molecular-weight liquid fluorescein used for soft lenses.[3] The high molecular weight inhibits absorption into a lower-water lens matrix. High-water lenses are susceptible to discoloration with fluorexon, however.

Pearl: Discoloration on a soft lens caused by fluorescein can sometimes be removed by soaking the lens in hydrogen peroxide.[4]

D. **Instillation** of fluorescein is usually on the inferior or superior sclera. The patient is instructed to look either up or down, while the moistened strip is touched on the sclera. The patient should blink one or two times to enhance mixing with the tear film. Touching the cornea with a strip can cause a small break in the epithelium and create an area of staining, confusing to the examiner. Applying fluorescein to the cornea should be avoided whenever possible.[5]

E. The **concentration** of fluorescein used largely depends on technique when using fluorescein strips. If the concentration varies wildly from patient to patient, the fluorescein patterns may confuse the practitioner because the patterns may change according to the concentration. A repeatable procedure such as saturating the strip and shaking off the excess before application can help maintain roughly the same concentration. Also, using the same type and brand of strip can decrease variability in concentration.[6]

F. For **viewing fluorescein patterns and staining,** magnification and a cobalt-blue filter or ultraviolet light for excitation are needed.

1. A **biomicroscope** has a cobalt filter for viewing fluorescein. It allows variable magnification and illumination.[7] The cornea produces a natural background fluorescence that can interfere with fluorescein pattern interpretation. Various filters help block out this background interference. Adding a yellow barrier filter such as a Kodak Wratten 12, Wratten 15, or Tiffen 2 photographic filter (adapted for contact lenses by Bausch & Lomb, Rochester, New York) to the observation system enhances viewing.[3] A Wratten 45 filter can be used in front of white light to replace a cobalt filter[6] (see Chapter 3).

2. A **Burton lamp** (Burton Medical Products, Chatsworth, California) is a hand-held lamp with a +5.00 D magnifier.[7] This lamp makes pattern evaluation faster because both eyes are visible within the magnifier. Lids are more freely manipulated using a slit lamp. Patients can also hold their heads up in a natural fashion. The white light of the Burton lamp can be used for low-magnification views of

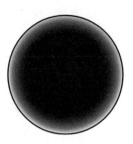 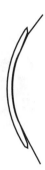

FIGURE 6.1 *Spherical alignment pattern. On the left is an alignment fluorescein pattern. The entire optic zone can be dark. The light areas around the lens periphery indicate adequate edge lift. On the right is a corresponding cross-sectional view of the cornea and lens. The lens and cornea are parallel to each other throughout the entire optic zone. There is clearance or edge lift along the periphery.*

the adnexa and conjunctiva.[8] An ultraviolet Burton lamp may not be as good as a slit lamp for reading patterns of lenses with ultraviolet inhibitors. The ultraviolet Burton lamp has a smaller spectral range than a slit lamp.[2] Filters can be used in front of the white light source to increase the spectral range. A Kodak Wratten 47, Wratten 47A, or Wratten 47B photographic filter over the white light source enhances the evaluation of a lens with an ultraviolet inhibitor.[3]

II. **Fluorescein patterns** provide a simple picture of a complex three-dimensional tear layer.[2] Fluorescein pools under the lens, where there are areas of **clearance,** or **vaulting.** The brighter the area, the thicker the tear film and the greater the amount of clearance. Areas of bearing and touch appear as dark areas in a fluorescein pattern.

Pearl: When reading fluorescein patterns, it is easier to identify the pattern from the amount of dark area rather than the amount of bright area.

A. **Central** and **peripheral areas** should be interpreted separately. The importance of evaluating these two areas separately increases with abnormal topographies such as keratoconus.

B. **Central fluorescein patterns** are read within the optic zone diameter (OZD).

1. **Alignment patterns** have an even amount of thin tear film under the spherical lens. Alignment is desired because it most closely parallels the cornea. The goal of most rigid contact lens fittings is alignment. Since the tear film is too thin to fluoresce, alignment usually appears as a large dark area across the entire OZ (Color Plate 6.1, Figure 6.1). It can also appear as a dim glow of very thin fluorescein-stained tears.

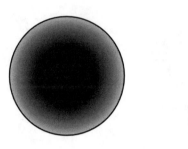 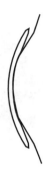

FIGURE 6.2   *Spherical flat pattern. On the left is a flat fluorescein pattern. The dark area encompasses the central area of the optic zone. There are light areas around the midperipheral areas and edges. On the right is the cross-sectional view of a flat-fitting lens. The lens and cornea contact each other (bearing or touch) in the center of the lens. There is clearance around the central bearing area.*

> *Pearl: The larger the dark area, the more aligned the pattern.*

2. **Flat-fitting** lenses have dark areas in the central portion and bright areas in the outer portion. Normally, the tear film does not abruptly change from light to dark. The tear film gradually thins toward the center of the lens with a flat fit. The fluorescence correspondingly fades as the tear film thins. Abrupt changes usually occur with changes in lens geometry (Color Plate 6.2, Figure 6.2). Lenses that fit too flat may distort the cornea. Excessively flat-fitting lenses usually do not center well and exhibit large amounts of movement.

3. **Steep-fitting** lenses may be comfortable but can adhere to the eye. Negative pressure can build up under a steep lens and have detrimental effects on the cornea. Steep fluorescein patterns have the greatest fluorescence under the central portion of the lens, where the tear film is the thickest. Dark areas are in the outer portion. Bright areas are in the central portion (Color Plate 6.3, Figure 6.3).

4. **Amounts** of flatness can be quantified. The smaller the dark areas, the flatter the lens. On the other hand, the larger the dark areas, the closer the lens is to alignment (Figure 6.4).

> *Pearl: Dark areas (apical touch) are much easier to quantify than amounts of apical clearance.*

C. **Peripheral patterns** usually indicate the edge clearance. The ideal axial clearance is 80 μm. Since the critical thickness for fluorescence is

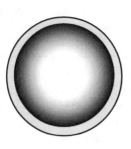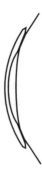

FIGURE 6.3 *Spherical steep pattern. On the left is a steep fluorescein pattern. The smaller dark areas surround the bright central area. Bright areas or pooling comprises the majority of the steep pattern. On the right is the cross-section of a steep lens. The lens touches in a peripheral ring around the optic zone.*

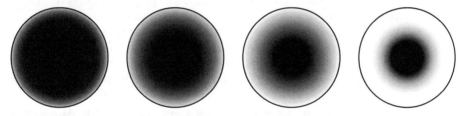

FIGURE 6.4 *Increasing flatness. The fit of a contact lens can be quantified on the flat side. Beginning on the left is an alignment pattern. The dark areas are at maximum. From left to right, the patterns represent a series of base curves that are progressively flatter. The lens on the right is an excessively flat lens. The dark areas are small and confined to the center. Edge lift, represented by pooling or clearance, encompasses most of the lens.*

60 µm, lack of a bright ring of fluorescein indicates insufficient clearance.[2] The width of the ring should be 0.4–0.5 mm.[9] Peripheral patterns have an opposite appearance to central patterns.

1. **Dark areas** usually indicate the lens is too steep for the peripheral cornea. The steepness of the peripheral system prevents a sufficient tear film from forming. A black arc of touch in the peripheral curve area means the peripheral cornea in that area is too flat for the lens. The peripheral curves may need flattening.[10,11]

2. **Bright** and **very wide areas** indicate a flat peripheral system, a flat base curve, or both. A very thick tear film is present. Areas of pooling in the periphery indicate a flat lens-to-cornea relationship. The peripheral cornea is steeper than the lens. The lens may need steepening of the peripheral system or base curve.

3. **Movement obstruction** in the periphery can be detected by manually pushing the lens into the superior, inferior, and lateral areas of

the cornea.[10] The lids should be held open during this procedure. Lid influence can confuse the results. Any dark areas detected in the periphery indicate an area of movement obstruction. Superior areas of touch can indicate the cause of an inferiorly positioned lens. If the superior portion of the cornea is too flat, lens excursion can be inhibited, and the lens will decenter inferiorly. The peripheral system may need to be flattened.[11] If the lens is riding inferiorly and there are no dark areas of obstruction superiorly, the edge may need thinning (**lenticulation**) (see Chapter 4). The upper lid may be pushing the lens down.

III. **Astigmatic fluorescein patterns** have different appearances than spherical patterns. The cornea has a flat meridian and a steep meridian with different curvatures. A spherical lens displays a different relationship with each of the two meridians in one fluorescein pattern. The appearance is characteristically different from a spherical pattern. Probably the best way to understand toric patterns is to consider the lens-to-cornea relationship of each principle meridian on its own.

   A. **With-the-rule (WTR), corneal alignment–bearing** areas appear as an **"H" type,** or classic **"dumbbell,"** pattern. This pattern is apparent with as little as 1 D of toricity.[7] The alignment dumbbell pattern appears when there is bearing along the entire flat meridian. Corneal topographic maps produced by videokeratography indicate that the flattest areas of the toric cornea form the shape of a dumbbell. Alignment is best defined by the observer as maximum darkness in the fluorescein pattern. On a toric cornea, maximum darkness occurs when there is bearing on the flattest areas of the cornea in the shape of a dumbbell (Figures 6.5–6.9).

   B. A **WTR cornea** and **flat** fluorescein pattern differ from those of a spherical cornea in the shape of bearing area. The central bearing area of a toric cornea is oval in shape rather than round. The axis of astigmatism usually coincides with the longer axis of the oval (Color Plate 6.4, Figures 6.10–6.14).

   C. A **WTR cornea** and **steep lens** look just like a spherical steep lens in the central area. Apical clearance appears in both a toric and spherical lens. The fluorescein pattern of a toric cornea differs with respect to the periphery of the OZD. A steep lens on a spherical cornea has a ring-touch or peripheral-bearing area. The bearing areas for a WTR cornea are along the flatter, horizontal axis. The steeper the lens, the smaller the bearing area (Color Plate 6.5, Figures 6.15–6.19).

   D. **Toric patterns** change with respect to fit. The bearing area moves from the central area in a flat fit toward the periphery in a steep fit. An aligned pattern shows the maximum amount of bearing area (Figure 6.20).

   E. **WTR lens movement** can be predicted by looking at the tear thickness. Tear lenses are rarely completely uniform in thickness. Tear thickness is

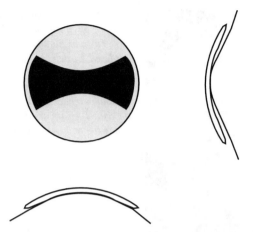

FIGURE 6.5   *With-the-rule cornea and alignment lens. The classic dumbbell pattern is shown on the upper left. On the right is a cross-sectional vertical, or 90-degree, view. Note that there is clearance above and below the central area. On the bottom is the horizontal, or 180-degree, meridian view. There is contact all along this meridian.*

most prominently displayed in the posterior views. The thickest areas are located along the 90-degree meridian for a WTR tear lens. Tear lens thickness also gives insight on lens movement. Lenses move in the direction of least mechanical resistance within the midperiphery.[11] Areas of dark, or bearing, offer the most resistance to lens movement. Areas where the tear lens is the thickest (which have clearance) offer the least resistance. Over a WTR cornea, the lens will move up and down along the thickest area of the tear lens, the 90-degree meridian (Figure 6.21).

   F.   An **against-the-rule (ATR) cornea** and alignment lens pattern appear almost the same as a WTR pattern, only rotated 90 degrees. The "dumbbell" is oriented vertically (Figures 6.22, 6.23).

  G.   An **ATR cornea** and flat lens look similar like a WTR flat pattern rotated 90 degrees. The axis of the bearing area is at 90 degrees (Figure 6.24).

  H.   An **ATR cornea** and steep lens appear like a WTR steep pattern rotated 90 degrees (Figure 6.25).

   I.   **Lens positioning** can considerably change the fluorescein pattern. A centered pattern will have a different appearance than a decentered pattern. An inferiorly positioning lens on a WTR cornea will exhibit excessive superior pooling[7] (Figures 6.26–6.28).

   J.   The **amount of toricity** affects the appearance of the pattern. The greater the toricity, the smaller the alignment area and the more apparent the dumbbell becomes.[6] The lower amounts of toricity appear rounder, more closely resembling a spherical alignment pattern. As the toricity increases (starting at around 1 D), the dark area develops into an oval or

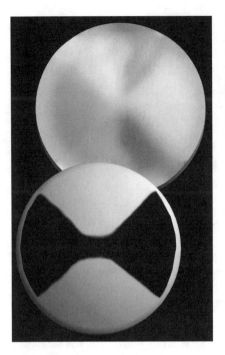

FIGURE 6.6 *A computer-modeled tear layer of a with-the-rule alignment pattern. The tear film has been lifted off the rendered cornea. At bottom is the front surface view typically seen in a fluorescein pattern. Behind the tear layer is the computer-rendered cornea. The holes in the tear layer are areas of touch or areas where the tears are too thin to fluoresce.*

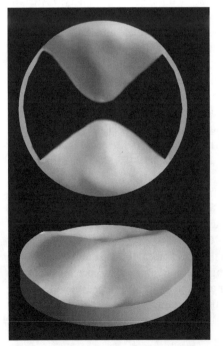

FIGURE 6.7 *A back surface view of a with-the-rule alignment tear layer. The three-dimensional tear layer has been isolated from the lens and cornea. It has been rotated to display different views.*

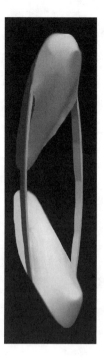

FIGURE 6.8 *The view of a with-the-rule tear layer from the vertical meridian. The rim around the tear layer represents adequate edge lift. The thickest portion of the tear film is along the 90-degree meridian.*

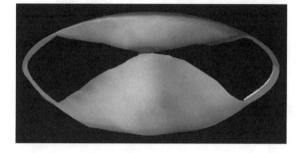

FIGURE 6.9 *Horizontal meridian view of the with-the-rule alignment tear layer.*

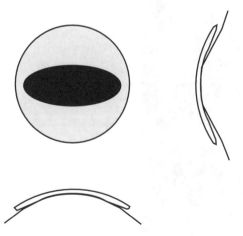

FIGURE 6.10 *With-the-rule cornea and flat lens. The oval pattern of a flat lens is shown on the left. On the right is a cross-sectional view of the 90-degree meridian showing contact in the central areas. The bottom left view is along the 180-degree meridian. As with the alignment pattern, there is contact all along this meridian.*

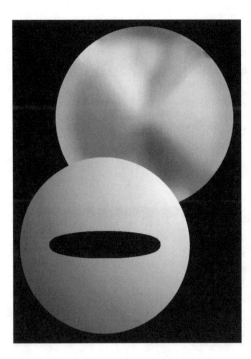

FIGURE 6.11   *Three-dimensional tear computer-rendered model of a with-the-rule flat pattern. The front surface view seen in the pattern is below the cornea. There is one large oval hole in the tear film that represents the area of touch.*

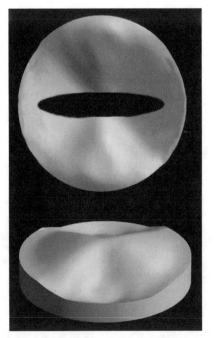

FIGURE 6.12   *Back surface view of with-the-rule flat tear layer.*

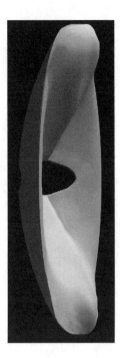

FIGURE 6.13   *Vertical meridian view of a with-the-rule flat tear layer.*

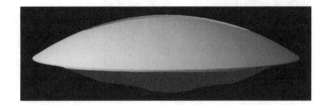

FIGURE 6.14   *Horizontal meridian view of a with-the-rule flat tear layer.*

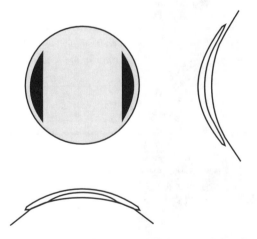

FIGURE 6.15   *With-the-rule cornea and steep lens. On the upper left is the steep lens fluorescein pattern. There are dark areas, or "horns," along the flat meridian. The rest of the lens has corneal clearance. The right view is along the vertical, or 90-degree, meridian. There is no touch along this meridian. On the bottom is the horizontal or 180-degree meridian. There are small contact areas in the periphery.*

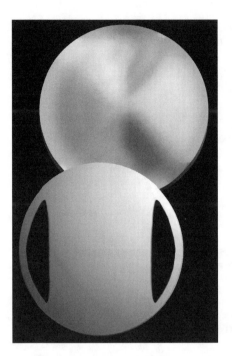

FIGURE 6.16   *A computer-modeled tear layer of a with-the-rule steep pattern is shown at the bottom. The tear film contains two holes, the dark bearing areas seen in the fluorescein pattern. The bearing areas touch on the outer portion of the dumbbell. The rendered with-the-rule cornea is shown above the computer-rendered tear film.*

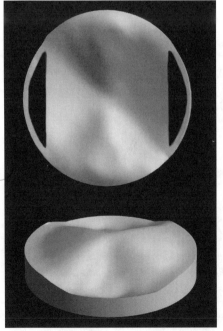

FIGURE 6.17   *Back surface view of a with-the-rule steep tear layer. The computer-modeled tear layer has been isolated from the lens and cornea. The back surface of the tear layer is shown at the top.*

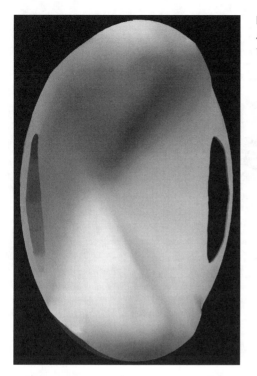

FIGURE 6.18 *A rotated view of the steep with-the-rule tear layer along the vertical meridian.*

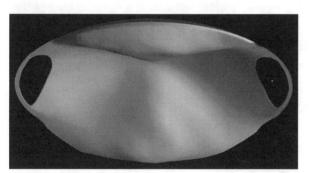

FIGURE 6.19 *Horizontal meridian view of a with-the-rule steep tear layer.*

FIGURE 6.20 *Changing toric patterns with respect to fit. In the center is a with-the-rule aligned fit. The pattern changes as the base curve changes. On the left is the with-the-rule flat pattern. On the right is the with-the-rule steep pattern. As the lens steepens, the dark area moves from the central area (flat lens) to the periphery (steep lens).*

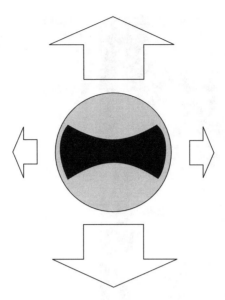

FIGURE 6.21   *With-the-rule lens movement. A spherical lens on a with-the-rule cornea will move up and down.*

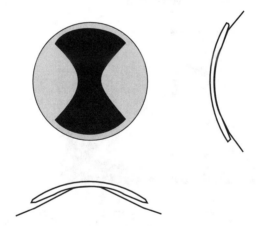

FIGURE 6.22   *Against-the-rule cornea and alignment lens. A spherical lens on an against-the-rule cornea has the "dumbbell" oriented vertically. On the right is the cross-section of the vertical meridian. There is bearing along the entire meridian. On the bottom is the horizontal view with bearing in the central area.*

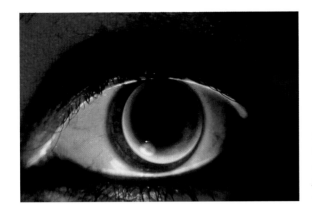

COLOR PLATE 6.1 *An alignment fluorescein pattern. (Courtesy of Tim Edrington, Southern California College of Optometry, Fullerton, California.)*

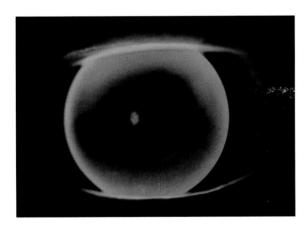

COLOR PLATE 6.2 *A fluorescein pattern reflecting flat fit. (Courtesy of Richard Lindsay, Victorian College of Optometry, Carlton, Victoria, Australia.)*

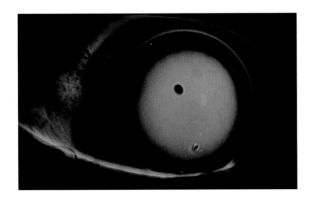

COLOR PLATE 6.3 *A fluorescein pattern reflecting steep fit. (Courtesy of Richard Lindsay, Victorian College of Optometry, Carlton, Victoria, Australia.)*

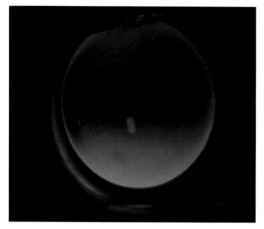

COLOR PLATE 6.4 *Flat lens on with-the-rule cornea fluorescein pattern. The lens is decentering laterally, creating a companion touch. Companion touch can be seen laterally or inferiorly. In this case, the companion touch is seen laterally. (Courtesy of Richard Lindsay, Victorian College of Optometry, Carlton, Victoria, Australia.)*

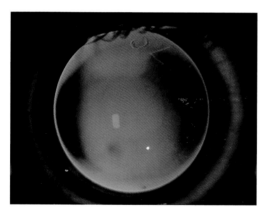

COLOR PLATE 6.5 *Steep lens on with-the-rule cornea fluorescein pattern. (Courtesy of Richard Lindsay, Victorian College of Optometry, Carlton, Victoria, Australia.)*

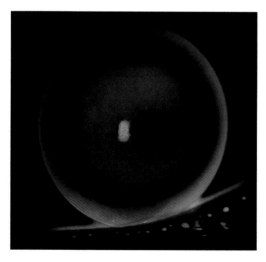

COLOR PLATE 6.6 *Three-point-touch fluorescein pattern. The lens has a central dark area surrounded by a peripheral bearing area. (Courtesy of Richard Lindsay, Victorian College of Optometry, Carlton, Victoria, Australia.)*

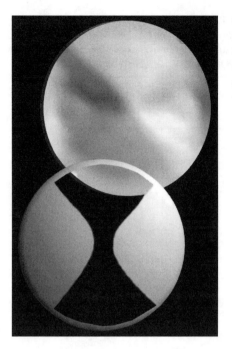

FIGURE 6.23 *Against-the-rule alignment tear layer. The computer-rendered tear model is shown at the bottom. The hole in the tear film forms the classic dumbbell pattern. The computer-rendered against-the-rule cornea is shown above.*

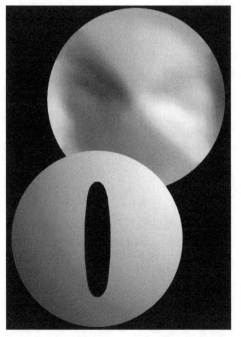

FIGURE 6.24 *Against-the-rule flat tear layer. A flat spherical lens on an against-the-rule cornea has an oval hole oriented along the flat vertical meridian.*

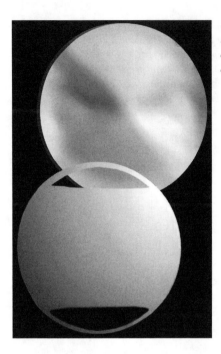

FIGURE 6.25   *Against-the-rule steep tear layer. A steep spherical lens on an against-the-rule cornea has two horns along the vertical meridian.*

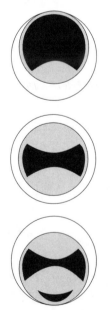

FIGURE 6.26   *With-the-rule lens positioning. Fluorescein patterns change appearance at different positions on the cornea. The top represents a superior-riding lens. The dark area in the superior portion of the lens is largely a result of upper lid pressure. In the middle is the centered lens. On the bottom is an inferior-positioning lens with companion touch.*

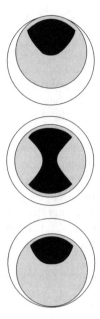

FIGURE 6.27   *Against-the-rule lens positioning. Positioning changes of an alignment lens on an against-the-rule cornea are shown. The top represents a superior-positioning lens. In the middle is the centered lens. On the bottom is an inferior-positioning lens.*

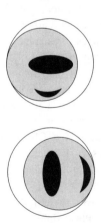

FIGURE 6.28   *Flat lens positioning. A flat lens has a tendency to laterally decenter. At the top is a with-the-rule flat lens decentering. The with-the-rule flat lens shows an oval bearing area with an inferior companion touch. At the bottom is a much more commonly seen against-the-rule flat lens decentering. The against-the-rule flat lens displays an oval oriented vertically with companion touch laterally.*

elliptic area. With more toricity, the dark area becomes more elongated and "horns" begin to appear. The "horns" become larger and more pronounced as the central elliptic area thins.

IV. **Keratoconus** has a characteristically different pattern because of the topography. An alignment, or **three-point touch,** pattern has a central dark area; a midperipheral light area, or clearance area; and a peripheral dark, or bearing, area. One point is the central dark area approximately 2–3 mm wide. The other two points are those of midperipheral touch, which are usually at 180 degrees to one another.[12,13] The pattern has a "bull's-eye" or "horseshoe" shape (Color Plate 6.6). The three-point touch is preferred by many practitioners for smaller or nipple-type cones. The **central dark area** is usually over the apex of the cone (see Chapter 17).

V. **Special considerations** concerning fluorescein patterns include false patterns, fluorescein on the front surface, and the effects of OZDs.

A. **False fluorescein patterns** have an opposite appearance of the true fitting relationship.

1. A **pseudoflat pattern** can appear with a steep-fitting lens because the fluorescein has not penetrated underneath the lens. The dye may accumulate only around the edges of the contact lens to form a false, flat-looking pattern.[7,14] Adding more fluorescein is the best way to determine if the pattern is false. Having the patient blink to increase flow under the lens is also helpful.

2. A **pseudosteep pattern** can appear with high-minus lenses made of fluorosilicone acrylate material. The edge thickness blocks the tear fluorescence. A brighter central fluorescence appears, leaving the impression of a steep pattern.[7]

B. **Front surface (F1) fluorescein** can sometimes confuse the appearance of the actual pattern. Fluorescein can stick to the front surface of an improperly wetting contact lens. Either the lens itself may be dirty or the patient's tear film may be inadequate. The lens will appear to be steep fitting because of the presence of dye on the front surface. Viewing the lens under higher magnification with a biomicroscope can help determine if the fluorescein is on the front surface. The best remedy is cleaning the lens and applying more dye. Checking the integrity of the tear film may also be warranted (see Chapter 16).

C. The **OZD** may have a pronounced effect on fluorescein patterns. A small OZD can appear flat with apical bearing. A large OZD of more 8.0 mm can appear steep or as a **three-point touch.**[2,5]

1. **Small OZDs** appear flat because of a smaller sag height.[5] The central portion of the lens touches on the apex surrounded by clearance. The lens may appear flat despite the fact that the base curve is steep.

2. **Large OZDs** appear to steepen because the sag height increases.[5] Apical clearance can be present even if the base curve is flat. There

is usually a black arc of touch at the edge of the optic zone accompanied by decreased lens movement.[11]

3. **Three-point touch** may appear with some large OZDs. Normally, corneal curvature flattens toward the periphery. A large zone demonstrates this flattening effect by showing clearance in the midperiphery. In some cases, this pattern bears some resemblance to a keratoconic cornea. The greater the flattening effect, the more likely it is that this three-point pattern will appear in normal eyes.[2]

VI. **Static** and **dynamic** are two ways of describing a pattern. **Static patterns** appear when the lens is centered on the cornea. Most references to fluorescein patterns depict static patterns. **Dynamic patterns** occur when the lens moves freely on the eye. In clinical situations, fluorescein patterns are read under dynamic conditions. Dynamic patterns are shown in the video on the accompanying **CD-ROM** (CD-ROM: RGP fluorescein patterns).

REFERENCES

1. Sabell AG. The History of Contact Lenses. In AJ Phillips, J Stone (eds), Contact Lenses (3rd ed). London: Butterworth, 1989;1–33.

2. Young G. Fluorescein in rigid lens fit evaluation. ICLC 1988;15:95–100.

3. Schnider CM. Dyes. In JD Bartlett, SD Jaanus (eds), Clinical Ocular Pharmacology. Boston: Butterworth–Heinemann, 1995;389–407.

4. Barr JT. What you need to know about solution interactions. CL Spectrum 1994;9(8):15–21.

5. Moss HI, Brungardt TF. Fluorescein Studies: Corneal Contact Lenses. Topeka, KS: Duffens Contact Lens Company, 1963.

6. Caffrey B. A better way to do sodium fluorescein staining. CL Spectrum 1994;9(2):56.

7. Bennett ES. Basic Fitting. In ES Bennett, BA Weissman (eds), Clinical Contact Lens Practice. Philadelphia: Lippincott, 1991(23);1–22.

8. McMonnies CW. After-Care Symptoms, Signs, and Management. In AJ Phillips, J Stone (eds), Contact Lenses (3rd ed). London: Butterworth, 1989;703–736.

9. Schnider CM. An option overlooked: make room in your practice for RGP extended wear. Rev Optom 1995;132(4):51–59.

10. Caroline PJ, Norman CW. A blueprint for RGP design. CL Spectrum 1991;6(11):15–19.

11. Caroline PJ, Norman CW. A blueprint for RGP design. Diagnostic lens fitting and fluorescein pattern interpretation: part III. CL Spectrum 1992;7(1):35–39.

12. Arias VC, Liberatore JC, Voss EH, et al. A new technique of fitting contact lenses on keratoconus. Contacto 1959;3:393–415.

13. Edrington TB. Contact Lens Management of Keratoconus. In CA Schwartz (ed), Specialty Contact Lenses: A Fitter's Guide. Philadelphia: Saunders, 1996;142–151.

14. Mandell RB. Trial Lens Method. In RB Mandell (ed), Contact Lens Practice. Springfield, IL: Thomas, 1988;243–264.

Chapter 7

Modification and Verification

Jerry R. Paugh and Milton M. Hom

I. **Modification** in the office is one of the contact lens practitioner's powerful capabilities. Patients truly appreciate the immediate service and convenience.[1] Sending the lenses back to the laboratory for modifications can be unnecessarily time consuming. Most modifications take a short 5–10 minutes.[2]

II. The **tools** and **equipment** needed for modification require a modest investment. Tools are available separately or bundled with the modification unit.

   A. The **modification unit** consists of a motor-driven spindle within a steel or plastic splash bowl. Average spindle speeds are 1,200–1,600 rpm. Varying the spindle speed for softer permeable materials is helpful. Newer materials probably need 1,000 rpm or less.[2]

   B. The **polishing compounds** used should be specifically made for gas-permeable lenses. One compound is **Boston Lens Cleaning Polish** (Bausch & Lomb, Rochester, New York).[1,2] These polishes usually come as a powder that is mixed with distilled water. Replacing the distilled water with a soft lens cleaner makes the polish more viscous. A more viscous solution will stay on the tools longer. Ammoniated **Silvo,** traditionally used for polymethyl methacrylate lenses, is contraindicated for rigid gas-permeable lenses.[1]

   C. **Lens attachment devices,** or **lens holders,** include suction-cup holders, spinners, and tools using double-sided tape. Both suction-cup holders and spinners are hand-held. Lens holders are mounted on the spindle.

      1. **Suction-cup holders,** also called **"greenies,"** have interchangeable concave and convex ends to grip the front or back surface of the lens. Water is needed to wet the holder and enable lens adhesion. The lens needs to be centered as perfectly as possible on the holder. The suction cup can flex the lens and produce undesirable results (lens warpage) if the lens is not positioned properly on the holder. One way to avoid creating irregular diameters and optical zone diameters (OZDs) is to frequently remove the lens and rotate and remount it.[3,4]

2. **Spinners** use either suction or double-sided tape to attach the lens. The lens freely spins during modification procedures to help avoid distorting the optics.[1]

3. **Lens-holder tools** require double-sided tape, not suction, to attach the lens.[1] Accurate centering is imperative when the lens is attached to the tool. Once mounted, different tools are easily applied to the lens.

III. **Modification procedures** that can be performed in the office are diameter reduction, peripheral curve adjustment, edge profile changes, polishing, and power adjustment.

A. **Diameter reduction** uses most of the skills necessary for adequate lens modification. After the lens is cut down, peripheral curves are added, and the edge profile is shaped. The lens can be mounted on the spindle or hand-held.

1. The **lens-holder tool** is mounted on the spindle, and the lens is attached with double-sided tape. A hand-held razor blade, Swiss file, or emery board is used to reduce the lens diameter. The lens should be kept wet while it is cut. The blade, file, or board is held perpendicularly to the lens edge and rolled to shape the edge.[2] A moleskin-covered wooden strip will also reduce the diameter, but not as quickly. The wooden strip is useful to shape the edge, however.[1]

2. A **diamond-impregnated tool,** or **abrasive stone conical tool,** is mounted on the spindle, and the lens is hand-held. The tool is a 60- to 90-degree abrasive cone. The lens is rocked back and forth in the spinning cone with plenty of water for lubrication.[1,5,6]

B. **Peripheral curve adjustment** or **fabrication** is performed with radius tools, or laps. A minimum set includes the following sizes: 7.6 mm, 7.8 mm, 8.0 mm, 8.2 mm, 8.4 mm, 8.6 mm, 8.8 mm, 9.0 mm, 9.3 mm, 9.6 mm, 10.0 mm, 10.5 mm, 11.2 mm, and 12.0 mm.[1,2] Adhesive tape is attached to the lap for abrasiveness. Adhesive tape adds 0.2 mm thickness, and velveteen adds another 0.4 mm to the radius. For example, an 8.8-mm tool becomes a 9.0-mm tool with adhesive tape. Polish is applied to the lap every 5–10 seconds. The lens is touched down on the lap while it is rotated in the opposite direction of the spindle. The lens can be held at 30 degrees to the vertical. If a spinner is used, the lens is held at a 45- to 60-degree angle. Another method of peripheral curve adjustment is holding the lens vertical to the lap and rotating it in a figure-eight fashion. After the peripheral curves are applied, a blend is added. Normally, the radius of the blend should be midway between the two peripheral curves. Depending on the pressure and contact time, the blend can be light, medium, or heavy.[2] The blend of the lens can be checked with a magnifier.

C. **Edge profile changes,** or **edge shaping,** is done with a cone tool. The edge is thinned by adding an **anterior bevel.**[5] The lens is placed into the cone and rocked slightly back and forth, alternating between left and right. Polish is frequently applied to the cone. Every 10 seconds, the anterior bevel of the edge should be checked. A 90-degree cone is normally used. A 60-degree cone adds a narrower bevel. Cones of 105 or 120 degrees add a wider bevel.

D. **Polishing** smooths the surface of the lens. An uneven or reshaped edge needs polishing. Light surface scratches and deposits need surface polishing.

    1. **Edge polishing** can be done with the fingers or with an adhesive tape sling while the lens is mounted on the spindle. **Finger polishing** is very effective and easy to perform. The lens-holder and double-sided tape hold the lens concave side up in place while the lens spins on the spindle. The pad of the index finger and thumb apply light pressure to finger polish the edge. Edge polishing with **adhesive tape** includes slinging 2–4 inches of a strip of adhesive tape around the spinning lens edge. A variation of this method is using the tape to "shoeshine" the lens edge. Apply polish frequently to either the fingers or tape when polishing the edge.[1] Another method of edge polishing is polishing with a series of velveteen-covered laps varying from 40 to 180 degrees.[5]

    2. **Hand-held polishing methods** include polishing the lens on a flat sponge or a sponge with a hole. A spinner or suction-cup holder is used to hold the lens. Polish is liberally and frequently applied to the sponge or large pad.

        a. The lens is attached with the back surface out to a suction-cup holder and polished on a **flat sponge.** The lens is held at a 40- to 60-degree angle to the sponge. It is touched down on the 9 o'clock position while the lens is rotated. Moving the lens in a circle will round out a sharp edge[6] (Figure 7.1). The flat sponge can also be covered with velveteen. A spinner can be used to hold the lens.[1,2]

        b. The lens is attached to a suction cup with the back surface out and polished on the **central hole of a sponge.** It is moved vertically up and down in the hole for 30–60 seconds.[1]

    3. **Concentric polishing procedure** entails stepping the lens through a series of velveteen-covered laps. The lens is placed front surface down through the 90-, 60-, and 40-degree laps. Then the lens is placed back surface down on the 180-, 140-, 90-, 60-, and 40-degree laps.[5]

Pearl: Choice of polishing surface varies with the modification. Abrasive surfaces, such as diamond, cut very fast and rough. Softer surfaces, such as velveteen, remove material slowly but smoothly. Using adhesive tape takes longer to remove material but leaves a smoother surface than velveteen. A sponge does not remove material well but leaves a very polished surface.

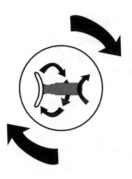

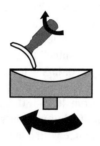

FIGURE 7.1   *Edge polishing. The lens is held at a 40- to 60-degree angle to the pad and rotated in a circular fashion. Make certain that not just one section of the edge is rounded. Different sections of the edge can be touched on the pad by rotating the lens and holder along their axis. Above is the view looking down on the pad and lens. Below is the side view.*

4. **Surface polish** removes light scratches and deposits. **Deposits** can be removed by rubbing the surfaces between the fingers with polish. A cotton swab can also be used.[7] Light scratches are removed by surface polishing on a sponge tool.

    a. The **back, concave surface** of a lens is very difficult to polish without distorting the optics. To polish the back surface periphery, the lens is touched down on a sphere-shaped or inverted cone sponge tool at a 30-degree angle.[1,6] The lens is rotated in the opposite direction of the spinning sponge tool. For polishing the central optic zone, the lens is touched down at 90 degrees (straight down or vertical).[1]

        Pearl: *It is much easier to distort the optics of a higher-Dk material (more than 60).[4] High-Dk materials are usually softer and more heat-sensitive by nature.*

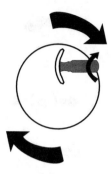

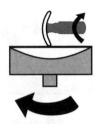

FIGURE 7.2 *Peripheral polishing of the front surface. The lens is held nearly parallel to the pad. The lens and holder need to be rotated along their axes to ensure complete coverage of the periphery. Above is the view looking down on the pad and lens. Below is the side view.*

    b. The **front, convex surface** commonly has the most scratches because of patients "scooping" the lens from the case.[6] A flat sponge tool is used. The periphery can be polished by holding the lens almost parallel to the pad for 10 to 20 seconds. Remember to rotate the lens to avoid distorting the optics[1,6] (Figure 7.2). The midperiphery is polished by touching the lens down onto a flat sponge at a 45-degree angle midway between the center and edge of the pad. The lens should be moved side to side across the midperiphery of the pad (Figure 7.3). For polishing the central zone, the lens is pushed straight down into the center of the pad 10–12 times for 1 second at a time.[1] Touch very lightly because this is the same procedure that adds minus to the lens (Figure 7.4). The edge can then be polished by holding the lens almost parallel to the pad and rotating at the 9 o'clock position in a circular fashion. The front and back portions of the edge will be buffed[6] (Figure 7.5).

    Pearl: *Use plenty of polish. The lens should be kept wet with polish during modification.*[4]

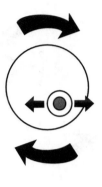

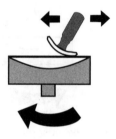

FIGURE 7.3 *Midperipheral polishing of the front surface. The lens is held at an angle to the pad and moved side to side. Above is the view looking down on the pad and lens. Below is the side view. Notice that the lens is at an approximate 60-degree angle.*

E. **Power adjustments** are made with a flat sponge or toepad.

1. **Minus addition** entails removing plastic from the center of the lens. Realistically, 0.12–0.50 D can be added easily without distortion.[6] The convex surface is vertically touched on the periphery of the flat sponge and rotated opposite to the spindle.[2] Leave the lens on the pad for 10–15 seconds at a time before checking power.[6] With a toepad, the lens is mounted on a spinner and touched near the apex. The lens is first touched on the edge to start it spinning. The lens is then pushed into the sponge to remove the plastic from the center.[1] The simplest method is adding minus **manually.** The convex surface of the lens is lightly rubbed into a hand-held polishing pad or flat sponge with an index finger. The lens is moved in a figure-eight pattern. This method is very easy and offers great control.

2. **Plus addition** consists of removing the plastic from the periphery of the lens. An experienced modifier can add 0.12–0.37 D without distortion.[6] On a flat sponge, the lens is pushed into the center of

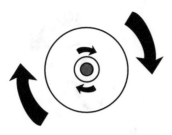

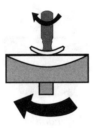

FIGURE 7.4 *Front surface central zone polishing. The lens is touched lightly while being held vertical to the pad. The lens must be rotated frequently. Above is the view looking down on the pad and lens. Below is the side view.*

the pad. With a toepad, the lens is positioned to remove plastic from the periphery.[1,2]

Pearl: Edge polishing, front surface polishing, and adding minus are the easiest and most commonly performed modification procedures in the office.

IV. It is necessary to master **verification** and inspection of the lenses.

    A. The **base curve radius** is measured with either a radiuscope or keratometer.

        1. The **radiuscope** is based on the same principles as the **optic spherometer,** an instrument used to measure curvatures of microscope objective.

            a. The **Drysdale principle** is used to determine radius of curvature. A microscope projects a real image of the target (spokes) onto the contact-lens surface. The projected target is reflected back, forming an aerial image. The distance between the real image and the aerial image is the radius of curvature of the contact lens.[5]

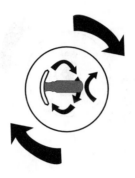

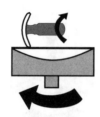

FIGURE 7.5   *Edge touchup. The lens is held parallel to the pad and moved in a circular fashion. The lens and holder are rotated along their axis at the same time. Above is the view looking down on the pad and lens. Below is the side view.*

    b. The **procedure of measuring base curve radius with a radiuscope** begins by placing the lens concave surface up onto the stage with a drop of water. The drop is added to block out the front surface of the lens.[7] Place the microscope close to the stage and focus in on the spokes. This is the real image of the target. It may be necessary to reposition the stage to make sure the lens is centered within the beam of light.[8] Set the reading on zero. Move the objective away from the stage with the focusing knob. The aerial image of the spokes will appear as the image of the light filament is passed. The radius is read when the aerial image is in focus.[9] The radius is the distance between the real and aerial images.[5]

 2. The **keratometer** can measure the radius by placing the lens in the same position as the eye would be. The keratometer can measure a convex curvature (cornea) as well as a concave curvature (base curve radius).[6] Different devices to hold the lens can be used.[9]

 3. **Warpage** of the lens usually shows as a small amount of toricity with the radiuscope or keratometer. The aerial image of the radiuscopic mires or spokes will not have an equal focus.[10] With the keratometer, the principal meridians will have unequal curvatures, indicating toricity. Warpage can then be confirmed if no associated toricity is measured with the lensometer.

B. **Lens power** is best measured with a **lensometer** in the same manner as a with spectacle lens. The contact lens is measured, cleaned, and dried against the lens stop. **Back vertex power** is measured with the concave surface down, or "cup down," against the lens stop. **Front vertex power** is measured with the concave surface up, or "cup up," against the stop. Front vertex power is the **standard of measurement** for contact lens powers. Indicating whether the power is front or back vertex is especially important for high plus lenses. The back vertex power for a high plus lens is usually greater than the front vertex power. Prism is measured by looking at the amount of mire decentration. The concentric rings in the ocular tell the amount of prism in the lens.[7,9]

C. **Diameter and OZD** are commonly measured with a **magnifier,** or **reticule.** The lens is held concave side down against the flat window of the magnifier. As you look through the ocular, the scale in the eyepiece magnifies and measures the lens. The OZD can also be inspected and measured. Many times, the OZD is not readily apparent. The lens needs to be viewed against a variable bright background such as a window or fluorescent tube. Moving the lens and magnifier slightly from side to side can help to reveal the transition. The heavier the blend, the more difficult it is to measure the OZD. Roundness should be checked by measuring the diameter or OZD along the various meridians. If no blend is present, the peripheral curve widths can also be measured. A **V-channel gauge** is another device used to measure diameter. A lens is allowed to slide into the channel by gravity.[10] When the lens stops, the diameter can be read off the adjacent scale.[9] The lens and V-channel gauge must be cleaned and dried to slide properly.[10] A V-channel gauge is more prone to errors in measurement than the reticule.

D. **Thickness** is best measured in the office with a thickness gauge. The lens is placed concave side up between the rod and plunger and measured on the gauge.[9,10]

E. **Edges** are very difficult to evaluate. They can be inspected with a **stereomicroscope** and **projection magnifier.**[10]

   1. **Edge inspection** should cover the entire circumferential surface. The lens is first held convex toward the light and rotated 360 degrees. Then the lens is held convex to the light and rotated. The edge should have an even thickness, with the apex closer to the back than the front surface.[11]

   2. Another method of inspection is placing the lens against the **palm,** concave side down, and pushing across. If there is any resistance to

movement or audible sounds are made, the edge needs polishing, reshaping, or both.[9]

F. **Surface quality,** such as presence of scratches and deposits, can be seen with the magnifier or reticule.

G. **Material** can be determined by specific gravity. Using the **Opti-MIS system,** the contact lens practitioner can determine the lens material by running it through a series of three solutions.[7] Whether the lens floats or sinks in each solution determines the material.[10]

REFERENCES

1. Bennett E, Egan DJ. Modification. In ES Bennett, RM Grohe (eds), Rigid Gas-Permeable Contact Lenses. New York: Professional Press, 1986;189–224.
2. Morgan BW, Bennett ES. Modification. In ES Bennett, BA Weissman (eds), Clinical Contact Lens Practice. Philadelphia: Lippincott, 1991(27);1–19.
3. Vehige JG. Gas-Permeable Material Modification Fabrication Procedures. Pamphlet.
4. Bennett E. Should you be modifying your RGP lenses? CL Spectrum 1994;9(12):13.
5. Mandell RB. Modification Procedures. In RB Mandell (ed), Contact Lens Practice. Springfield, IL: Thomas, 1988;475–501.
6. Paugh JP. Modifications Made Simple. Pamphlet.
7. Lee WC. Contact lens modifications. CL Forum 1987;12(12):41–48.
8. Mandell RB. Contact Lens Instruments. In RB Mandell (ed), Contact Lens Practice. Springfield, IL: Thomas, 1988;913–953.
9. Henry VA, Bennett ES. Inspection and Verification of Rigid Gas-Permeable Contact Lenses. In ES Bennett, BA Weissman (eds), Clinical Contact Lens Practice. Philadelphia: Lippincott, 1991(26);1–11.
10. Mandell RB. Inspection and Verification. In RB Mandell (ed), Contact Lens Practice. Springfield, IL: Thomas, 1988;352–387.
11. Barr J, Stepphen R. Tips to improve your contact lens inspections. CL Spectrum 1995;10(5):26.

Chapter 8

Rigid Gas-Permeable Lenses for Astigmatism

Timothy B. Edrington

I. **The optimal rigid contact lens design** is determined by applying a nonflexing, spherical base curve, rigid diagnostic lens to the patient's eye and performing a spherocylinder over-refraction (OR). Based on the corneal toricity, fitting characteristics, and OR cylinder, the simplest acceptable lens design is selected, designed, and ordered. The flow chart in Table 8.1 is a guideline for selecting the most appropriate rigid lens design for the patient. The lens designs in Table 8.1 are listed in descending order of preference based on factors such as simplicity of design; optical characteristics; cost; and ease of fabrication, analysis, modification, and duplication. Prescribe the first rigid lens design in the table that satisfies the needs of your patient based on corneal toricity and residual OR cylinder. Spherical rigid contact lens design is presented in Chapter 4. This chapter introduces toric rigid lens designs.

   A. The use of a **nonflexing diagnostic lens** is advised so that flexure does not alter the residual cylinder measured. If a rigid lens flexes or warps on an against-the-rule cornea, the OR increases in against-the-rule cylinder by the amount of lens flexure. If a rigid lens flexes on a with-the-rule cornea, the OR increases in with-the-rule cylinder (or can beneficially decrease against-the-rule cylinder) by the amount of lens flexure.

   B. The ideal diagnostic rigid lens material to minimize "on-the-eye" flexure is polymethyl methacrylate (**PMMA**). Generally, flexure increases as the material increases in permeability.[1] Rigid lenses with a thinner center or overall thickness flex more than thicker designs. Mid-Dk rigid gas-permeable (RGP) contact lenses can flex clinically significant amounts with center thicknesses of 0.15 mm or less.

II. A **base curve toric,** spherical front surface rigid lens design is indicated when 1.50 D or more of corneal toricity is present and a residual OR cylinder of more than 0.75 D is obtained with a diagnostic rigid sphere on the eye. The residual cylinder needs to be at or near the same axis as the corneal toricity,

Table 8.1   Rigid Contact Lens Design Flowchart

Rigid Gas-Permeable Lens Design	Residual Cylinder in Over-Refraction (D)	Corneal Toricity (D)
Spherical	≤0.75	≤2.50
Base curve toric	≥0.75 at same axis as K toricity	≥1.50
Spherical power effect bitoric	<0.75	≥1.50
Cylinder power effect bitoric	≥0.75	≥1.50
Front surface toric	≥1.00	≤1.00

and the amount of the residual cylinder needs to be approximately **one-half** the amount of the corneal toricity.

A.   **Design** a base curve toric rigid lens according to the following "recipe":

1.   **Step 1. Verify** that a base curve toric is the most appropriate RGP lens design.

2.   **Step 2. Design your standard spherical RGP contact lens,** and alter the parameters according to the following steps:

3.   **Step 3.** Determine the ideal amount of **base curve toricity** using the corneal toricity measured by keratometry. For against-the-rule corneas, select the base curve toricity equal to the patient's corneal toricity to enhance lens centration. For with-the-rule corneas, the base curve toricity should be approximately 0.50 D less than the corneal toricity to enhance tear exchange. For a base curve toricity that is less than the amount of the corneal toricity, the base curve toricity needs to be at least two-thirds the amount of the corneal toricity to minimize unwanted lens rotation.[2]

4.   **Step 4. Select base curves** such that the mean value of the toric base curves is equal to the spherical design base curve. The average of base curves prescribed should be approximately 0.75 D flatter than the average keratometry value for an interpalpebral positioning toric lens design. The fitting relationship can be confirmed by fluorescein pattern analysis.

5.   **Step 5. Select contact lens powers** such that the mean value is equal to the spherical design lens power and the difference between the two powers is 3/2 the amount of the prescribed base curve toricity.

6.   **Step 6. Order remaining parameters** in the same way as for a spherical design, except specify that the secondary curve is toric by the amount of the ordered base curve toricity.

EXAMPLE: BASE CURVE TORIC

Given

Keratometry	43.00 @ 080/45.50 @ 170
Subjective refraction (vertexed)	–2.00 –3.75 × 080 (20/15)
Diagnostic rigid contact lens	43.75 D base curve/–2.50 D power
Over-refraction	–0.25 –1.25 × 080 (20/15)
Fluorescein pattern	Apical clearance by 2.50 D/2.50 D against-the-rule toricity

Step 1.   Determine the most appropriate RGP lens design for the given patient data. A spherical RGP lens design would not be acceptable because of the residual astigmatism (–1.25 × 080) obtained through the diagnostic OR. However, the cornea is more than 1.50 D toric, the OR cylinder is at the same axis as the corneal toricity (axis 80), and the OR cylinder is approximately one-half of the corneal toricity. Therefore, a base curve toric, spherical front surface RGP design is indicated.

Step 2.   Design a spherical RGP contact lens based on the patient data given:

Base curve	43.50 D
Power	–3.12 D
Overall diameter	9.0 mm
Optic zone diameter	7.4 mm
Secondary curve radius	8.60 mm
Third curve radius	12.00 mm
Third curve width	0.2 mm
Center thickness	0.12 mm

Step 3.   Determine the ideal amount of base curve toricity. In this case, the base curve toricity is prescribed equal to the corneal toricity (2.50 D) because the cornea is against-the-rule.

Step 4.   Select base curves such that their mean value is equal to the spherical design base curve. In step 3, we determined that a base curve toricity of 2.50 D is indicated; therefore, the base curves would be 42.25 and 44.75 D (mean value of 43.50 D). An apical alignment fitting relationship is expected and should be confirmed by fluorescein pattern analysis.

Step 5.   Select the contact lens powers such that the mean value is equal to the spherical design lens power and the difference between the two powers is 3/2 the amount of the prescribed base curve toricity. Three-halves of the difference between the base curve toricity (2.50 D) is 3.75 D, and the spherical design power is –3.12 D. Therefore, the powers for the base curve toric are –1.25 and –5.00 D (mean value of –3.12 D).

Step 6.   Order remaining parameters, specifying a secondary curve toric by the amount of the base curve toricity. This will result in a spherical optic zone. Therefore, the final prescription is as follows:

Base curves and powers	44.75 D/–5.00 D
	42.25 D/–1.25 D
Overall diameter	9.0 mm
Optic zone diameter	7.4 mm
Secondary curve radius	8.60 mm/Secondary curve ordered toric by 2.50 D
Third curve radius	12.00 mm
Third curve width	0.2 mm
Center thickness	0.17 mm

EXAMPLE: BASE CURVE TORIC

Given

Keratometry	41.87 @ 180/45.87 @ 090
Subjective refraction	+1.75 –5.50 × 180 (20/15)
Diagnostic rigid contact lens	43.50 D base curve/+0.25 D power
Over-refraction	–0.25 –1.50 × 180 (20/15)
Fluorescein pattern	Apical clearance by 0.37 D/4.00 D with-the-rule toricity

Step 1.   Determine the most appropriate RGP lens design for the given patient data. A spherical RGP lens design would not be acceptable due to the residual OR cylinder and the high amount of corneal toricity. A base curve toric, spherical front surface, rigid lens would be indicated because there is adequate corneal toricity to minimize lens rotation and the OR cylinder is at or near the axis of the corneal toricity. The OR cylinder is also approximately one-half of the corneal toricity.

Step 2.   Design a spherical RGP contact lens based on the patient data given:

Base curve	43.12 D
Power	–0.25 D
Overall diameter	9.0 mm
Optic zone diameter	7.4 mm
Secondary curve radius	8.70 mm

Third curve radius	12.00 mm
Third curve width	0.2 mm
Center thickness	0.19 mm

Step 3.   Determine the ideal amount of base curve toricity. In this case, the base curve toricity is prescribed 0.50 D less than the corneal toricity (i.e., 3.50 D toric) to enhance the tear exchange because the cornea is with-the-rule.

Step 4.   Select base curves such that their mean value is equal to the spherical design base curve (43.12 D). In step 3, we determined that a base curve toricity of 3.50 D is indicated; therefore, the base curves would be 41.37 and 44.87 D (mean value of 43.12 D). An apical alignment fitting relationship is expected and should be confirmed by fluorescein pattern analysis.

Step 5.   Select the contact lens powers such that the mean value is equal to the spherical design lens power and the difference between the two powers is 3/2 the amount of the prescribed base curve toricity. Three-halves of the difference between the base curve toricity (3.50 D) is 5.25 D, and the spherical design power is –0.25 D. Therefore, the powers for the base curve toric are +2.37 and –2.87 D (mean value of –0.25 D).

Step 6.   Order remaining parameters specifying a secondary curve toric by the amount of the base curve toricity. This will result in a spherical optic zone. Therefore, the final prescription is as follows:

Base curves and powers	44.87 D/–2.87 D
	41.37 D/+2.37 D
Overall diameter	9.0 mm
Optic zone diameter	7.4 mm
Secondary curve radius	8.70 mm/Secondary curve ordered toric by 3.50 D
Third curve radius	12.00 mm
Third curve width	0.2 mm
Center thickness	0.24 mm

B.   Clinically, the **1-2-3 rule** is used when considering the use of a base curve toric, spherical front surface, rigid contact lens. The 1-2-3 rule is based on approximations of the optical effects of this design with PMMA material. Optically, a PMMA contact lens ordered with a base curve toricity of 2 D will create a change in OR cylinder, or on-eye effect, of 1 D. When the contact lens powers are measured by lensometry, the 2 D base curve toric lens will exhibit 3 D of cylinder.[3] This on-eye effect refers to the change in OR cylinder relative to the residual cylinder obtained through a spherical diagnostic contact lens. The on-eye effect and cylinder power measured by lensometry with an RGP lens material of lower index of refraction are slightly less than those of PMMA.

C. **Lens rotation** with a base curve toric RGP contact lens can be minimized when there is sufficient corneal toricity. A corneal toricity of 1.50 D or more is desired to stabilize lens rotation. The toricity of the base curve should be selected to be within the range of two-thirds to the full amount of corneal toricity. If this is not done, excessive lens rotation can induce unwanted OR cylinder and subsequent reduced visual acuity.

D. Whenever indicated, it is preferable to prescribe a toric base curve, spherical front surface lens design instead of a bitoric RGP. Even though a bitoric lens can be designed to entirely correct the residual error and provide for an optimal base curve-to-cornea fitting relationship, opt for a base curve, spherical front surface toric lens design. Unlike with a bitoric design, the power can easily be adjusted by modification and the front surface polished when indicated. Also, the optics of a bitoric RGP lens are usually not as crisp as those of a base curve toric, spherical front surface contact lens.

E. **Do not specify the power for the steep meridian** when you order a base curve toric. If a power is specified, most laboratories bill the practitioner for a more expensive bitoric RGP lens. When the lens is received from the laboratory, expect the gross difference between the two lensometry powers to be approximately 3/2 the amount of the base curve toricity. The power in the steep meridian will be more minus than the flat meridian's power. In the examples, the steep meridian power is specified for illustration purposes.

F. **Center thickness** is prescribed based on the overall diameter and the power of the base curve toric lens in the most plus meridian.

G. A toric base curve or bitoric **diagnostic lens set** is extremely beneficial for interpreting fluorescein patterns of patients with high amounts of corneal toricity.

III. A **bitoric rigid lens design** is indicated when a patient presents with 1.50 D or more of corneal toricity and residual cylinder through a spherical rigid lens would not be adequately corrected by a base curve toric design.

A. **To design** a bitoric using a spherical diagnostic rigid contact lens, the following "recipe" can be used:

1. **Step 1.** Verify that a **bitoric** is the most appropriate RGP lens design.

2. **Step 2.** Place **keratometry** and **vertexed subjective refraction** findings on an optical cross.

3. **Step 3.** Determine the ideal amount of **base curve toricity.** For against-the-rule corneas, select the base curve toricity to equal the

corneal toricity to enhance lens centration. For with-the-rule corneas, the base curve toricity should be approximately 0.50 D less than the corneal toricity to enhance tear exchange. For a base curve toricity less than the corneal toricity, the base curve toricity should be at least two-thirds the amount of the corneal toricity to minimize unwanted lens rotation.

4. **Step 4.** **"Subtract"** tear lens values from keratometry and vertexed subjective refraction values. The result gives you the bitoric base curves and contact lens powers.

5. **Step 5.** **Order** remaining parameters the same as for spherical design, except specify that the secondary curve be fabricated toric by the amount of the prescribed base curve toricity.

EXAMPLE: BITORIC (USING SPHERICAL DIAGNOSTIC CONTACT LENS)

Given

Keratometry	42.75 @ 080/44.25 @ 170
Subjective refraction (vertexed)	−1.75 −3.25 × 080 (20/15)
Diagnostic rigid contact lens (sphere)	42.75 D base curve/−1.37 D power
Over-refraction	−0.50 −1.75 × 080 (20/15)
Fluorescein pattern	Apical alignment /1.50 D against-the-rule toricity

Step 1. Determine the most appropriate RGP lens design for the given patient data. A spherical RGP lens design would not be acceptable due to the amount of residual OR cylinder (1.75 D). A base curve toric, spherical front surface lens that is toric by the full amount of the corneal toricity (1.50 D) would correct approximately one-half (0.75 D) of the OR cylinder. This would leave the patient with 1.00 D of residual astigmatism. A bitoric lens can then be prescribed if the corneal toricity is greater than or equal to 1.50 D.

Steps 2, 3, and 4. Place keratometry and vertexed subjective refraction findings on an optical cross. Determine the ideal base curve toricity. A base curve toricity of 1.50 D (equal to the corneal toricity) is prescribed to enhance lens centration on the against-the-rule cornea. This creates a spherical tear lens. "Subtract" desired tear lens values from the keratometry and subjective refraction findings. A −0.75 D sphere tear lens is selected to achieve an interpalpebral, alignment fitting lens.

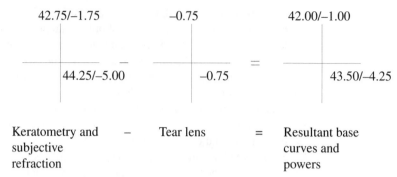

42.75/–1.75		–0.75		42.00/–1.00
44.25/–5.00	–	–0.75	=	43.50/–4.25
Keratometry and subjective refraction	–	Tear lens	=	Resultant base curves and powers

The resultants are the base curves and contact lens powers for the bitoric prescription. Note that for base curve determination, the resultant is flatter if a minus tear lens is desired.

Step 5. Order remaining parameters, specifying the secondary curve toric by the amount of the base curve toricity. This will result in a spherical optic zone. Therefore, the final prescription is as follows:

Base curves and powers	43.50 D/–4.25 D
	42.00 D/–1.00 D
Overall diameter	9.0 mm
Optic zone diameter	7.4 mm
Secondary curve radius	8.75 mm/Secondary curve ordered toric by 1.50 D
Third curve radius	12.00 mm
Third curve width	0.2 mm
Center thickness	0.17 mm

EXAMPLE: BITORIC (USING SPHERICAL DIAGNOSTIC CONTACT LENS)

Given

Keratometry	40.87 @ 180/44.62 @ 090
Subjective refraction	+3.00 –2.50 × 180 (20/15)
Diagnostic rigid contact lens (sphere)	42.25 D base curve/+3.62 D power
Over-refraction	– 0.50 –1.25 × 090 (20/15)
Fluorescein pattern	Apical clearance/3.75 D of with-the-rule toricity

Step 1. Determine the most appropriate RGP lens design for the given patient data. A spherical RGP lens design would not be acceptable because of

the residual OR cylinder (1.25 D) and the high amount of corneal toricity (3.75 D). A base curve toric, spherical front surface lens is not acceptable because the OR cylinder axis is not at or near the axis of the corneal toricity. A bitoric lens can be prescribed if the corneal toricity is greater than or equal to 1.50 D.

Steps 2, 3, and 4.   Place keratometry and subjective refraction findings on an optical cross. Determine ideal base curve toricity (3.25 D toric to create a 0.50 D toric tear lens because the cornea is with-the-rule) and "subtract" the ideal tear lens value from the keratometry and subjective refraction values. A mean tear lens of –0.75 D is selected to achieve an interpalpebral, alignment fitting relationship.

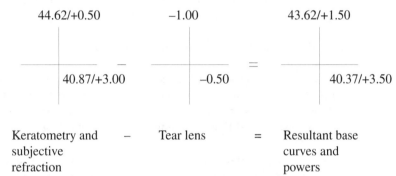

The resultants are base curves and contact lens powers for the bitoric prescription. Note that for base curve determination, the resultant is flatter if a minus tear lens is desired.

Step 5.   Order remaining parameters specifying a secondary curve toric by the amount of the base curve toricity. This will result in a spherical optic zone. Therefore, the final prescription is as follows:

Base curves and powers	43.62 D/+1.50 D
	40.37 D/+3.50 D
Overall diameter	9.0 mm
Optic zone diameter	7.4 mm
Secondary curve radius	9.10 mm/Secondary curve ordered toric by
	3.25 D
Third curve radius	12.00 mm
Third curve width	0.2 mm
Center thickness	0.27 mm

Pearl: *Order toric RGP lenses with a warranty.*

B. A practitioner can select **other tear lens** values to customize the fitting relationship. Fluorescein pattern assessment with the prescribed lens will allow the practitioner to fine-tune the fit. The original lens should be ordered with a warranty to minimize the lens cost in the event the lens needs to be reordered.

C. Even though a bitoric can always be designed to provide an optimal OR with no residual cylinder and an ideal lens-to-cornea fitting relationship, a **base curve toric** should be ordered when indicated. A base curve toric, with its spherical front surface, can be easily polished or have additional power added. Also, a base curve toric is less expensive and optically superior to a bitoric rigid lens design.

Pearl: Polishing or adding power to base curve toric, spherical front surface lenses is an easy, in-office modification.

D. **Mandell and Moore** have developed an easy-to-use form for designing bitorics.[4]

IV. **An SPE bitoric** is indicated when there is 1.50 D or more of corneal toricity and an OR with a spherical rigid diagnostic lens reveals an acceptable amount of residual cylinder—that is, refractive astigmatism is entirely or almost entirely corneal.[5]

A. **To design** an SPE bitoric **using an SPE bitoric diagnostic set,** the following "recipe" can be used:

1. **Step 1. Select an SPE bitoric diagnostic lens** with a base curve toricity of approximately the same amount as the corneal toricity if the cornea is against-the-rule. If the cornea is with-the-rule, select a diagnostic lens with a base curve toricity less than the corneal toricity by approximately 0.50 D. The average or mean base curve of the diagnostic contact lens should be approximately 0.75 D flatter than the average keratometry reading.

2. **Step 2. Perform a spherocylinder OR.** Note: if OR cylinder is 0.75 D or greater, prescribe a cylinder power effect (CPE) bitoric contact lens.

3. **Step 3. Evaluate the fluorescein pattern.**

4. **Step 4. Add** equivalent dioptric sphere of OR to the lens power of each meridian of the diagnostic SPE bitoric lens.

5. **Step 5.** If indicated by fluorescein pattern interpretation of apical relationship or tear lens toricity, **alter the base curves.** If changes to base curves are made, the contact lens power in the same meridian must be altered by the amount of the dioptric change in base curve.

EXAMPLE: SPE BITORIC

Given

Keratometry   42.75 @ 090/44.75 @ 180

Step 1. Select a diagnostic lens 0.75 D flatter than the average keratometry value with base curve toricity equal to corneal toricity. In this case, the average K = 43.75 D, average K – 0.75 D = 43.00 D, and the corneal toricity is 2.00 D against-the-rule. Therefore, the ideal diagnostic base curves are 42.00 D × 44.00 D.

Diagnostic SPE contact lens selected:

$$\frac{44.00\ D/-2.00\ D}{42.00\ D/plano\ D}$$

Step 2. OR: –1.50 D sphere (20/15)

Step 3. Fluorescein pattern: apical alignment/no toricity.

Step 4. Add equivalent sphere of the OR (–1.50 D) to powers of the diagnostic contact lens in both meridians as follows:

$$\frac{44.00\ D/-3.50\ D}{42.00\ D/-1.50\ D}$$

Remember that powers in step 4 are correct only for the diagnostic contact lens base curves.

Step 5. Alter base curves if indicated by fluorescein pattern. This is not necessary for this example. Therefore, the final prescription for base curves and powers is as follows:

$$\frac{44.00\ D/-3.50\ D}{42.00\ D/-1.50\ D}$$

Order the remaining lens parameters in the same manner as for a spherical design, except specify that the secondary curve is toric by the amount of the ordered base curve toricity.

EXAMPLE: SPE BITORIC

Given
Keratometry   42.00 @ 180/46.00 @ 090

Step 1. Select a diagnostic lens 0.75 D flatter than the average keratometry value with base curve toricity one-half diopter less than corneal toricity. In this case, average K = 44.00 D, average K – 0.75 D = 43.25 D, and corneal toricity

= 4.00 D with-the-rule. Therefore, the ideal diagnostic base curves are 41.50 D × 45.00 D. Note: The desired base curve is 3.50 D toric to enhance tear exchange.

Diagnostic SPE bitoric contact lens selected:

$$\frac{45.00 \text{ D/}-3.50 \text{ D}}{41.50 \text{ D/plano D}}$$

Step 2.   OR: +2.50 –0.25 × 180 (20/15).

Step 3.   Fluorescein pattern: apical touch by 0.25 D/0.50 D with-the-rule toricity

Step 4.   Add equivalent sphere of OR (+2.37 D in this case) to powers of the diagnostic lens in both meridians:

$$\frac{45.00 \text{ D/}-1.12 \text{ D}}{41.50 \text{ D/}+2.37 \text{ D}}$$

Remember that powers in step 4 are correct only for the diagnostic contact lens base curves.

Step 5.   Alter base curves as indicated by fluorescein pattern. Since the base curves in both meridians are to be steepened by 0.25 D, you must correspondingly increase contact lens power by –0.25 D in both meridians. Therefore, the final prescription for base curves and powers is as follows:

$$\frac{45.25 \text{ D/}-1.37 \text{ D}}{41.75 \text{ D/}+ 2.12 \text{ D}}$$

Order the remaining lens parameters in the same manner as for a spherical design, except specify that the secondary curve is toric by the amount of the ordered base curve toricity.

B.   One of the most **common indications** for prescribing an SPE bitoric is a patient with a moderate amount (1.50 D or more) of corneal toricity successfully wearing a spherical PMMA or low-Dk RGP contact lens. If the practitioner upgrades the patient to a more permeable material and duplicates the parameters of the habitual contact lens, the new lens tends to flex on the eye, creating unwanted cylinder in the OR.

   1.   If the fit and power of the habitual spherical rigid lens are optimal, the parameters can be altered to prescribe an SPE bitoric design. For example:

Keratometry	41.75 @ 090/43.75 @ 180
Spherical habitual	
rigid contact lens	42.00 D base curve/–2.50 D power
SPE bitoric design	43.00 D/–3.50 D
	41.00 D/–1.50 D

Note that the average values of the SPE bitoric base curves (42.00 D) and powers (–2.50 D) are maintained the same as for the spherical habitual low-Dk RGP lens. Starting with the optimal spherical base curve and power, the practitioner decides on the ideal amount of base curve toricity based on corneal toricity (see section II.A.3). Using the spherical design base curve and power for the mean values, the practitioner uses the desired base curve toricity difference between the prescribed base curves and powers. This SPE design will result in the same spherocylinder OR as with the spherical rigid lens, but the SPE bitoric lens will tend to position more centrally. Also, flexure is not a clinical concern with toric back surface rigid contact lenses. With a rigid sphere design, the lens may bend or flex over the "fulcrum" of the cornea caused by the corneal toricity. With a toric back surface, this "fulcrum" effect is negated because the lens-to-cornea fitting relationship becomes similar to that of a spherical base curve on a spherical cornea.

    2. Another option to minimize lens flexure with a mid- to high-Dk RGP is to prescribe a lid attachment spherical design.[6]

C. A **12-lens SPE bitoric diagnostic set** listed in Table 8.2 is recommended by the author. This diagnostic set can be fabricated in any rigid lens material. PMMA is preferred due to its machinability, dimensional stability, durability, and low cost. The set listed is a 3.00 D toric design in order to fit a wide range of corneal toricities. Other amounts of base curve toricities can be ordered to augment this basic set.

V. A **CPE bitoric** is indicated when 1.50 D or more of corneal toricity is present and an OR with a spherical rigid diagnostic lens reveals an unacceptable amount (0.75 D or more) of residual cylinder.

A. First rule out the possibility of prescribing a base curve toric design.

B. **To design a CPE bitoric using an SPE bitoric diagnostic set,** the following "recipe" can be used:

    1. **Step 1. Select an SPE bitoric diagnostic lens** that has a base curve toricity of approximately the same amount as the corneal toricity if the cornea is against-the-rule. If the cornea is with-the-rule, select a diagnostic lens with a base curve toricity less than the corneal toricity by approximately 0.50 D. The average or mean base curve of the diagnostic contact lens should be approximately 0.75 D flatter than the average keratometry reading.

Table 8.2   Spherical Power Effect (3.00 D) Bitoric Diagnostic Lens Set

42.00 D (8.04 mm)/–3.00 D
39.00 D (8.65 mm)/plano D
42.50 D (7.94 mm)/–3.00 D
39.50 D (8.54 mm)/plano D
43.00 D (7.85 mm)/–3.00 D
40.00 D (8.44 mm)/plano D
43.50 D (7.76 mm)/–3.00 D
40.50 D (8.33 mm)/plano D
44.00 D (7.67 mm)/–3.00 D
41.00 D (8.23 mm)/plano D
44.50 D (7.58 mm)/–3.00 D
41.50 D (8.13 mm)/plano D
45.00 D (7.50 mm)/–3.00 D
42.00 D (8.04 mm)/plano D
45.50 D (7.42 mm)/–3.00 D
42.50 D (7.94 mm)/plano D
46.00 D (7.34 mm)/–3.00 D
43.00 D (7.85 mm)/plano D
46.50 D (7.26 mm)/–3.00 D
43.50 D (7.76 mm)/plano D
47.00 D (7.18 mm)/–3.00 D
44.00 D (7.67 mm)/plano D
47.50 D (7.11 mm)/–3.00 D
44.50 D (7.58 mm)/plano D

Note: All secondary curves are toric by 3.00 diopters. Other recommended parameters include 9.0 mm overall diameter, 7.4 mm optic zone diameter, and 0.19 mm center thickness.

2. **Step 2. Perform a spherocylinder OR.**
3. **Step 3. Evaluate the fluorescein pattern.**
4. **Step 4.** Place diagnostic lens base curves and corresponding powers on an **optical cross,** with the flat base curve corresponding to the meridian of most plus contact lens power.
5. **Step 5.** Place OR raw powers on an **optical cross.**
6. **Step 6. Arithmetically add** OR power to diagnostic lens power for each meridian. The powers obtained correspond only to the diagnostic contact lens base curves.

7. **Step 7.** If indicated by fluorescein pattern interpretation of apical relationship or tear lens toricity, **alter the base curves.** If changes to base curve are made, the contact lens power must be altered by the amount of the dioptic change in the base curve.

EXAMPLE: CPE BITORIC

Given
Keratometry   42.50 @ 090/44.50 @ 180

Step 1.   Select a diagnostic lens 0.75 D flatter than the average keratometry value with base curve toricity equal to corneal toricity. In this case, the average K = 43.50 D, average K – 0.75 D = 42.75 D, and corneal toricity = 2.00 D against-the-rule. Therefore, the ideal diagnostic base curves are 41.75 D × 43.75 D.

Diagnostic SPE bitoric contact lens selected:

$$\frac{43.75 \text{ D}/-2.00 \text{ D}}{41.75 \text{ D}/\text{plano D}}$$

Step 2.   OR: –0.50 –1.75 × 090 (20/15)

Step 3.   Fluorescein pattern: apical alignment/no toricity

Steps 4, 5, and 6.   Place diagnostic contact lens base curves and corresponding powers on an optical cross. Place OR raw powers on a separate optical cross. Add corresponding powers on optical crosses.

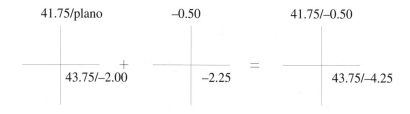

41.75/plano	–0.50	41.75/–0.50
43.75/–2.00	–2.25	43.75/–4.25

Diagnostic SPE   +   Over-refraction   =   Resultant base
bitoric rigid   curves and
contact lens   powers

Remember that obtained powers are correct only for the diagnostic contact lens base curves.

Step 7.   Alter base curves if indicated by fluorescein pattern analysis. This is not necessary for this example. Therefore, the final prescription for base curves and powers is as follows:

$$\frac{43.75\ D/–4.25\ D}{41.75\ D/–0.50\ D}$$

Order the remaining lens parameters in the same manner as for a spherical design, except specify that the secondary curve is toric by the amount of the ordered base curve toricity.

EXAMPLE: CPE BITORIC

Given
Keratometry   41.00 @ 180/45.50 @ 090

Step 1.   Select a diagnostic lens 0.75 D flatter than the average keratometry value with a base curve toricity one-half diopter less than corneal toricity to enhance tear exchange on a with-the-rule cornea. In this case, the average K = 43.25, average K – 0.75 D = 42.50 D, and corneal toricity = 4.50 D with-the-rule; therefore ideal base curve toricity is 4.00 D. Ideal diagnostic base curves are 40.50 D × 44.50 D.

Diagnostic contact lens selected:

$$\frac{44.50\ D/–4.00\ D}{40.50\ D/plano\ D}$$

Step 2.   OR: +3.75 –2.00 × 090 (20/15)

Step 3.   Fluorescein pattern: apical touch by 0.25 D/0.50 D with-the-rule toricity

Steps 4, 5, and 6.   Place diagnostic contact lens base curves and corresponding powers on an optical cross. Place OR raw powers on a separate optical cross. Add corresponding powers on optical crosses.

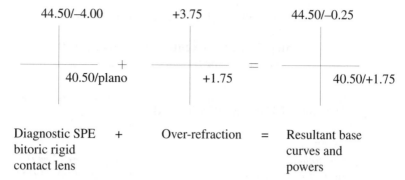

Diagnostic SPE	+	Over-refraction	=	Resultant base
bitoric rigid				curves and
contact lens				powers

Remember that obtained powers are correct only for the diagnostic contact lens base curves.

Step 7. Alter base curve as indicated by fluorescein pattern. Since the base curve in each meridian is to be steepened by 0.25 D, you must correspondingly increase contact lens power by –0.25 D in both meridians. Therefore, the final prescription for base curves and powers is as follows:

$$\frac{44.75\ D/-0.50\ D}{40.75\ D/+1.50\ D}$$

Order the remaining lens parameters in the same manner as for a spherical design, except specify that the secondary curve is toric by the amount of the ordered base curve toricity.

VI. A prism-ballasted, **front surface toric** lens is indicated when a patient has a low amount of corneal toricity (not more than 1.00 D) and an unacceptable amount of residual cylinder (1.00 D or more) in the OR with a spherical rigid diagnostic lens on the eye—that is, refractive astigmatism is primarily internal and the cornea is spherical or minimally toric.
  A. **To design** a prism-ballasted, **front surface toric** the following "recipe" can be used:
      1. **Step 1. Verify** that a prism-ballasted, **front surface toric** is the most appropriate RGP lens design.
      2. **Step 2. Design** your standard spherical RGP contact lens, and alter parameters according to the following steps:
      3. **Step 3. Order** the cylinder component (amount and axis) of the diagnostic lens OR.
      4. **Step 4. Calculate** the spherical component of **contact lens power** such that the equivalent sphere of your spherical order is maintained.
      5. **Step 5. Specify prism** to stabilize rotation.

6. **Step 6.** Instruct the laboratory to **allow for** 10–15 degrees of **nasal rotation.**
7. **Step 7. Increase center thickness** by 0.10 mm for each prism diopter prescribed.

EXAMPLE: FRONT SURFACE TORIC

Given

Keratometry	43.62 @ 180/44.12 @ 090
Subjective refraction	–2.00 –1.25 × 090 (20/15)
Diagnostic rigid contact lens	43.00 D base curve/–0.50 D power
Over-refraction	–0.50 –1.75 × 090 (20/15)
Fluorescein pattern	Apical touch by 0.12 D/0.50 D with-the-rule toricity

Step 1. Determine the most appropriate RGP lens design for the given patient data. A spherical RGP lens would not be acceptable due to the amount of residual astigmatism obtained through the spherical design. There is insufficient corneal toricity (in this case, 0.50 D) to prescribe a base curve toric or bitoric lens design. The resulting rotational instability would decrease visual performance. A front surface toric with a spherical base curve would be indicated due to the low amount of corneal toricity and the unacceptable amount of residual astigmatism.

Step 2. Design a spherical RGP contact lens based on the patient data given.

Base curve	43.12 D
Power	–2.00 D
Overall diameter	9.0 mm
Optic zone diameter	7.4 mm
Secondary curve radius	8.60 mm
Third curve radius	12.00 mm
Third curve width	0.2 mm
Center thickness	0.15 mm

Step 3. Order the cylinder component of the diagnostic contact lens OR (in this case, –1.75 × 090).

Step 4. Calculate the spherical component of power such that the equivalent sphere is maintained. If the power of the spherical design is –2.00 D, the power prescribed is as follows: –1.12 –1.75 × 090 (maintains a –2.00 D equivalent sphere).

Step 5.   Specify 1 Δ prism to stabilize rotation.

Step 6.   Instruct the laboratory to allow for approximately 12 degrees nasal rotation.

Step 7.   Increase the center thickness calculated for the spherical order by 0.10 mm for each prism diopter prescribed.

Center thickness of sphere	0.15 mm
1 Δ × 0.10 mm	+0.10 mm
Center thickness with prism	0.25 mm

The final prescription is as follows:

Base curve	43.12 D
Power/axis	−1.12 −1.75 × 090
Overall diameter	9.0 mm
Optic zone diameter	7.4 mm
Secondary curve radius	8.60 mm
Third curve radius	12.00 mm
Third curve width ·	0.2 mm
Center thickness	0.25 mm
1 Δ/allow for 12 degrees nasal rotation	

B.   Whenever a front surface toric, spherical base curve rigid contact lens is indicated, first consider fitting the patient with a **toric soft contact lens.** It is difficult to achieve rotational stability with prism-ballasted, front surface toric RGP contact lenses. Fifteen degrees mislocation of a 1.75 D cylinder would result in approximately 0.87 D of induced residual cylinder at an axis oblique to the prescribed axis.[7]

> ***Pearl:*** *Front surface toric indicated? First consider a toric soft lens.*

C.   **To minimize** rotational undershoot or overshoot, the following remedies could be considered:
  1. **Increase the prism** to 1.5–2.0 Δ. This necessitates increasing the overall thickness of the lens, possibly resulting in increased lens awareness and a more inferior-positioning lens.
  2. **Truncate** the lens to stabilize rotation. Truncation can be ordered or performed by in-office modification. If the lens is ordered round, truncation can be reserved to fine-tune lens rotation on dispensing or follow-up care.

VII. **It is beneficial to analyze rigid contact lenses** in order to verify parameters and to determine the lens design.

  A. **If lensometry reveals cylinder,** the lens is a base curve toric, bitoric, or front surface toric design. Spherical and minimally warped rigid lenses will not reveal cylinder on lensometry. If cylinder is present but no prism is measured by lensometry, assume that the lens is a base curve toric or bitoric design. Radiuscope measurements will differentiate between them. If prism is present, it is assumed that the lens design is a front surface toric, spherical base curve design. This is confirmed by the radiuscope measurement of a spherical base curve.

   1. When analyzing a **base curve toric, spherical front surface rigid lens,** the difference between radiuscope readings (converted to diopters) in the two major meridians will be two-thirds (or slightly more) of the difference between the two gross lensometry readings in the corresponding meridians. For example:

Radiuscope readings	7.94 mm (42.50 D) and 7.50 mm (45.00 D)
Lensometry readings	–1.25 D and –5.00 D

      There is a 2.50 D difference between the two base curve findings and a 3.75 D difference between the two gross lensometry power readings. The ratio between base curve toricity and power difference is 2:3. Therefore, the lens is a base curve toric, spherical front surface design. Keratometry or overkeratometry readings of the front surface would reveal that it is spherical. The 2:3 ratio is most appropriate for PMMA material (index of refraction = 1.49). Most of the current RGP contact lens materials have a lower index of refraction (n), causing the relationship to be closer to 2:2.75.

   2. When analyzing an **SPE bitoric rigid contact lens,** the difference between radiuscope readings (converted to diopters) will equal (1:1 ratio) the difference between the two gross lensometry readings. For example:

Radiuscope readings	8.16 mm (41.37 D) and 7.56 mm (44.62 D)
Lensometry readings	+2.25 D and –1.00 D

      There is a 3.25 D difference between both the base curve findings and the gross lensometry power readings. Therefore, the lens is an SPE bitoric.

3. If the ratio between the differences in radiuscope readings (converted to diopters) and gross lensometry readings is not 1:1 or approximately 2:3, the lens is a **CPE bitoric.** For example:

Radiuscope readings	8.28 mm (40.75 D) and 7.67 mm (44.00 D)
Lensometry readings	−2.50 D and −6.50 D

There is a 3.25 D difference between base curve findings. If the difference in lensometry powers was approximately 4.87 D (3/2 × 3.25 D), the lens would be a base curve toric design. If the difference in lensometry powers was 3.25 D, the lens would be an SPE bitoric design. Since neither of the two above scenarios is true, the lens is a CPE bitoric design.

4. If lensometry reveals prism *and* a cylinder, suspect a **prism-ballasted, front surface toric rigid lens with a spherical base curve.** To verify, measure the base curve radius. If spherical, it is a front surface toric lens design. During lensometry, the prism is rotated to the base-down position and the power is measured and recorded in the same manner as spectacles, that is, sphere, cylinder, and axis. The axis measured is relative to the prism base-down location. The prescription generally compensates for 10–15 degrees of nasal rotation when placed on the eye. Therefore, the cylinder axis measured relative to the prism located base-down will not agree exactly with the subjective refraction cylinder axis. It will be 10–15 degrees different depending on whether it is a right or left lens. For example:

Radiuscope reading	7.87 mm (42.87 D sphere)
Lensometry readings	−2.75 −1.25 × 090 (1.0 Δ located base down)

Assuming the practitioner allowed for 12 degrees nasal rotation, the axis of the above lens would be correct if an axis of 102 were prescribed for the right eye or an axis of 78 were prescribed for the left eye.

B. **Radiuscope mires** should be in focus for all of the above rigid lens designs. For lens designs with a toric back surface (base curve torics and bitorics), it might be necessary to minimally rotate the radiuscope lens well to sharpen the focus of the legs of the mire. Other reasons why radiuscope mires might be out of focus include water on the back surface of the lens or a dirty lens back surface.

C. **Lensometry mires** will be in focus when analyzing a base curve toric, spherical front surface rigid lens. It might be necessary to minimally rotate the lens on the lensometer stop to sharpen the focus of the meridian being analyzed. Lensometry mires are generally less in focus, but readable, when analyzing a bitoric lens. It is often difficult to obtain exact power and axis endpoints when analyzing a front surface toric, spherical base curve rigid lens.

D.   **Figure 8.1 is a flow chart** to assist in analyzing rigid toric contact lenses.

REFERENCES

1.   Miller WL, Andrasko G. An analysis of flexure characteristics of the Boston Rx material. CL Forum 1989;14(8):57–59.
2.   Edrington T, Stewart B, Woodfield D. Toric base curve rotation on toric corneas [guest editorial]. J Am Optom Assoc 1989;60(3):162.
3.   Sarver MD. Calculation of the optical specifications of contact lenses. Arch Am Acad Optom 1963;40(1):20–28.
4.   Mandell RB. Contact Lens Practice (4th ed). Springfield, IL: Thomas, 1988;302–303.
5.   Sarver MD, Kame RT, Williams CE. A bitoric gas permeable hard contact lens with spherical power effect. J Am Optom Assoc 1985;56(3):184–189.
6.   Herman JP. Flexure of rigid contact lenses on toric corneas as a function of base-curve fitting relationship. J Am Optom Assoc 1983;54(3):209–213.
7.   Snyder C. A review and discussion of crossed cylinder effects and over-refractions with toric soft contact lenses. ICLC 1989;16(4):113–118.

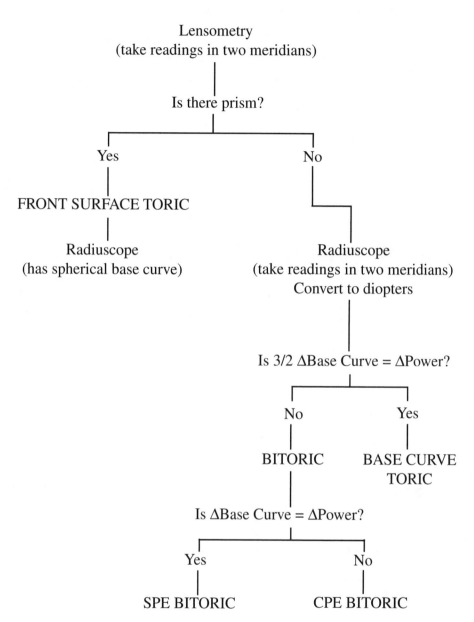

FIGURE 8.1 *Toric rigid contact lens analysis flow chart. The Δ symbol refers to differences in base curve or lens power readings. (Courtesy of Pauline Ilsen, O.D.)*

Chapter 9

Rigid Gas-Permeable Lens Care and Patient Education

Milton M. Hom

I. **Rigid gas-permeable (RGP) lens care systems** are necessary for proper maintenance of RGP lenses. The eye and contact lens are under a constant barrage of microorganisms.[1]

II. **Preservatives** are antimicrobials, which are added to contact lens solutions to ensure there is no spoilage after they are opened. Preservatives are necessary to make solutions safe and effective. In high enough concentrations, most preservatives cause toxic reactions, but lower concentrations provide insufficient disinfection. The manufacturer's challenge is to formulate the solution that provides effective disinfection without producing sensitivity reactions. There are several preservatives in use today for RGP lens solutions.

   A. **Benzalkonium chloride (BAK)** is an effective quaternary ammonium compound commonly used for RGP lens disinfection. It is a cationic detergent with a positively charged hydrophilic nitrogen end and a long hydrocarbon hydrophobic tail. It is not used for soft lenses because of binding and absorption into the lens matrix. Studies conflict as to whether BAK binds to RGP lenses in significant quantities. Actual uptake studies have provided mixed results. BAK is positively charged and will bind to the lens surface in a fashion similar to that of chlorhexidine. BAK also has a hydrophobic end that can attract the hydrophobic ends of other BAK molecules. BAK can, in fact, layer itself onto the surface, causing reactions and poor wetting.[2,3] Some experts contend, however, that the number of sites where BAK can attach itself is extremely small. There are also reports of suspected BAK-induced reactions.[4] BAK is used for its strong antimicrobial effectiveness. Compared with chlorhexidine, BAK has superior effectiveness against *Candida albicans* and *Serratia marcescens*.[5]

B. **EDTA** or its salt, **edetate disodium,** is used as a chelating agent for calcium ions.[6] They are both used in disinfecting solutions because they enhance the bacterial action of BAK, especially against *Pseudomonas*.[7,8] EDTA is also commonly used in soft lens solutions.

C. **Chlorhexidine gluconate (CHG)** is an effective disinfectant commonly used in RGP solutions.[7] CHG has limited effectiveness against yeast and fungi.[8] Unlike soft lenses, chlorhexidine does not bind readily to RGP lenses and has much lower sensitivity rates. CHG molecules are positively charged and have an electrostatic attraction to the negatively charged lens surface. A solution such as **Boston Conditioner** (Bausch & Lomb [B&L], Rochester, New York) has competing hydrophilic components for the same sites, however, reducing the amount of binding.[3]

D. **Polyaminopropyl biguanide (PAPB)** has lower sensitivity rates and greater disinfection efficacy than chlorhexidine.[9,10] PAPB has better effectiveness than chlorhexidine over *S. marcescens*. *Serratia* secretes an exotoxin that irritates the eye and stimulates mucus secretion. RGP patients developing discomfort, redness, lens awareness, and excessive mucus may be suffering from *Serratia* toxins.[10] Switching to a PAPB system may dramatically improve comfort. Sensitivities to PAPB have been reported. PAPB is used in soft lens solution as **DYMED**. The concentration in RGP solutions is 30–50 times that found in soft lens solutions.[8]

E. **Thimerosal** is a slow-acting disinfectant to which patients are often sensitive.[7] Once commonly seen in soft lens solutions, thimerosal's use in soft lens solutions has been curtailed in recent years (see Chapter 13).

F. **Benzyl alcohol** was used in the past as a solvent for contact lens materials and is now used in contact lens solutions.[11] When combined with a surfactant, benzyl alcohol provides effective microbial action against **biofilms;** however, when used alone, it does not work well against bacterial biofilms. Both *Pseudomonas aeruginosa* and *S. marcescens* produce biofilms that bind the bacterial cells into a colony, shield the colony from harmful chemicals, and trap nutrient particles. Biofilms are composed of predominantly anionic polysaccharides. *Pseudomonas* biofilms are amorphous, whereas *Serratia* produces dense biofilms.[11–13] Preservatives that are normally effective against bacteria do not work well against bacteria that produce biofilms.[13]

G. **Chlorobutanol** has a different antimicrobial effect than other preservatives. It is converted to epoxide by the bacteria and becomes lethal to the microorganism.[6] Chlorobutanol is, however, toxic to the cornea.[14] It was used in polymethyl methacrylate (PMMA) solutions in the past, but it is rarely used in solutions today.

III. A **wetting and soaking solution** may be the only solution an RGP lens wearer remembers to use. Patients may believe they can do without daily cleaning and enzyming, but they will not do without the solution needed to soak the lens and apply to the eye. After daily cleaning, the lens is usually soaked overnight in the wetting and soaking solution. In the morning, the solution is also used for lens application. Wetting and soaking solutions serve several functions, including enhancement of surface wettability, disinfection, and cushioning.[7] Notable differences in relative acidities, buffering capacities, viscosities, osmolalities ("saltiness"), refractive indices, and wetting angles may occur among solutions.[15] Since there are differences between the systems, trying another system may be the best plan for a patient experiencing intolerances to the system he or she is using.

A. **Cushioning,** which is related to viscosity and viscoelasticity, provides comfort to the patient when applying lenses. Solutions with higher viscosity are preferred over those with low viscosity. High viscosities can become too thick, however, and leave a residue on the lens and lid. High viscosities can also blur vision and hinder lid movement. On the other hand, if the solution's viscosity is too low, the solution dissipates rapidly from the lens surface.[16] Optimal viscosity for comfort and cushioning is 35–40 centipoise.[17]

B. **Boston Advance Comfort Formula** (B&L) is preserved with PAPB.[9,18] PAPB was used for its antimicrobial action against *S. marcescens.*[10]

C. **Boston Conditioning Solution** (Original) by B&L is preserved by chlorhexidine.[9] **B&L Wetting and Soaking** contains chlorhexidine and EDTA.

D. **WET-N-SOAK Plus** by Allergan (Irvine, California) is preserved by BAK and EDTA.[18]

E. **Claris Cleaning and Soaking Solution** by Menicon (Clovis, California) is preserved with benzyl alcohol.[19]

F. The **ComfortCare** system by Allergan is a daily cleaner, disinfectant, and enzyme cleaner. The lenses are placed into a Hydramat II (Allergan), a unit that hydrodynamically cleans the lenses with ComfortCare GP Wetting and Soaking Solution. A daily cleaner tablet with a surfactant and enzyme is added. ComfortCare GP Wetting and Soaking Solution contains chlorhexidine.[18,20]

G. **Soaclens** by Alcon Laboratories (Fort Worth, Texas) is preserved with thimerosal. When compared with other solutions, it shows initially reduced on-eye wetting angles.[21]

IV. **Daily cleaning** should be performed immediately after lenses are removed. The lens is placed in the palm of the hand with several drops of cleaner and rubbed with a circular motion for 15–20 seconds on each side.[7] The lenses should not be cleaned between the fingers because warpage can occur.[22] The lenses are rinsed and placed in the wetting and soaking solution.

A. **Surfactant cleaners** remove contaminants from the lens surface. **LC-65** and **Resolve GP** by Allergan are such cleaners.[18]

B. **Abrasive cleaners** contain particulate matter that shears deposits from the lens surface. Abrasive cleaners are more effective than nonabrasive cleaners for deposit removal. They can, however, produce small surface scratches and induce minus power.[9,23]

1. **Opti-Clean Cleaner II** and **Opti-Free Daily Cleaner** by Alcon use polymeric beads to provide abrasiveness.[18] **Opti-Clean** has a very large particle size and may be best used to control deposit buildup.[24]

2. **SLC** by Permeable Technologies (Morganville, New Jersey) uses small particles, which appear almost sandy or gritty. Small particle sizes may be better than large ones in eliminating filming or hazing.[24]

3. **Boston Cleaner** and **Boston Advance Cleaner** are both abrasive cleaners made by B&L. Boston Cleaner contains both small and large particles. A combination of particle sizes may work best for multiple types of deposits. Boston Advance has been optimized for the lipid deposits seen with fluorosilicone acrylate (FSA) lenses. Advance has an additional nonionic surfactant meant for lipid and oil-based contaminants. The particle sizes have also been reduced compared with those in the original Boston Cleaner. Smaller sizes help to maintain the highly polished surface characteristic of FSA lenses.[24,25]

V. **Multiaction RGP solutions** combine cleaning and wetting in one solution. **Boston Simplicity** (B&L) eliminates the need for a separate saline rinse after cleaning. The lenses are soaked for 4 hours after rubbing. Soaking the lenses in enzyme solution is not necessary. The solution contains a betaine surfactant and silicone glycol wetting agent. Simplicity is preserved with chlorhexidine, EDTA, and PAPB.[26]

VI. **Wetting agents** are needed for RGP lenses because the polymer has naturally hydrophobic properties.[6] RGP lenses are primarily hydrophobic with small wetting zones.[2]

A. **Polyvinyl alcohol (PVA)** is a wetting agent that has both lipophilic and hydrophilic groups. The lipophilic groups bind to the lens surface, enabling the hydrophilic groups to bind water more effectively. PVA is colorless, water-soluble, and nonviscous and does not settle when left standing.[6,16] It has good spreading and wettability on the lens and ocular surfaces.

B. **Methylcellulose** is another wetting agent that adds more viscosity than PVA. Unfortunately, methylcellulose retards epithelial regeneration, whereas PVA does not.[8]

C. **Boston Reconditioning Drop** (B&L) contains PVA and polyelectrolytes. The polyelectrolytes are positively charged and are attracted to the RGP surface. Moisture retention is enhanced because the wetting agents are highly hydrophilic.[16,27] The two components together provide excellent wetting. Boston Reconditioning Drop is preserved by chlorhexidine.[18]

VII. **Enzymes** are often required by silicone acrylates but usually not by fluoropolymers.[28] **ProFree GP** by Allergan is made of papain and can be used once a week. **Opti-Zyme** by Alcon contains pancreatin[18] (see Chapter 13).

VIII. **Complications** and **crossover problems** do exist. Three types of motivations account for most use of inappropriate cleaners: conscious (shopping for bargains), unconscious (becoming confused about which solution to use), and creative (searching for better products). Patient misuse or switching solutions can lead to three categories of problems: sensitivity reactions, toxic reactions, and poor efficacy.[29]

Pearl: Alcohol, acetone, sodium hydroxide, gasoline, or lighter fluid will damage RGP lenses. Wine, Coca-Cola, or cognac will not.[30]

A. **Sensitivity reactions** occur when the eye reacts to certain components in the solution. The symptoms are discomfort, lens intolerance, and infiltrative keratitis. The offending agent can be avoided by switching solutions.

   1. **Boston Advance** (B&L) solutions have been known to cause adherent lenses and superficial punctate keratitis (SPK) when patients switch from Boston (Original) conditioner solution.[30] The solution has since been reformulated to avoid these reactions. Boston Advance (0.0015% PAPB) is significantly more toxic to rabbit corneal epithelium than B&L's Boston Conditioning (0.006% CHG) or WET-N-SOAK Plus (0.003% BAK).[31]

   2. **Chlorhexidine** has been known to cause limbal conjunctival cysts. The associated signs and symptoms are red, irritated eyes and staining.[32] The reaction is an allergic or hypersensitive reaction.

B. **Toxic reactions** are characterized by very mild symptoms presenting with much more severe objective clinical findings. Patients can report vague dryness or intermittent mild discomfort. The clinical signs are staining, corneal disruption, and lens adherence.

   1. **BAK** chemical keratitis has been reported with RGP lenses. The patient experienced red, irritated eyes and hazy vision. A diffuse keratitis was seen in both eyes. Other symptoms and signs include more rapid drying between blinks and greater mucus adhesion.[3]

   2. **Superficial corneal epithelial desquamation** is caused by BAK-preserved solutions. Even wetting drops containing BAK produce more severe staining than drops without BAK.[33] Switching the patient to solutions not preserved with BAK solves the problem.[4]

C. A **morning RGP lens ritual** or morning cleaning is not as effective as cleaning the lenses in the evening after lens wear; therefore, leaving the cleaning to the next morning is not recommended. It is better to clean the lenses immediately after removal while the deposits on the lenses are still fresh and easier to loosen up. Because an overnight soak also conditions the lenses, rinsing the conditioner away by cleaning in the morning precludes enhancing comfort.

D. **"Left lens syndrome"** occurs when one lens has a greater amount of deposits than the other. The right lens tends to be favored when cleaning; patients tend to first clean the right lens carefully and then clean the left lens quickly. The left lens has greater buildup and needs more frequent replacement. Equal care and effort should be applied to both lenses.

E. **Self-modification** by overuse and excessive pressure with abrasive cleaners can change the power of the lens. Gentle cleaning with the "pinkie" finger is recommended for patients who have had this problem.

F. **Case contamination** can be avoided by rinsing out and air drying the case daily. Every week, the case should be scrubbed. Dispensing less durable deep-welled flat packs encourages frequent case replacement. With longer-lasting lens cases, biofilm may accumulate in the case, providing an optimal medium for bacterial growth.

G. **Rewetting** with saliva should discouraged. Numerous bacteria harmful to the eye reside in the mouth. Some authors discourage patients from using saliva by telling them that even urine would be preferred over saliva as a rewetting solution because it contains less destructive bacteria.[30] Patients should carry a small bottle of rewetting solution with them.

H. **"First-day nonwetting syndrome"** consists of poor initial wetting when the lenses are dispensed to the patient.[34,35]

   1. **Manufacturer-related causes** of first-day nonwetting syndrome are residual pitch, solvent exposure, and improper finishing or polishing.[36] Use of a laboratory cleaner such as **Fluoro-solve** (Paragon Vision Sciences, Mesa, Arizona) or **Boston Laboratory Cleaner** (B&L) is sometimes effective.[37]

   2. **Organic causes** could be surface contamination or tear film bioincompatibility.[36]

       a. **Emollient contamination** is the leading cause of patient-related nonwetting. Lanolin in cosmetics, soaps, and dermatologic products is transferred to the lens when handling. The tear film will bead over large areas of smeared lanolin. Cleaning the lenses well and soaking for 24–48 hours before dispensing is recommended to avoid nonwetting. An overnight surfactant soak with Menicon's **Claris Cleaning and Soaking Solution** may work well. Hand-washing with optical soaps may be necessary.

       b. Poorly manufactured contact lens cases may transfer **hydrophobic oils** used in the manufacturing process to lenses.[34,36]

   3. **Solution incompatibility** with lens material can cause lens awareness, dryness, burning, itching, deposits, and blurred vision. There may be associated injection, epithelial edema, SPK, and poor wetting. Switching solutions is recommended.[36]

I. **Deposits** are commonly seen on silicone acrylate surfaces. Abrasive cleaners and enzymes can help remove deposits. The deposits come from the contact lens pellicle.

   1. **Pellicle formation** occurs within 1 minute of lens application to the eye. The lens is enveloped by a protective coating of mucus and

protein originating from the tear film. The pellicle lubricates the lens surface and allows better movement. It also causes deposits and soilage, however.

2. **Plaquelike deposits** form on the posterior surface, anterior surface, and anterior bevel of the lens. Surface plaque is a gelatinous accumulation of bacteria, tear mucin, and protein. The plaque accumulates in layers.[24,38] Bacteria is commonly found adhering to lens deposits.[38]

3. **Poor efficacy** sometimes occurs when first-generation RGP lens cleaners are used on FSA lenses. Oily films and deposits occur frequently on FSA lenses. Newer lipid-specific surfactants are better than first-generation cleaners, which were focused on proteins. One such cleaner is **Boston Advance Cleaner.** Sometimes, laboratory cleaners are indicated for severe cases.

IX. **Patient education** on a regular, ongoing basis is necessary to ensure compliance with proper lens care procedures.

A. **Application** and **removal** are best done with the fingers rather than using a **suction cup device.** Difficult situations can develop if the patient loses the suction cup device.[39]

1. **Hand washing** before handling lenses is a necessity.[7]

2. **Application** of lenses with **two hands** entails placing the lens on the index finger and using the middle finger to hold down the lower lashes. The other hand holds the upper lashes open. While the patient fixates with the other eye, the lens is gently placed onto the cornea. A variation is using only **one hand.** The lids are held apart by the index and ring finger while the lens is placed with the middle finger.[39]

3. **Removal** of lenses with **one hand,** or using the **scissors method,** entails holding the upper lid margin with the middle finger and the lower lid margin with the ring finger. The patient looks nasally while the lids are pulled temporally. **The two-hand** method is similar, but instead of using the middle and ring fingers of one hand, the index fingers of both hands are used.[39]

B. **Recentering** the lens should be performed if the lens becomes lodged on the bulbar conjunctiva. The patient should be reassured that the lens cannot get lost behind the eye. First, the lens should be located. Using a mirror is extremely helpful. The fingers can use the lid margin to manipulate the lens onto the cornea. The lens edge farthest from the cornea should be pushed by the lid margin.[39]

C. **Handling** should be done carefully. RGP lenses are easily **scratched** because of the material softness. Handling care is important to avoid **warping** or even **inverting** the lens. Lenses should not be bent or flexed between the fingers. If the lens is inverted, vision may be blurred and the lens will be uncomfortable to wear. Significant edge stand-off would be seen with a biomicroscope, and distorted optics would be seen with the radiuscope. The lens can be reinverted carefully, but a replacement may be needed.[7]

D. **Cleaning** and **disinfection** entail manually cleaning the lens with a surfactant, then rinsing and soaking with the wetting and disinfection solution. An enzyme can be used once a week for silicone acrylates. Wetting drops are used as needed.

Pearl: Do not use water from the faucet to rinse RGP lenses. Tap water rinses are the common denominator for Acanthamoeba *infections and RGP lenses. Rigid lenses permit greater adherence by* Acanthamoeba *than soft lenses.[40,41]*

1. **Cases** should be ribbed and deep-welled.[7] Cases should be replaced on a regular basis because of microbial and biofilm concerns.
2. **Solution reuse** and "topping off" should be discouraged.[30] Patients like to reuse solutions for economic reasons. Unfortunately, solutions are designed for one-time usage. Used solution should be thrown out of the case and replaced with fresh solution.

E. The **wearing schedule** can begin with 4 hours the first and second days. Every 2 days, another 1 hour is added until a maximum of 14 hours is reached.[7] Some experts prefer a much shorter adaptation period of 3 days. Under a shorter adaption period, patients are expected to reach 6–8 hours of wear within the first 2 days.[42]

Pearl: Removing, rinsing, and reapplying the lenses can enhance wear for the adapting patient.[42]

F. **Adaptation** is similar to that for PMMA lenses.

Pearl: Normally, RGP lens comfort is the worst the first minute after the lenses are put on. It usually becomes more comfortable from that moment on.

1. **Normal symptoms** are tearing, minor irritation; intermittent blurred vision; photophobia; redness; and sensitivity to wind, smoke, and dust.[7]
2. **Abnormal symptoms** are great amount of pain, seeing severe halos, severe redness, and blurred vision with spectacles after taking off lenses that lasts for more than an hour (**spectacle blur**).

G. **Compliance** is important to ensure safe, comfortable lens wear. Fill-in-the-blank printed materials and videotapes are helpful. Rather than the doctor dictating instructions to the patient, a mutual-participation relationship is preferred in which the patient is totally responsible for contact lens care based on education and suggestions from the practitioner and in which the doctor is flexible and allows the patient to assume control.[43] The patient should be able to understand the words the doctor uses, and the information should be as specific and concise as possible.

Pearl: *Maintain a friendly, flexible manner when addressing compliance matters. Make suggestions, not commands, to the patient.*[43]

REFERENCES

1. Fleiszig SM, Fletcher EL, Lowe R. Microbiology of Contact Lens Care. In ES Bennett, BA Weissman (eds), Clinical Contact Lens Practice. Philadelphia: Lippincott, 1992(36);1–29.
2. Hoffman WC. Ending the BAK-RGP controversy. ICLC 1987;14:31–35.
3. Rosenthal P, Chou MH, Salamone JC, et al. Quantitative analysis of chlorhexidine and benzalkonium chloride adsorption on silicone/acrylate polymers. CLAO J 1986;12(1):43–50.
4. Sterling JL, Hecht AS. BAK-induced chemical keratitis? CL Spectrum 1988;3(3):62–65.
5. Bevington R, Cole T, Davis H, et al. Evaluation of BAK in a soaking/disinfecting RGP regimen. CL Spectrum 1988;3(3):30–39.
6. Mandell RB. Lens Care and Storage. In RB Mandell (ed), Contact Lens Practice (4th ed). Springfield, IL: Thomas, 1988;326–351.
7. Bennett ES. Lens Care and Solutions. In ES Bennett, RM Grohe (eds), Rigid Gas-Permeable Contact Lenses. New York: Professional Press, 1986;225–246.
8. Bennett ES. Lens Care and Patient Selection. In ES Bennett, VA Henry (eds), Clinical Manual of Contact Lenses. Philadelphia: Lippincott, 1994;41–88.
9. Bennett ES, Grohe RM, Snyder C. Lens Care and Patient Education. In ES Bennett, BA Weissman (eds), Clinical Contact Lens Practice. Philadelphia: Lippincott, 1993(25);1–17.
10. The new generation of RGP solutions meets increasing demands. CL Spectrum 1990;5(1):45–50.
11. Feldman GL. Benzyl alcohol—new life as an ophthalmic preservative. CL Spectrum 1989;4(5):41–42.
12. Feldman GL, Krezanoski JK, Ellis B, et al. Is benzyl alcohol effective against biofilms on RGPs? CL Spectrum 1992;7(3):29–33.
13. Feldman GL, Krezanoski JK, Ellis B, et al. Control of bacterial biofilms on rigid gas-permeable lenses. CL Spectrum 1992;7(10):36–39.
14. Collin B, Grabsch BE, Carroll N, et al. Corneal endothelial changes due to chlorobutanol. ICLC 1985;1(6):435–439.
15. Carney LG, Hill RM, Barr JT, et al. Rigid lens care solutions: how different are they? CL Spectrum 1988;3(11):78–80.
16. Greco A. Lubricating drops for hard and soft contact lenses. ICLC 12(4):205–210.
17. Herskowitz R. Biocompatibility of rigid gas-permeable care systems. CL Spectrum 1993;8(7):37–40.
18. White P, Scott C. Contact lenses and solutions summary. CL Spectrum 1994(suppl);9(12):1–24.

19. Lowther GE, Pole J, Biolo M. Comparison of two care systems when used with low-Dk and high-Dk silicone/acrylate materials. ICLC 1990;17:276–279.

20. Anderson B, Christensen B, Ebling R, et al. A new care regimen for fluorosilicone acrylate lenses. CL Spectrum 1993;8(9):46–49.

21. Yeager MD, Benjamin WJ. Care regimens and initial wetting of a silicone/acrylate surface in vivo. ICLC 1987;14:58–61.

22. Grohe RM. RGP handling techniques. CL Spectrum 1991;6(10):49–50.

23. Bennett ES, Henry VA. RGP lens power change with abrasive cleaner use. ICLC 1990;17:152–153.

24. Grohe RM, Caroline PJ. Surface Deposits on Contact Lenses. In ES Bennett, BA Weissman (eds), Clinical Contact Lens Practice. Philadelphia: Lippincott, 1992(24);1–12.

25. Ames KS. The surface characteristics of RGP lenses. CL Spectrum 1991;6(6):45–48.

26. One-bottle RGP regimen debuts. CL Spectrum 1995;10(10):5.

27. Raheja MK, Ellis EJ. Achieving new levels of RGP comfort. CL Spectrum 1995;10(10):45.

28. Gasson A, Morris J. Care Systems. In A Gasson, J Morris (eds), The Contact Lens Manual. Oxford, England: Butterworth–Heinemann, 1992;234–244.

29. Ames KS. RGP solutions—will you or your patient decide? CL Spectrum 1995(suppl); 10(5):2–4.

30. Connelly S, Morgan B, Norman C, et al. Your most perplexing RGP lens complications—solved! CL Spectrum 1995;10(2):23–30.

31. Begley CG, Waggoner PJ, Hafner GS, et al. Effect of rigid gas-permeable contact lens wetting solutions on the rabbit corneal epithelium. Optom Vis Sci 1991;68(3):189–197.

32. Pole JJ, Malinovsky VE. Conjunctival cyst with chlorhexidine sensitivity. ICLC 1987;14:78.

33. Imayasu M, Moriyama T, Ichijima H. The effects of daily wear of rigid gas-permeable contact lenses treated with contact lens care solutions containing preservatives on the rabbit cornea. CLAO J 1004;20(3):183–188.

34. Bourassa S, Benjamin WJ. RGP wettability: the first day could be the worst day! ICLC 1992;19:25–34.

35. Benjamin WJ. The patient's first impressions of high-Dk RGP lenses. ICLC 1992;19:273–275.

36. Grohe RM, Caroline PJ. RGP non-wetting lens syndrome. CL Spectrum 1989;4(3):32–44.

37. Kremer JL, Bennett ES. Rigid Lens Care and Compliance. In ES Bennett (ed), Contact Lens Problem Solving. St. Louis: Mosby 1995;19–34.

38. Fowler SA, Korb DR, Finnemore VM, et al. The surface of worn siloxane-PMMA gas-permeable lenses: a scanning electron microscope study. CLAO J 1987;13(5):259–263.

39. Atkinson KW, Port MJA. Patient Management and Instruction. In AJ Phillips, J Stone (eds), Contact Lenses (3rd ed). London: Butterworth Publishers, 1989;299–332.

40. Shovlin JP. *Acanthamoeba* keratitis in rigid lens wearers: the issue of tap water rinses. ICLC 1990;17:47–49.

41. Kelly LD, Long D, Mitra D. Quantitative comparison of *Acanthamoeba castellanii* adherence to rigid versus soft contact lenses. CLAO J 1995;21(2):111–113.

42. Schnider C. The initial comfort factor. CL Spectrum 1995;10(8):16.

43. Marren SE. Negotiating compliance with contact lens care. ICLC 1990;17:63–66.

PART III

Soft Lenses

Chapter 10

Soft Lens Design, Fitting, and Physiologic Response

Adrian S. Bruce and Simon A. Little

I. **Soft lenses** may be characterized by certain general features.
   A. Soft lenses are the most popular contact lens wear modality, accounting for some 88% of lens wearers.[1] In the United States alone, there are more than 75 companies manufacturing at least 185 types of lenses.[2]
   B. Soft lenses offer certain **advantages.**
      1. Soft lenses are **immediately comfortable,** and adaptation time is short due to minimal movement and less tearing compared with rigid gas-permeable (RGP) lenses.
      2. Soft lenses are suitable for long or short wearing times and **variable wearing** schedules.
      3. These lenses are relatively **inexpensive,** which makes them suitable for planned-replacement systems. Lenses can often be dispensed from an inventory.
      4. Apparent eye color can be changed with soft lenses.
      5. Soft lenses cause minimal corneal distortion, so spectacle blur is rare.
      6. The **large optic zone** makes for minimal flare.
      7. There is less foreign body trapping than with RGP lenses.
      8. Soft lenses are good for **sporting activities,** since they are rarely dislodged.
      9. They are a good option when a spheric refractive error is associated with a toric cornea.
   C. Soft lenses also have certain **limitations.**
      1. They may be inadequate for correcting low astigmatism.
      2. They have a relatively **short life,** since they are fragile and subject to rapid accumulation of surface deposits.
      3. Ongoing lens care takes a significant amount of time—at least 5 minutes per day in daily wear. This may seem trivial, but **noncompliance** is a very common problem. Lens cleaning and disinfection are essential. The results of noncompliance with care systems may be devastating.

   4. It is difficult to verify soft lens parameters.
   5. Soft lenses offer only limited oxygen transmissibility. As a result, they may present difficulties with extended wear or when used to correct high ametropia.
   6. Compared with RGP lenses, soft lenses have limited postlens tear exchange.

II. Several soft lens modalities are available, including the following:

   A. **Conventional daily wear lenses** are those that have a replacement interval of more than 6 months.[1] A more traditional definition is a lens that is worn until change is necessary due to deteriorating lens performance, lens loss, or lens damage.

      1. Conventional daily wear lenses offer certain **advantages** over other lens modalities. They can be custom-fitted in a wide range of spheric, toric, and multifocal designs in materials of low, medium, or high water content. Lens cost alone is lower overall per year to the patient than the cost of disposable or frequent-replacement lenses (excluding cost of care systems).

      2. Conventional daily lenses also present certain **disadvantages.** They require complex care systems that include protein-remover tablets. They are associated with a higher overall rate of adverse reactions than disposable lenses. The majority of conventional daily wear lenses are manufactured by lathe-cutting, which is the most labor-intensive and hence the most expensive per lens of the available methods.

      3. There has been a **decrease** in use of this lens modality since 1990. Conventional soft contact lenses were worn by 51% of soft contact lens wearers in 1994. In 1990, the figure was closer to 100% (Table 10.1).

   B. **Planned,** or **frequent, replacement** systems use conventional daily wear lenses, but they have a nominated replacement interval rather than relying on serendipity. Common replacement intervals are annual, semi-annual, and quarterly. Conventional care and maintenance systems are used.

   Pearl: All soft lenses should be replaced at least annually.

      1. Planned-replacement lenses have certain **advantages** over conventional daily wear lenses.
         a. Using planned-replacement lenses, it is possible to avoid the effects of **lens deterioration,** such as those due to deposition of protein, lipid, and mucin, while retaining full parameter availability. Another effect of lens deterioration is decreased visual acuity.[3]
         b. They encourage compliance with instructions regarding lens wear and the lens care system, since the patient has regular appointments for both aftercare and lens replacement.

Table 10.1 Some Representative Brands and Lens Types in the Major Hydrogel Lens Categories

Company	Conventional Spheres	Disposable and Multipack Spheres	Conventional Toric	Disposable and Multipack Toric	Daily and Hi-Dk Disposable	Multifocal[a] and Opaque Tint
Bausch & Lomb (Rochester, New York)	Optima 38%[b] B&L70 70%	Medalist Optima FW 38% SeeQuence 38% (2 wk)[b] SofLens 66 66%	Optima Toric Core and Select 45% FW Toric 70% prism ballast	Medalist Toric 70% (1–3 mos) prism ballast Soflens 66 Toric 66% (2 wk)	Soflens One Day 70% (daily) PureVision 36% Hi-Dk (monthly)	PA1 38% aspheric Occasions 38% (1 mo) concentric
Biocompatibles International (Farnham, UK)	Proclear Sphere 62% (Note: Low dehydration)	Proclear 62% (Note: Low dehydration) (1 mo)	Proclear Tailor Made Toric 62% (Note: Low dehydration)	—	—	—
CIBA Vision (Duluth, Georgia)	Cibasoft STD 38%[c] Cibasoft 38%[c]	Focus Monthly 55%[c] Focus 2 weekly 55%[c]	Torisoft 38%[c] double slab off	Focus Toric 55% prism ballast (1 mo)	Focus Dailies 69% (daily) Night & Day 24% Hi-Dk (monthly)	Spectrum 55%[b] concentric Illusions Opaque 38%
CooperVision (Fairport, New York)	Cooperclear 38% Vantage 43%[b] Permalens 71%	Preference 43% (1 mo)[b]	HydraSoft Toric 55% prism ballast	Preference Toric 43% (3 mos)	—	Vantage Accents 43%
Johnson and Johnson Vistakon (Jacksonville, Florida)	—	Acuvue 2 58% (2 wk)[b] Surevue 58% (2 wk)[b]	—	Acuvue Toric 58% (Note: thin design)	1*Day Acuvue 58% (daily)	Acuvue Bifocal 58% multi-concentric (2 wk)

Table 10.1 (continued)

Company	Conventional Spheres	Disposable and Multipack Spheres	Conventional Toric	Disposable and Multipack Toric	Daily and Hi-Dk Disposable	Multifocal[a] and Opaque Tint
Ocular Sciences/Hydron (South San Francisco, California)	Zero 6 38%[c] Zero 4 38%[b] Edge III 55%	ProActive 38%[c] (1–3 mos) Hydron Biomedics 38% or 55%[b] (2 wk)	Hydron Ultra T RP toric prism ballast	—	—	Echelon 38% aspheric with phase plate
Wesley-Jessen (Des Plaines, Illinois)	SOFT MATE B 45% Hydrocurve II 55%[c] CSI Clarity Daily Wear 39%[c] Durasoft 2 38%[c] Durasoft 3 55%[c]	Gentle Touch 65% (1 mo) Precision UV 74% (2 wk) Fresh Look 55% (2 wk)[b]	Hydrocurve 3 55% toric prism ballast CSI Clarity Toric 39% Durasoft 2 Optifit 38% Durasoft 3 Optifit 55% thin zones	Durasoft 3 Optifit Toric 55% (also available in opaque colors)	—	Hydrocurve II bifocal 45%[c] aspheric Natural Touch Opaque 38% Durasoft 3 colors 55% Fresh Look Colors and Colorblends 55% (2 wk)[b]

Note: This table illustrates the diversity of lens designs available. Note that only seven manufacturers are shown here, although there are more than 75 contact lens companies in the United States alone.[2] Furthermore, many manufacturers have more lens designs than those shown.

[a]Consider also monovision fitting using standard lenses.

[b]Interval for standard visibility tint.

[c]Interval for optional cosmetic tint.

      c. Patients may find it convenient to have a spare pair of lenses in the event of lens loss.

  2. Planned-replacement lenses also have possible **advantages** over disposable lenses.

      a. A **wide variety of parameters** is available. Regular lens replacement may be the only option for patients requiring complex, expensive lenses.

      b. If solution costs are not considered, planned lens replacement may be **less expensive** for the patient than disposable lenses. Replacement intervals are rarely more frequent than quarterly due to the prohibitive expense, however. Lens stockpiling is not possible, as only one or two pairs of lenses are supplied at one time.

  3. There are two approaches to selecting a replacement interval.

      a. Some practitioners prefer a **patient-dependent replacement interval.** Soft lens deterioration varies between patients, and Bleshoy et al. recommend that lens replacement frequency be determined by monitoring the patient in the first few weeks or months of lens wear.[4] It may be difficult to convince patients to replace lenses that appear to be in good condition and are not associated with adverse signs or symptoms, however. The replacement frequency of soft lenses is often determined by the ratio of cost to benefit.

      b. Another approach is the **fixed-replacement interval.** Bleshoy et al. also recommended that group II lenses (high water content, nonionic) should be replaced every 3 months and group IV (high water content, ionic) each month to maintain optimal lens performance.[4] Other studies have found average lens lives of 6 months for group IV lenses and 11 months for group I (low-water-content, nonionic) lenses.[5]

    Pearl: *If the new lens feels much better than the one it replaced, it was supplied too late.*[6]

C. **Hydrogel disposable lenses** were first considered in 1980, when Tripathi and coworkers analyzed deposition on soft contact lenses and concluded that an inexpensive, disposable lens that could be replaced weekly to biweekly would be a beneficial modality for many patients.[7] In addition, disposable lenses reduce the amount of lens maintenance required, reducing the cost and compliance burden on the patient.[8]

  1. **Two-week disposable hydrogel lenses** became possible with the introduction of molding technology, which brought the unit cost of lenses down enough to permit disposing of lenses rather than protein-cleaning them. A second advance was innovative multiple packaging of lenses, which allows convenient replacement schedules, since the patient need not return to the practitioner for every new pair of lenses. Disposable lenses have the advantage of the patient always having spare lenses.

2. **Daily disposable lenses** were a logical development, since this modality means that lenses do not need to be cleaned or disinfected each night. There is no care system, and even a lens storage case is no longer required. McLaughlin states that the Food and Drug Administration defines disposable, in terms of contact lenses, as using once, which may mean 1 week of extended wear or 1 day of daily wear.[9] Daily disposable lenses appear to reduce or eliminate many of the problems that may occur with conventional soft lenses, as well as providing maximum convenience for the patient.[10,11]

Pearl: A lens a day keeps adverse responses away (apologies to the apple adage).

3. **Disposable lenses** have some advantages over conventional and frequent-replacement lenses.
   a. The practitioner maintains an **inventory** of lenses, so the patient can generally keep the first trial pair to wear home.
   b. **No protein-remover tablets** are used in either 2-week disposable or daily disposable lens, which reduces the cost and is more convenient for the patient.
   c. **No cleaning or disinfecting solutions or lens storage case** is required for daily disposable lenses. This reduces potential sources of contamination and avoids a substantial cost to the patient. Although solution reactions are already rare, this source of complications is negated.
   d. **Convenience** may be enhanced as the care system is simplified. Daily disposables suit daily wear patients who do not want to clean and disinfect lenses every day. In addition, part-time wearers do not have to worry about long-term lens storage.
   e. **Compliance** can be enhanced because the patient must meet the eye care provider at least every 6 months for an aftercare visit to order a new set of disposable lenses. The patient who purchases replacement lenses from a pharmacy or by mail order does not have this advantage, of course.
   f. Disposables produce **physiologic advantages** as well. Reduced deposits improve success for giant papillary conjunctivitis patients.[11] Because they need not be so durable, disposable lenses can be made thinner, which enhances oxygen transmissibility and comfort. One study found that dis-

posable lenses **reduced myopia progression** compared with conventional hydrogel lenses.[12]

g.   A **handling tint** is frequently included as a standard feature.

4.   To assess the economic factors one must consider the real versus the apparent cost.

   a.   The **costs** involved in lens care may be **hidden.** Patients may appear to prefer conventional lenses over disposable lenses, because the apparent cost per year is lower. Apparent cost is usually based only on the lens cost, however. Care and maintenance solution costs are "hidden," since patients are free to buy solutions as they use them during the year.

   b.   **Lens costs** can be estimated for daily, biweekly, and annual (conventional) replacement lenses. At $30 for a box of 30 lenses, daily replacement lenses cost approximately $720 per year. At $23 for a box of six lenses, biweekly replacement lenses cost approximately $184 per year. Conventional hydrogel lenses cost approximately $70 per year.

   c.   Solution costs can be estimated based on a daily consumption of 5 ml of disinfection solution for storage of lenses in a flat lens case, 5 ml for irrigation or rub and rinse of lenses, 1 ml of cleaner, and a weekly enzyme cleaning. On this basis, the maintenance of conventional and disposable lenses may cost approximately $3 and $1.10 per week ($156 and $57 per year), respectively. (This assumes that a multi-action solution is used for both disinfection and cleaning for disposable lenses.)

   d.   Overall costs in the United States for biweekly disposable and conventional hydrogel lenses appear comparable based on the above calculations. At present, however, there is a price premium associated with the extra convenience of daily replacement lenses.

5.   Disposable lenses have certain potential disadvantages (see also section II.B.2).

   a.   **Quantity of manufacturing** is affected. A patient who switches from conventional daily wear to daily disposable lenses requires about 360 times as many lenses per year. This requires a huge increase in manufacturing capacity. For this reason, fewer lens parameters are available, and not all patients can be fitted.[6]

   b.   **Lens-parameter repeatability** is generally good. Port found that the back optic zone radius (BOZR) varied by a maximum of 0.13 mm for NewVues (CIBA Vision, Duluth, Georgia) lenses of the same nominal parameters (8.8/14.0/various powers).[13] Lens thickness may be a source of variability, although this not easy to measure in practice.

  c. **Acuvue** (Vistakon, Jacksonville, Florida) lenses can have a significant number of **minor edge defects,** although only one study has claimed them to be clinically significant.[14] By comparison, no edge defects were found with SeeQuence lenses (Bausch & Lomb [B&L], Rochester, New York).[15]

D. **Silicone-hydrogel extended wear disposable lenses**
  1. The first examples of a new generation of disposable lenses were introduced in 1999, intended primarily for extended wear.
     a. The key breakthrough, made independently by two companies, was the development of hybrid silicone-containing hydrogel materials. The inclusion of silicone allows oxygen transmissibility values in excess of 100, considered sufficient for overnight lens wear with the majority of patients.
     b. Since silicone is hydrophobic, the silicone-hydrogel materials are surface modified by a plasma batch process in order to ensure *in vivo* wettability.
     c. A water content of 20–40% gives sufficient water transmissibility to ensure rapid recovery from any lens adherence after overnight wear. The aqueous phase of the tear film is able to penetrate the lenses, replenish the postlens tear film, and thereby restore lens movement with blinks. There are anecdotal reports that these low water content materials also reduce symptoms of dryness in some patients.
     d. The two new high-Dk lenses, Night & Day (CIBA Vision) and PureVision (Bausch & Lomb), are not identical. The Night & Day lens is a fluorosilicone-hydrogel (FDA group I) with nominal water content of 24% and Dk/t (–3.00) of 175. The PureVision is a silicone-hydrogel (FDA group III) with a nominal water content of 36% and Dk/t (–3.00) of 110.
     e. Both lenses are monthly disposable lenses, initially approved for 30-day extended wear in Europe and 7-day extended wear in the United States. The regular replacement will help to minimize any inflammatory, allergic, or mechanical complications related to lens deposition.
     f. Lens cost is slightly higher than hydrogel daily wear disposable lenses, but the patient needs to clean and disinfect the lenses only occasionally or not at all, thereby minimizing the cost of lens maintenance. However, lubricating drops may need to be instilled by the patient on waking each morning.

Pearl: The monthly replacement, high Dk, hydrogel-containing contact lenses are expected to keep to a minimum the incidence of microbial keratitis in extended wear; however, noninfectious inflammatory reactions may still occasionally occur.

E. **Tinted lenses** of various kinds are available.
1. **Handling tints** (visitint) are usually of 10% density, which does not have any cosmetic effect on eye color.[16] They are becoming more commonly prescribed, particularly because they are standard on many disposable lenses. Such tints are particularly recommended for hypermetropic or presbyopic patients who have near-focusing difficulties.
2. **Enhancement tints** can be used to modify apparent iris color for cosmetic reasons when a patient has a lightly colored iris. These lenses are usually tinted over a diameter equal to the horizontal iris diameter, usually 11.0–11.5 mm, and the tint includes the pupil zone. Colors are additive to the iris color, so, for example, an aqua tint covering a light green iris might produce a medium blue.
3. **Opaque tints** can serve several purposes, although they may also have limitations.
    a. They can change the apparent iris color. **Durasoft Colors** (Wesley-Jessen, Des Plaines, Illinois) were the first opaque tints, which offer a realistic change of eye color for patients with a dark iris. The key characteristic is the matrix of opaque dots, which allows some of the natural iris color to be seen and prevents the "bulbous" look of a fully opaque tint.
    b. Opaque lenses induce a slight loss in sensitivity across the entire visual field, usually less than 1 dB.[17] People whose jobs require that they be in poorly lighted areas should be counseled about going into unfamiliar dimly lit areas wearing opaque lenses.
    c. **Comfort** may be slightly reduced with opaque lenses, possibly due to surface irregularities where the colorant is located.[18]
4. **Ultraviolet-blocking lenses** are effective, although naturally only the cornea is protected; the lenses are not a replacement for sunglasses. These lenses absorb an average of 90% of ultraviolet light across the band. They are useful for patients taking medication with the side effect of photosensitization and for those working outdoors. Precision UV is an example in a disposable modality.[19]
5. **"Night club" lenses** are designed to be flashy and conspicuous.
6. **Custom hand-painted lenses** may be required if the patient's eye is disfigured.
7. **Occluder lenses** have an opaque pupil for cases of intractable diplopia.
F. Toric lenses are discussed in Chapter 12.
G. Extended-wear lenses are discussed in Chapter 15.
H. Bifocal lenses are considered in Chapter 18.

III. **Soft lens fitting and evaluation** require some skill and experience.
   A. The **optimal lens fit** can be evaluated in terms of a number of parameters.
   1. **Lens movement** is considered important, as it promotes postlens tear film exchange and mixing. Movement is quantified as the vertical change in lens position before and after a normal blink. Lens movement of less than 0.1 mm can be considered inadequate, and movement of more than 1.0 mm is excessive. Lathed lenses that fit well show about 0.3 mm of movement.[20]

   Pearl: It is easy to overestimate lens movement when viewing with a slit lamp. A handy guide is to remember that a 14.0-mm lens on a 12.0-mm cornea has moved 1.0 mm if the lens edge traverses the limbus.

   2. The **push-up test** has been advocated as an indicator of lens mobility that is independent of the patient's eyelid blink dynamics.[20] The examiner pushes the lens superiorly by manipulating the patient's inferior eyelid margin. A lens that fits well can moved easily using the push-up test.
   3. **Centration** of a soft lens is assessed as optimal if the lens edge shows uniform and symmetric overlap onto the sclera in all meridians. Furthermore, if the lens is decentered, such as with the push-up test, it should regain optimal centration in less than 1 second.
   4. **Lag on upgaze and version movement** is readily evaluated by observing the change in lens centration in eye positions other than primary gaze. A normal amount of lag could be 0.3–0.7 mm. Excessive lag is associated with poor centration and zero lag occurs if there is lens adherence.
   5. **Tear exchange and the postlens tear film** may be evaluated clinically using observation in specular illumination with the biomicroscope. High magnification (30× or more), a wide angle of observation (more than 60 degrees), and a narrow slit beam (0.1 mm) are needed.[21] An optimal lens fit requires an aqueous postlens tear film, which is observed as amorphous or nonpatterned in specular reflection. Patterned or colored postlens tear film appearances are taken to indicate reduced tear exchange.[22]
   6. The **comfort** of a soft lens is considered optimal if the patient has only slight awareness of the lens's presence. Excessive awareness may indicate excessive lens movement or poor centration, and no sensation at all may indicate lens adherence. Lens defects can be reported as a foreign body sensation; incompatible care solutions may be reported as stinging on lens insertion.
   7. Stable vision also relates to good lens centration and movement and to good **prelens tear film stability** (greater-than-normal interblink interval).

Table 10.2 International Standards Organization Contact Lens Terminology

Term	Abbreviation	Common Previous Terms
Back optic zone radius	BOZR	Base curve (radius), central posterior curve, posterior central curve radius, back central optic radius
Back optic zone diameter	BOZD	Optic zone diameter, posterior optic zone diameter
Total diameter	TD	Lens diameter, diameter
Back vertex power	BVP	Refractive power
Oxygen transmissibility	Dk/t	Dk/L

    8. **Keratometer mires** can be examined on the anterior lens surface to detect any lens distortion on the eye. Any mire irregularity would be considered abnormal.

  B. Selection of a lens for fitting requires the choice of a number of parameters. Some relevant lens parameters are summarized in Table 2.

    1. The **BOZR** of a hydrogel lens is usually selected as 0.6–0.8 mm flatter than the average corneal curvature measured with keratometry. If a lens BOZR is too flat for the cornea, lens centration may be poor.[23] Changing the BOZR of the current generation of soft lenses does not significantly alter lens movement, however.[20,24] If the lens BOZR is too steep, the lens may not conform properly to the eye during wear.

    2. **Aspheric back curves** are used in some soft lenses, such as the CIBA Weicon (CIBA Vision), which is available in Flat (FL) and Steep (ST) curvatures. The lens curvature is slightly flatter peripherally than centrally to more closely match the average corneal shape. For such lenses, the manufacturer usually has recommendations as to which lens curvature to trial-fit in the first instance.

    3. **Total diameter (TD)** is usually selected as about 2.0 mm greater than the patient's horizontal visible iris diameter. A lens that is too large will tend to show low amounts of movement and may have inadequate tear exchange. A lens that is too small may move excessively, show poor centration, and be less comfortable to wear.

    4. Lenses are made from a variety of **materials** and with varying percentages of **water content**. The wide range of hydrogel lens materials available is discussed in Chapter 11. Historically, a low-water-content material was the material of choice owing to its durability and ease of manufacture. More recently, mid-water-content and high-water-content materials have become popular, as they are available in disposable lens modalities and have improved oxygen transmissibility. The disposable lens materials often have a standard visibility tint and may have UV blocking and an inversion indicator.

Table 10.3   Oxygen Transmissibility (Dk/t) of Hydrogel Lenses[a]

Lens	Average Dk/t[b] Power of		
	-8.00	-3.00	+6.00
38% U3, Cibasoft, CSI	8	10	6
56% Acuvue, Spectrum, Hydrocurve II	16	18	11
73% Permaflex, Precision UV	26	28	22
PureVision (Bausch & Lomb)	~100	110	N/A
Night & Day (CIBA Vision)	~160	175	N/A

[a]The average Dk/t values show the variation with center thickness, power, and lens design but should be used only as guides. Lenses with low Dk/t (<12 Barrer/cm) are likely to cause hypoxic changes during daily wear; lenses with moderate Dk/t (12–35 Barrer/cm) are likely to cause hypoxic changes during extended wear.
[b]Oxygen transmissibility (Dk/t) of a contact lens is directly proportional to the oxygen permeability of the lens material (Dk, Barrer) and inversely related to the lens average thickness (L, cm).

5. The **oxygen transmissibility** (Dk/t) of a contact lens material is directly proportional to the oxygen permeability of the lens material (Dk, Barrer) and inversely related to the lens average thickness (L, cm). The Dk unit Barrer is calculated with the following formula[25]:

$$\text{The Dk unit Barrer} = \frac{[\text{cm}^2 \text{ ml (STP) O}_2] \times 10^{-11}}{[\text{sec ml mm Hg}]}$$

An alternative term for the Dk unit is "Fatt units," in honor of Irving Fatt's work in this area. Carbon dioxide transmissibility is directly related to the oxygen transmissibility for both soft and hard lenses, being numerically 7 and 21 times greater for RGP and soft lenses, respectively.[26] Representative lenses are listed in Table 10.3.

Pearl: If a lens has acceptable oxygen transmissibility, the carbon dioxide transmissibility will also usually be sufficient.

a. The oxygen transmissibility of lenses is defined as follows: low, less than 12 Barrer/cm; moderate, 12–34 Barrer/cm; and high, 35–100 Barrer/cm. Low-Dk/t lenses are mainly older-design lenses or high-powered lenses.

b. Under **open-eye conditions,** or daily wear, lenses of moderate Dk/t (12–34 Barrer/cm) are usually suitable. Furthermore, under open-eye conditions, a contact lens with a Dk/t of 24 Barrer/cm or more can allow a corneal oxygen partial pressure of 75 mm Hg, which is sufficient to avoid all detectable hypoxic changes in most patients. Contact lenses with a slightly lower Dk/t, of 12–20 Barrer/cm, are also generally acceptable. During open-eye lens wear, the pCO_2 in the anterior cornea will vary depending on the transmissibility of the lens, rising to a maximum of about 40 mm Hg with a gas-impermeable lens.[27]

   c. Under **closed-eye conditions,** or extended wear, a high Dk/t lens (more than 34 Barrer/cm) is required. Holden and Mertz determined that Dk/t values of more than 70 Barrer/cm are required to prevent corneal swelling for closed-eye lens wear.[28] They suggested that an adequate oxygen transmissibility may be 34 Barrer/cm, for corneal swelling of 8% or less during closed-eye wear. During eye closure, corneal pCO_2 is always approximately 40 mm Hg because this is the tension in the tarsal conjunctiva.

6. Different lens designs and materials may not have comparable performance despite similar lens diameters and BOZRs.[24] In one study, an 8.8 Acuvue fit was equivalent to an 8.4 NewVue despite similar diameters and thicknesses.[29]

7. **Back vertex power** affects lens thickness profile and average thickness. Consequently, many lens attributes are affected, including Dk/t, fitting, and handling. Contact lens power differs significantly from spectacle lens power for powers greater than 4.00 D. The required contact lens power is calculated from the following formula:

$$F = \frac{F'_v}{[1 - (d \cdot F'_v)]}$$

where F = back vertex power of contact lens at the eye (D), F'_v = back vertex power of spectacle lens (D), and d = vertex distance in meters. The equation can also apply to rigid gas-permeable lenses (see Chapter 4).

Pearl: Whereas the standard low-water-content lens (hydroxyethyl-methacrylate) allows sufficient oxygen transmission in low to moderate myopia, mid- or high-water-content lenses should be fitted for high minus (more than –4.00) or plus (more than +1.00 D) prescriptions.[30]

8. Lenses of **different thicknesses** have different advantages and disadvantages.
   a. The majority of current lenses are made as thin as practical to maximize oxygen transmissibility.
   b. A drawback of thin lenses is that if they are too thin, it is more difficult for the patient to handle them and they have a shorter

life. Thinner lenses also tend to support a thinner postlens tear film and consequently have less movement with blinks.[31] If a lens is excessively thin, the result can be desiccation staining of the cornea.

    c. As a guide, low-water-content lenses may have a center thickness as low as 0.04–0.06 mm, mid-water-content lenses 0.07–0.09 mm, and high-water-content lenses 0.10–0.14 mm.

  9. In summary, **different brands of lenses and modalities** will suit different patients. Disposable lenses are the lens modality of choice for the majority of patients for reasons of convenience and better ocular health. For patients with moderate myopic or any hypermetropic prescriptions, a **thin mid-water-content lens** such as Acuvue or CIBA Focus 2 weekly may be an optimal design.[32] Conventional custom made lenses have a role for patients with a refraction or corneal curvature outside the normal range. Daily disposable and high-Dk extended wear silicone-hydrogel materials are new lens types, offering greater convenience for many patients. A patient prone to tear evaporation or with marginal dry eye may benefit from a Biocompatibles Proclear disposable lens, or use of the Benz 45G material in a convenient custom made hydrogel lens. Patients who are exposed to the sun a great deal may benefit from the ultraviolet blocker in lenses such as the Precision UV and Acuvue.

C. **Tear film and blinking** have an effect on fitting. Lens movement can be affected by interactions between the lens and upper lid, which depend on the lubricative properties of the prelens tear film, the surface quality of both lens and lid, and the nature of the blink. Furthermore, the postlens tear film appears to influence lens movement, since hypotonic solutions can thin the postlens tear film and cause lens adherence.[33]

  1. **Lens settling** is a postinsertion equilibration process. The tear film trapped behind the soft lens appears to be squeezed out by the initial blinking, leading to a reduction in lens movement.[34,35] Reflex tearing on lens insertion may also affect lens movement, leading to a transitory reduction.[36]

  2. Initial **lens movement** immediately on insertion is not usually representative of normal movement. Evaluating movement after **5 minutes** of wear adequately predicts movement after 8 hours of wear for lenses with water contents of 38% and 67%.[37]

  3. **Eye closure** can also affect lens movement. Periods of eye closure as short as 15 minutes can reduce lens movement to near zero.[38] The reduction of lens movement appears to be due to a thinning of the postlens tear film.

  4. **Air movement** at the anterior surface of the lens can lead to a reduction in lens movement due to postlens tear film thinning.[39]

5. The **water flow conductivity** of the lens may be a parameter that controls tear film effects on lens movement. The flow conductivity is a function of the material pore size and lens thickness, and high-water-content materials have increased values.[40] Holden and colleagues noted that the lack of water in a flexible material such as silicone may be responsible for its tendency to adhere to the eye.[41]

D. Several procedures can be used for lens **verification and inspection.**

   1. **Lens integrity** may be checked using a projection microscope, or a slit lamp when the lens is on the eye. Check for edge defects, central defects, etc.

   2. Coffee filters are good for lint-free blotting of soft lenses when verifying **lens power.**[42]

   3. A variety of electronic-mechanical gauges have been used to measure soft **lens thickness,** to an accuracy of about 1 μm (0.001 mm). More recently, Bachman has suggested the use of a hand-held ultrasonic pachymeter for one eye measurement of soft lens thickness.[43]

   4. **Water content** may be measured using a hand refractometer.[44]

   5. It is impractical for the practitioner to verify each disposable lens, but the patient can check each new lens before inserting it.

IV. **Fitting by physiology** is the term used by Efron and Holden[45] to designate the role of lens design and fitting in ocular complications in lens wear. Some ocular complications of contact lens wear observed at follow-up visits can be viewed as an indication for changing lens design for a given mode of wear. Such ocular changes fall into eight categories of signs and symptoms (Figure 10.1). In this section physiologic changes are grouped according to the underlying cause to assist in understanding of the development and recovery of each condition, highlight similarities among allied conditions, and aid the selection of appropriate management strategies. This section is an adaptation of a review by Bruce and Brennan, with some additional recent references cited.[46]

A. A decreased availability of oxygen (**hypoxia**) and an increase in carbon dioxide (**hypercapnia**) may occur during contact lens wear and can be an indication for contact lens refitting. Normally there is a flow of oxygen into the anterior corneal surface and an efflux of carbon dioxide. The partial pressure gradients for oxygen and carbon dioxide are the key to gas movement across the cornea (Table 10.4). When the eyelid is closed during sleep, the palpebral vascular supply becomes the site of gas exchange.

   1. Signs of a **reduced epithelial aerobic metabolism** are usually manifest in the epithelium itself. They arise from possible underlying microscopic physiologic changes, such as a reduction in mitotic cell activity, loosening of tight junctions, decreases in numbers of hemidesmosomes, and separation of corneal epithelial cells. The surface cells may become more fragile, and there may be a slight epithelial thinning. The most obvious clinical manifes-

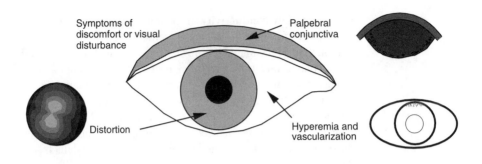

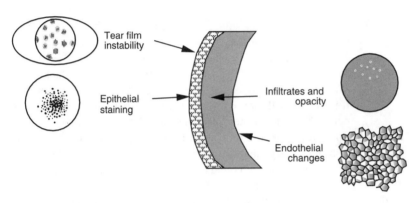

FIGURE 10.1   *Eight categories of signs and symptoms indicating that contact lens refitting may be necessary. (Reprinted with permission from AS Bruce, NA Brennan. A Guide to Clinical Contact Lens Management: Signs, Symptoms, Diagnosis, and Management [2nd ed]. Duluth, GA: CIBA Vision, 1995.)*

Table 10.4   Oxygen and Carbon Dioxide Partial Pressures

	Oxygen Partial Pressure (pO_2)	*Carbon Dioxide Partial Pressure (pCO_2)*
Corneal surface, open eye	155 mm Hg	~0 mm Hg
Corneal surface, closed eye	55 mm Hg	40 mm Hg
Anterior chamber (open and closed eye)	55 mm Hg	40 mm Hg

tation of hypoxic changes to epithelial physiology is surface disruption, as seen via fluorescein staining. A graphic summary of ocular changes listed in this section is shown in Figure 10.2.

Pearl: *Fluorescein staining is a ubiquitous sign in contact lens wear, with many possible causes; however, the configuration of staining is likely to give a clue as to the nature of the cause.*

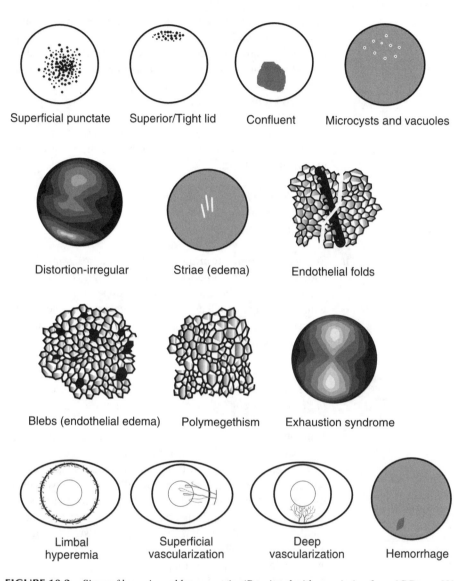

FIGURE 10.2 *Signs of hypoxia and hypercapnia. (Reprinted with permission from AS Bruce, NA Brennan. A Guide to Clinical Contact Lens Management: Signs, Symptoms, Diagnosis, and Management [2nd ed]. Duluth, GA: CIBA Vision, 1995.)*

a. **Superficial punctate keratitis** is characterized by premature shedding of small groups of surface cells as well as disruption of the ocular surface mucus layer. Hypoxia can produce central punctate staining, including both moderate short-term hypoxia, for example from polymethyl methacrylate (PMMA) lens overwear, and chronic long-term hypoxia, such as that caused by thick low-water-content lenses or extended wear of hydrogel lenses. Mild superficial punctate keratitis in contact lens wear may not be diagnostic of an underlying problem.

   Pearl: A patient with epithelial fluorescein staining is generally asymptomatic, since the injury threshold of the cornea is less than the touch threshold.

b. **Superior arcuate staining** is staining in a horizontal linear pattern close to the superior limbus. This sign is more likely in patients with tight or low-positioning upper lids and patients with thicker hydrogel lenses, possibly because of reduced oxygen availability to the superior region of the cornea. It can also occur in the region of the cornea corresponding to the lens bevel.

   Pearl: Even in daily contact lens wear, the superior cornea is in "extended wear" if covered by the upper lid.

c. **Epithelial abrasion** is seen as severe central fluorescein staining resulting from overwear of PMMA or closed-eye wear of low-oxygen-transmissibility hydrogel contact lenses. If the lens has become adherent to an epithelium already weakened by hypoxia, the abrasion will have sharply demarcated edges and may be several millimeters in diameter. These are acute conditions, and the patient may experience significant discomfort or pain. The lesion is not usually infected, however, and stromal infiltration is not present.

d. **Microcysts** and **vacuoles** appear as translucent cysts in the epithelium, 0.01–0.1 mm in diameter. Since they are microscopic in size, only careful biomicroscopic examination using the technique of retroillumination will show the cystic formations. Microcysts are smaller and less regular in shape than vacuoles, but the functional distinction is uncertain. Although very uncommon in contact lens daily wear, these formations are relatively common in extended wear of lenses of low to moderate oxygen transmissibility, such as mid-water-content hydrogel lenses. It takes 6–8 weeks of extended wear with hydrogel lenses before microcysts appear.

Pearl: One clue to the presence of microcysts or vacuoles may be scattered punctate fluorescein staining.

e. In terms of **management,** significant epithelial staining of these types is usually an indication for a 24-hour discontinuation of lens wear, to allow the epithelial surface to heal, and possibly for review of healing of the lesion by the practitioner. Mild staining may be managed by reducing wearing time (e.g., to less than 10 hours per day) or ceasing extended wear. If the staining is chronic, even if slight, modification of lens parameters to increase Dk/t is advisable. Superior arcuate staining may require an improvement to peripheral lens Dk/t, whereas central staining may indicate the need to improve central corneal oxygenation.

Pearl: Unlike ocular changes with other causes, ocular changes related to hypoxia and hypercapnia tend to affect only the cornea, and there are few associated symptoms.

2. **Stromal edema** arises within hours of the onset of hypoxia, the degree being related to the severity of the hypoxia. An inflow of water into the stroma (edema) can arise due to an accumulation of lactate in the stroma, secondary to a hypoxia-related increase in anaerobic metabolism via the Embden-Meyerhof biochemical pathway of the epithelial cells.

   a. **Corneal thickness** is not simple to measure clinically, although ultrasonic and optic techniques are available. The edema response begins within half an hour of lens insertion and generally peaks within 3 hours. Corneal swelling in people using daily wear lenses (Dk/t ranging from 7 to 18 Barrer/cm) typically ranges from 1.5% to 5.0%.[28] With extended wear of hydrogel lenses (Dk/t = 15 Barrer/cm or higher), overnight edema averages 10–12%.[47] It is worth noting that corneal thickness measurements can also be influenced by reflex hypotonic tearing or by a physical thinning of the stroma in long-term wear. Also, there is marked individual variability in the degree of corneal swelling response.

   b. **Corneal distortion** is an uncommon complication of hydrogel lens wear, although it can occur as a result of poor RGP lens fitting or wear of low Dk/t RGP lenses or PMMA lenses. Such distortion is known as "spectacle blur" or "corneal warpage" and is manifested as a change in the spectacle refraction and central corneal curvature.

c. **Stromal striae** are visible as fine, white vertical lines in the posterior stroma of the cornea, if stromal edema of 6% or higher is present. Thus, striae are not present with most current-generation daily-wear hydrogel lenses for myopia (Dk/t greater than approximately 7 Barrer/cm). However, striae remain a useful diagnostic indicator of corneal edema for plus-powered hydrogel lenses, such as those prescribed for monovision, or soon after eye opening with extended-wear lenses.

d. Using biomicroscopy, posterior **stromal folds** appear as dark lines in the endothelial specular reflection and appear to represent a buckling of the posterior stroma and endothelial layer. They appear when stromal edema exceeds 10% and thus rarely occur with daily wear of rigid or hydrogel contact lenses. With extended wear of hydrogel lenses (Dk/t of 15–20 Barrer/cm), however, posterior folds can be apparent on eye opening.

e. In terms of **management,** if **stromal edema** is noted at follow-up examination, increasing lens Dk/t to at least 15 Barrer/cm for daily wear and at least 34 Barrer/cm for extended wear is recommended.[28] In the case of plus-powered hydrogel lenses, this may require a change to high-water-content material or a RGP lens design. If a change to lens fitting is not desired, then other strategies may also be useful, such as reducing wearing hours per day or inserting lenses later after eye opening in the morning.

3. **Stromal acidosis** can arise from hypercapnia as well as hypoxia. Respiratory acidosis can occur when a gas-impermeable lens prevents carbon dioxide efflux from the corneal stroma (hypercapnia). Metabolic acidosis can occur if there is a decrease in the pH of the stroma due to accumulation of stromal lactate. Normal human corneal stromal pH under closed-eye conditions is 7.39 ± 0.01, a level similar to that of the blood. Under open-eye conditions, human stromal pH rises about 2%, and it may decrease as much as 5% during wear of an oxygen-impermeable contact lens. This condition is a relatively uncommon indication for lens refitting.

a. Under the biomicroscope, **endothelial edema** appears as circumscribed defects in the endothelial specular reflection. It has also been termed **"blebs,"** "events," and "pseudoguttata." Application of a contact lens to the unadapted eye can cause a sudden-onset but transient endothelial edema response. It occurs within 10 minutes of lens insertion, peaks after approxi-

mately half an hour, and may last for several hours. The initial
bleb response to contact lens wear does not result in cell loss,
and a change in lens fitting is not required.

b. **Endothelial polymegethism** is a greater-than-normal varia-
    tion of cell size in the corneal endothelial mosaic, observed
    with the biomicroscope or the clinical specular microscope.[48]
    It is graded by the coefficient of variation of cell area, which is
    the standard deviation divided by the mean. A normal en-
    dothelium has a coefficient of approximately 25%, but it may
    be as high as 46% in a patient who has had 20 years of oxy-
    gen-impermeable daily lens wear or 5 years of hydrogel ex-
    tended wear.

c. **Corneal exhaustion syndrome** is a condition associated with
    the presence of marked endothelial polymegethism. Patients with
    high refractive errors necessitating fitting of thick lenses and pa-
    tients fitted for extended wear who have worn lenses for 10 years
    or more are probably most susceptible to developing the condi-
    tion. Other signs are intolerance to lens wear and blurred, fluctu-
    ating vision due to fluctuations in refractive error.[49]

d. **Corneal hypoesthesia** is not easy to measure quantitatively in
    the clinical situation. One technique is based on using a fine
    nylon thread of adjustable length and stimulating a peripheral
    corneal location. Low-Dk/t hydrogel or rigid lenses are most
    commonly implicated. Affected patients are naturally asymp-
    tomatic, so corneal hypoesthesia is an uncommon indication
    for lens refitting.

e. **Polymegethism, corneal exhaustion syndrome, or corneal
    hypoesthesia** is an indicator of the need to refit with a lens of
    moderate to high Dk/t, or to cease extended wear.

4. Under certain circumstances, lens wearers may experience **hyper-
    emia** of the limbal capillaries and **vascularization** of the superfi-
    cial cornea or deep stroma.

a. The **normal limbus** is a vascular transition zone containing
    blood vessels, whereas the cornea itself is avascular. It is ap-
    proximately 1 mm in width, although it is often wider in the
    vertical meridian, particularly superiorly. The limit of the lim-
    bus can be located as the limit of the translucent conjunctival
    overlay using the technique of marginal retroillumination.[50]

b. **Limbal hyperemia** is a dilation of existing limbal capillaries. It
    is a common chronic bilateral complication of hydrogel con-
    tact lens wear, and patients are asymptomatic. Low-water-
    content hydrogel lenses cause greater limbal hyperemia than
    high-water-content lenses, since low-water-content lenses have
    a lower oxygen transmissibility in the periphery.[31] Hyperemia

is also more likely with long wearing times or overnight wear. A second potential cause of limbal hyperemia is a "tight" or immobile hydrogel lens where the lens edge occludes the superficial limbal blood vessels.

Pearl: Limbal hyperemia, fluorescein staining, and the presence of microcysts have been found to be the best biomicroscopic indicators of corneal hypoxia in hydrogel extended wear.[51]

c. **Superficial vascularization** is penetration of blood vessels into the superficial cornea, and such vessels can be observed as continuous with the limbal vessels. The superior limbus is most susceptible. Stark and Martin defined vascularization as vessel penetration greater than 1.5 mm.[52] It is uncommon in hydrogel lens daily wear, but a higher prevalence has been noted for aphakic or therapeutic hydrogel extended wear. Corneal vascularization is of concern because it makes the cornea more susceptible to inflammation or hemorrhage.

Pearl: Since vascularization can develop in the absence of symptoms, routine follow-up examinations are the only means of detecting this condition.

d. **Deep stromal vascularization** is the rarest of the vascular changes associated with contact lens wear, but it is also potentially the most serious. Vision can be profoundly affected in some cases due to associated opacities. Risk factors include chronic hypoxia and stromal edema, previous surgery for aphakia, corneal disease, injury or infection, extended wear of low-Dk/t lenses, and toxic solution preservatives.

e. An **intracorneal hemorrhage** at the subepithelial level is an uncommon sequelae to superficial corneal vascularization. It has been most often related to aphakic hydrogel lenses.

f. An **intrastromal opacity** associated with vascularization is also a rare complication of lens wear, although one that may threaten vision. If related to corneal exhaustion syndrome, an opacity will be deep stromal, but avascular.[49]

g. **Mild limbal hyperemia** requires no management and is presently an unavoidable part of hydrogel lens wear. Marked hyperemia or any **vascularization** requires lens refitting to improve peripheral corneal oxygenation. Patients may be refitted with high-water-content or RGP lenses and may need to reduce wearing time or cease extended wear. Deep stromal vas-

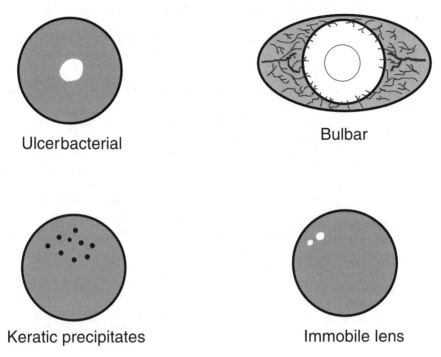

Ulcerbacterial

Bulbar

Keratic precipitates

Immobile lens

FIGURE 10.3   *Signs of infection. (Reprinted with permission from AS Bruce, NA Brennan. A Guide to Clinical Contact Lens Management: Signs, Symptoms, Diagnosis, and Management [2nd ed]. Duluth, GA: CIBA Vision, 1995.)*

cularization is a most serious complication, and immediate cessation of lens wear, rather than lens refitting, is indicated.

> ***Pearl:*** *In general, patients with a refractive error of more than –4.00 D or virtually any plus prescription should not be fit with a low-water-content lens.[31]*

B. The following discussion of **infection** is not considered in depth here, since there are causative factors in addition to the lens fitting and design. These factors include the patient's compliance with lens care instructions and contamination of the care solutions (see Chapter 13). A graphic summary of ocular changes listed in this section is shown in Figure 10.3.

   1. **Infection** is the most serious, but also one of the rarest, complications of contact lens wear. It can occur in all types of lens wear but has been most commonly associated with cosmetic extended wear. Even in extended wear, 99.9% of contact lens wearers do not contract a corneal infection.

2. A number of **ocular defense mechanisms** exist to help prevent infection.[53]
   a. **Blinking and tear flow** are among the front-line defenses. They operate by sweeping away bacteria before they can adhere to the cornea.
   b. **Mucus strands** are rolled across the cornea by blinking, and these tend to trap bacteria.
   c. **Desquamation of epithelial cells** is a regular occurrence, which helps remove bacteria that may have adhered.
   d. **Tear film antibacterial factors** act toward lysing bacteria. These include lysozyme, lactoferrin, transferrin, ceruloplasmin, beta-lysin, and cellular immune factors.
   e. The **acquired immune system of the eye** consists of immunoglobulin A, secretory IgA, and the complement system.
   f. The **natural immune system** consists of macrophages, neutrophils, and natural killer cells.
3. **Bacterial corneal infection** may produce any of several signs.[54]
   a. The presence of corneal **pain** of more than a transitory nature in a contact lens wearer is a warning sign of the possibility of a corneal infection. The pain may be exacerbated by lens removal and accompanied by redness, discharge, or decreased vision. Other possible causes are *Acanthamoeba* keratitis or an inflammatory reaction in extended wear (see the following sections).
   b. **Infective ulceration** is characterized by an epithelial defect with an underlying stromal excavation and infiltrate. These findings may be considered pathognomonic for corneal infection until proven otherwise. An infective ulcer is typically unilateral and the ulcer is likely to be central or midperipheral.
   c. Other possible associated signs are surrounding epithelial, stromal, and endothelial edema; stromal thinning; necrosis of the infiltrate; mucopurulent discharge; keratic precipitates; and an anterior chamber reaction.
   d. In terms of **management,** symptoms or signs are indications for immediate ophthalmic evaluation and lens wear should immediately be ceased (see Chapter 15).
4. *Acanthamoeba* **corneal infection** is a rare but particularly devastating cause of infection.
   a. Severe ocular **pain,** out of proportion to the manifest clinical signs, is a hallmark sign of infection. Early in the disease process, signs are frequently nonspecific and limited to an epitheliopathy or neurokeratitis. Later evidence of infection may include stromal infiltration in a ring pattern and scleritis. The infection tends to have a waxing and waning course.

    b. In terms of **management,** where possible, corneal scrapings are vital for confirmation of diagnosis. Early diagnosis is correlated with success in treatment, possibly because fewer *Acanthamoeba* cysts are present in the cornea early in the course of the disease. Other suggestions for lens fitting are in section IV.B.6.

5. **Bacterial immunologic reactions** also rarely occur.

    a. There are several sources of bacterial contamination. Bacteria may be harbored in the lid margins or in biofilm on the lens surfaces and produce substances toxic to the cornea.[55,56] Signs of blepharitis or meibomianitis may indicate that the lid margin is the source of organisms, such as *Staphylococcus*, that can secrete exotoxins. These conditions interrelate with general ophthalmologic conditions such as marginal keratitis, catarrhal ulcers, and blepharitis.

    b. Bacterial reactions may **present** in two forms: either acute inflammation reactions or low-grade, sterile, peripheral ulcers. Both acute inflammatory reactions and low-grade sterile peripheral ulcers have been observed as responses to hydrogel extended wear.[57]

    c. **Bulbar hyperemia** or a marked engorgement of the blood vessels over the entire bulbar conjunctiva is indicative of an acute inflammatory reaction. If the inflammatory response is less severe, the hyperemia may be adjacent to the corneal inflammatory response.

    d. **Peripheral corneal infiltrates** are focal white accumulations approximately 0.5–2.0 mm in diameter and located in the corneal epithelium or anterior stroma. The associated epithelium usually shows minimal fluorescein staining and no ulceration. Minor infiltrates may be asymptomatic or associated with a mild foreign-body sensation. Infiltrates in the immobile lens syndrome are usually associated with acute pain, however.

       A more gradual onset of inflammation over a period of contact lens wear may lead to breakdown of the overlying epithelium and subsequent ulceration, although the infiltrate remains sterile. Such infiltrates have been termed marginal keratitis, sterile ulcers, catarrhal lesions, marginal infiltrates, or sterile infiltration.

    e. Keratic precipitates are often present in an acute inflammatory reaction.

    f. Regarding **management,** suggestions for lens fitting are given in IV.B.6. Also see the section on culture-negative peripheral ulcer and contact lens acute red eye (Chapter 15).

Pearl: *Sterile peripheral infiltrates must be differentiated from infectious ulceration. Infectious infiltrates tend to be associated with significant pain, epithelial defect, discharge, anterior chamber reaction and a central location (the PEDAL mnemonic). If in doubt, treat as infectious.*[57]

6. **Lens-fitting technique** can be used to minimize the risk of infection.
   a. **Ensure adequate movement and postlens tear flow.** This helps clear bacteria, maintain a normal rate of epithelial desquamation, replenish the mucin layer, and circulate tear film antibacterial factors and nutrients for the epithelium.
   b. **Ensure adequate corneal oxygenation** via a lens with moderate Dk/t (daily wear) or high Dk/t (extended wear) to minimize epithelial defects and other metabolic alterations that increase susceptibility to bacterial adherence.
   c. **Minimize exposure of the eye to microbial contamination** by patient education on hygiene, avoiding the use of homemade saline or tap water, and attention to compliance with lens care systems. Other risk factors for *Acanthamoeba* infection are the contamination of lenses or solutions through contact with swimming pools, hot tubs, and freshwater ponds.
   d. Disposable lenses do not appear to alter the risk of infection when allowance is made for factors such as compliance with cleaning and disinfection systems.[58] Regular lens replacement does appear to reduce the incidence of inflammatory reactions, however.[59]
   e. **Minimize extended wear** since infections and inflammatory reactions are less common in daily wear.

C. The following discussion of **allergy and toxicity** is not considered in depth, since there are a number of causative factors in addition to lens fitting and design. These factors include the patient's compliance with lens care instructions and the chemical composition of the care solutions (see Chapter 13).

In addition, during recent years, there has been a dramatic reduction in the incidence of allergic and toxic reactions in lens wear. Planned-replacement regimens for hydrogel lens wearers have become very popular, thereby avoiding problems associated with a chronic buildup of lens deposits and biofilm. Less toxic disinfection solutions have been developed using high-molecular-weight preservatives that do not penetrate the lens matrix. Thus, the following signs are now relatively uncommon indications for lens refitting. A graphic summary of the ocular changes listed in this section is shown in Figure 10.4.

1. Solution preservatives, particularly **thimerosal,** may provoke an ocular immune reaction in sensitized persons. Leukocytic infil-

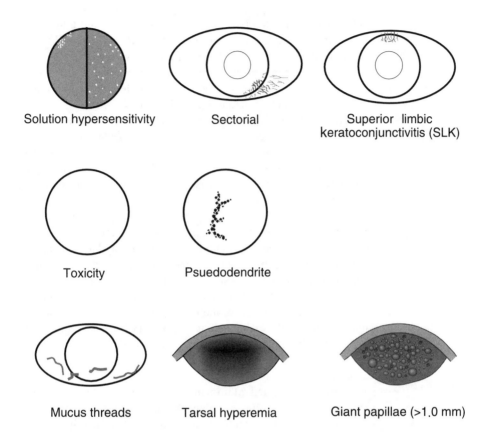

FIGURE 10.4 *Signs of allergy and toxicity. (Reprinted with permission from AS Bruce, NA Brennan. A Guide to Clinical Contact Lens Management: Signs, Symptoms, Diagnosis, and Management [2nd ed]. Duluth, GA: CIBA Vision, 1995.)*

tration is the key factor distinguishing a **hypersensitivity reaction** from a toxicity reaction (see next section). Sensitization may take months or years of exposure to the chemical. Sensitized patients show a rapid infiltrative reaction on re-exposure to the chemical, however. With changes in solution preservatives, reports have become very uncommon. The symptoms that often accompany a thimerosal allergic reaction are bilateral itching and conjunctival hyperemia. Diffuse epithelial punctate staining is usually present. Other possible signs are epithelial infiltrates, sectorial hyperemia, and contact lens–induced superior limbic keratoconjunctivitis.

2. **Toxicity reactions** (keratitis) are due to chemical trauma, and the effects are related to concentration and dosage. Disinfecting

chemicals can potentially bind or accumulate within a hydrogel lens, increasing the concentration of chemicals exposed to the eye. Modern high-molecular-weight preservatives and planned-replacement regimens have greatly reduced the incidence of such effects. Possible signs include stinging on lens insertion, punctate staining, and epithelial pseudodendrites.

3. **Giant papillary conjunctivitis** is an inflammation of the tarsal conjunctiva. With the trend away from thermal disinfection, and more recently with the advent of planned-replacement or disposable lenses, the condition has become less common. The etiology appears likely to be both a basophilic hypersensitivity reaction (delayed type IV reaction) and a mechanical trauma arising from a lens surface roughened by deposits. Possible signs are ocular itching on lens removal, lens intolerance, mucus threads, palpebral hyperemia, and papillae.

D. Hydrogel lenses, by their soft and pliable nature, rarely have significant **mechanical effects** on the ocular surfaces. Furthermore, the patient may be unaware of minor trauma if only superficial cells of the cornea or conjunctiva are affected. Also, note that lens deposits can cause a chronic form of mechanical irritation of the palpebral conjunctiva (see the discussion of giant papillary conjunctivitis, section IV.C.3). A graphic summary of ocular changes listed in this section is shown in Figure 10.5.

1. Under certain conditions, soft lenses can leave **imprints** on the cornea or conjunctival surface.

    a. Bulbar **conjunctival imprinting** may arise due to compression or chaffing of the lens edge. If compression is the cause, the soft lens will exhibit tight fitting and distal conjunctival vessels will become engorged adjacent to the lens edge.[60] **Conjunctival staining** associated with chaffing appears to be due to rough lens edges and is exacerbated by lens movement.[61] Conjunctival imprinting does not affect vision or comfort.

    b. **Corneal wrinkling** is a rare form of corneal distortion associated with wear of ultrathin high-water-content lenses. Although it can profoundly affect vision, the condition is fortunately fully reversible on lens removal. The corneal furrows are visible with keratometry, fluorescein pooling, and retinoscopy.

    c. **Lens defects** such as a central split in the lens can cause corneal staining, or they can cause an imprint if the lens defect is a subtle one. Patients usually report a marked foreign body sensation.

    d. **Management** of imprinting of the corneal or conjunctival surface is via lens refitting. Compression of the conjunctival surface is avoided by fitting a lens with a flatter BOZR. Chaffing of the conjunctival surface by rough lens edges is often asymptomatic, and a change of lens type may not be required.

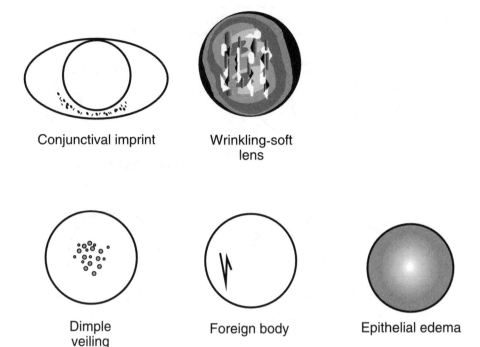

Conjunctival imprint

Wrinkling-soft
lens

Dimple
veiling

Foreign body

Epithelial edema

FIGURE 10.5 *Signs of mechanical effects of lenses. (Reprinted with permission from AS Bruce, NA Brennan. A Guide to Clinical Contact Lens Management: Signs, Symptoms, Diagnosis, and Management [2nd ed]. Duluth, GA: CIBA Vision, 1995.)*

Corneal wrinkling is managed by refitting with a soft lens of increased center thickness, lower water content, or both.

2. **Materials** can become trapped under the lens.

   a. **Dimple veiling** is created by air bubbles trapped under a lens. It is an uncommon complication of hydrogel lens wear, because of the close conformity of the lens to the corneal contour. The dimples are multiple, sharply demarcated, circular areas of fluorescein pooling. Symptoms are uncommon, and the condition is innocuous.

   b. **Foreign body tracks** are epithelial abrasions due to presence of foreign material under a lens. Fluorescein staining typically highlights a thin spiral track or linear streaks. The condition is painful until the foreign body is eliminated from the postlens tear film. As with dimple veiling, the condition is relatively uncommon in hydrogel lens wear.

   c. In terms of **management,** if dimple veiling occurs frequently, the hydrogel lens may require refitting with better alignment to corneal shape. Foreign body tracks are random events that do

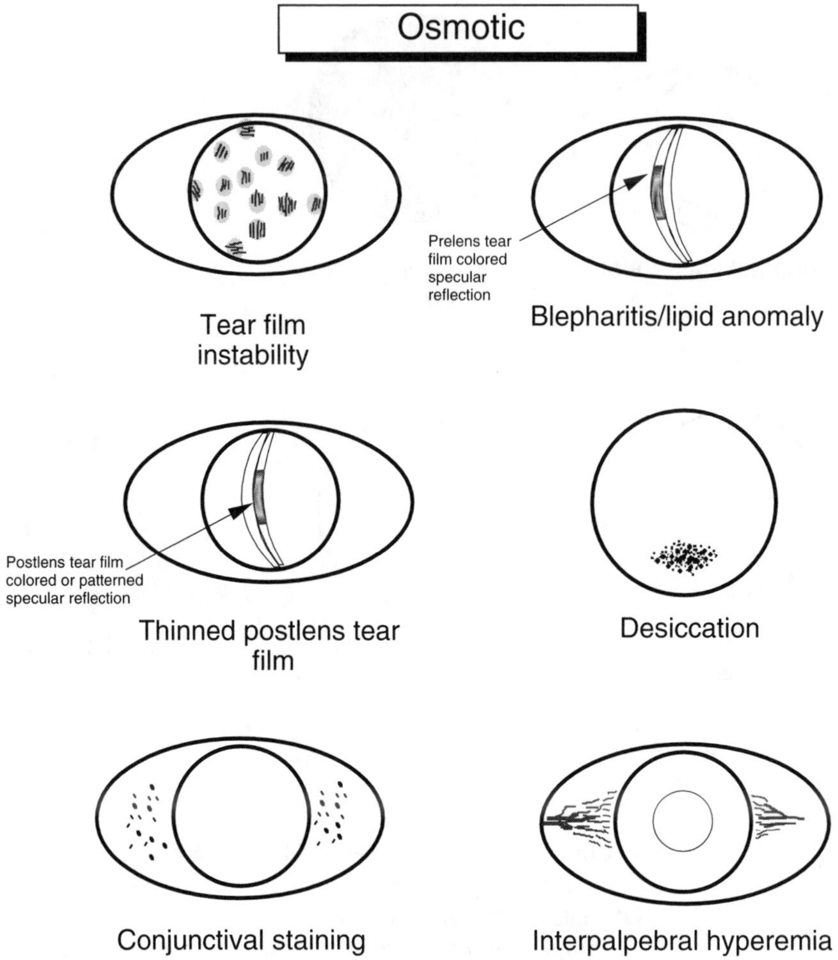

FIGURE 10.6   *Signs of desiccation. (Reprinted with permission from AS Bruce, NA Brennan. A Guide to Clinical Contact Lens Management: Signs, Symptoms, Diagnosis, and Management [2nd ed]. Duluth, GA: CIBA Vision, 1995.)*

not usually require lens refitting. If lens wear is discontinued the minor abrasion usually heals within 24 hours.

E. **Desiccation** is sometimes a problem. On application of a contact lens, the tear film is divided into the prelens tear film, postlens tear film, and preconjunctival tear layers. Compromise of any of these layers can have specific effects on lens wear. It is only relatively recently that tear film influences on soft lens fitting have been highlighted. A graphic summary of ocular changes listed in this section is shown in Figure 10.6.

1. One source of desiccation is **prelens tear film evaporation.** A hydrogel lens should support an adequate prelens tear film for the patient to have good comfort and vision during wear.

   a. The symptom of **ocular dryness** is the most common sensation reported by soft lens wearers. There is increased awareness of the lens, usually bilaterally, and the patient's wearing time is reduced.[62] Dryness has various causes, but tear deficiency is implicated. There may be a lack of lubrication between the eyelid and the lens and ocular surfaces, or the interpalpebral bulbar conjunctiva may be desiccated.

   b. **Reduced tear film stability** may be quantified by observing the prelens tear film breakup time using the keratometer mires or a reflected grid pattern. It is desirable that tear film stability be longer than the interblink interval, which is approximately 3 seconds in soft lens wearers.

   c. In terms of **management,** a poor prelens tear film may be an indication for replacing the lenses or changing the lens modality to frequent replacement or disposable lenses. This prevents lens deposits from accumulating. Possible alternative strategies include blinking exercises, tear supplements, or remediation of blepharitis, if present.

2. **Postlens tear film depletion** is a loss of water from the tear film layer located between the hydrogel lens and the cornea, leading to a thinning of that layer and a decrease in tear exchange. Typically, a thinned postlens tear film causes a hydrogel lens to be difficult to remove or be adherent to the eye.

   a. **Influences on the postlens tear film** include expulsion, evaporation, and osmotic flow. Expulsion indicates loss of the postlens tear film out under the edge of the lens with blinking or eye closure. Evaporation is a loss of the tear film at the anterior lens surface, which appears to draw aqueous from the postlens tear film anteriorly through the lens. Osmotic flow occurs when a hypotonic tear film (e.g., excess tearing or exposure to water) leads to flow of the postlens tear film into the cornea.

   b. **Postlens tear film patterns** may be observed, when the postlens tear film is thinned, using the biomicroscopic technique of specular reflection. Mottled or colored appearances are characteristic.[32] Conversely, a uniform amorphous appearance is indicative of an aqueous component in the postlens tear film. Particle movement visible in direct illumination is also evidence of an aqueous component to the postlens tear layer.

   c. **Desiccation staining** appears as coarse punctate epithelial erosions in the inferior or central cornea. Minor symptoms of dryness or discomfort may be reported. The mechanism of desiccation staining is thought to be lens dehydration leading to postlens tear film drying and, ultimately, epithelial desiccation.[32]

d. Regarding **management,** an adherent hydrogel lens may be removed from the eye by irrigation of the lens with normal saline or with gentle and repeated stroking of the lens edge with a finger tip. Thinned postlens tear film, desiccation staining, or both occur most often with ultrathin mid- or high-water-content lenses and may be remedied by increasing the lens center thickness or decreasing the water content. The patient may also need to avoid low-humidity environments and practice complete blinking.

3. The presence of the lens can prevent proper tear film formation because of a **surface anomaly,** a disruption to the normal surfacing action of the blink. Both the conjunctival epithelium and overlying mucus layer may be disrupted by desiccation.

a. **Conjunctival staining** due to desiccation is seen as scattered micropunctate defects in the interpalpebral zone; they can be viewed using a combination of illumination and barrier filters. It is usually a benign condition, and patients may be asymptomatic or have symptoms of dryness.

b. **Interpalpebral bulbar hyperemia** can be the patient's presenting complaint, and is most evident if the eyelids are retracted away from the globe. Low-grade interpalpebral hyperemia occurs with most lens wearers and in some cases is associated with desiccation of the conjunctiva.

c. In terms of **management,** a low-grade surfacing anomaly in hydrogel lens wear may not require refitting. Lenses should not have excessive deposits and should have adequate prelens tear film stability. A change to a lens with thinner edge design may be required, such as away from a toric lens or to a low-water-content material. If these measures fail then a reduction in wearing time, advice on environments, or tear supplements may be useful.

REFERENCES

1. Barr JT. A hopeful economy within the contact lens industry. CL Spectrum 1995;10(1):25–30.
2. Thompson TTT (ed). Tyler's Quarterly Soft Contact Lens Parameter Guide. Little Rock, AR: Tyler's Quarterly Publications, 1995.
3. Gellatly KW, Brennan NA, Efron N. Visual decrement with deposit accumulation on HEMA contact lenses. Am J Optom Physiol Opt 1988;65:937–941.

4. Bleshoy H, Guillon M, Shah D. Influence of contact lens material surface characteristics on replacement frequency. ICLC 1994;21:82–95.
5. Haig-Brown G. A clinical study of high-water-content contact lenses in the daily wear regime. Trans BCLA Clin Conf 1985;12–16.
6. Norman C, Wood W, Rigel L, et al. Seven steps to success with disposables. CL Spectrum 1995;10(2):33–40.
7. Tripathi RC, Tripathi BJ, Ruben M. The pathology of soft contact lens spoilage. Ophthalmology 1980;87:365–380.
8. Collins MJ, Carney LG. Compliance with care and maintenance procedures amongst contact lens wearers. Clin Exp Optom 1986;69:174–177.
9. McLaughlin R. Are planned replacement contact lenses "better" than disposables? CL Spectrum 1995;10(7):35–37.
10. Kame RT, Farkas B, Lane I, et al. Patient response to disposable contact lenses worn on a daily disposable regimen. CL Spectrum 1993;8(6):45–49.
11. Nilsson SEG, Soderqvist M. Clinical performance of a daily disposable contact lens: a 3-month prospective study. J Br CL Assoc 1995;18(3):81–86.
12. Edmonds CR. Myopia reduction with frequent replacement of Acuvue lenses. ICLC 1993;20:195–199.
13. Port MJA. NewVues disposable lens: back optic zone radius variations. CLJ 1992;20(3):6–9.
14. Efron N, Veys J. Defects in disposable contact lenses can compromise ocular integrity. ICLC 1992;19:8–18.
15. Snyder C, Hammack GG. Disposable hydrogel lens quality: commentary and clinical report. ICLC 1994;21:79–81.
16. Bruce A, Dain S, Holden BA. Spectral transmittance of tinted hydrogel contact lenses. Am J Optom Physiol Opt 1986;63:941–947.
17. Good GW, Ricer CS. Effect of opaque iris contact lenses upon visual field testing. CL Spectrum 1993;8(3):33–40.
18. Steffen RB, Barr JT. Clear versus opaque soft contact lenses: initial comfort comparison. ICLC 1993;20:184–186.
19. Ghormley NR. Precision UV: a new ultraviolet-blocking disposable soft lens. ICLC 1995;22:3–4.
20. Young G. Soft lens fitting reassessed. CL Spectrum 1992;7(12):56–61.
21. Bruce AS, Brennan NA. Clinical observations of the post-lens tear film during the first hour of hydrogel lens wear. ICLC 1988;15:304–310.
22. Little SA, Bruce AS. Postlens tear film morphology, lens movement and symptoms in hydrogel lens wearers. Ophthalmic Physiol Opt 1994;14:65–69.
23. Bruce AS. Influence of corneal topography on centration and movement of low water content soft contact lenses. ICLC 1994;21:45–49.
24. Roseman MJ, Frost A, Lawley ME. Effects of base curve on the fit of thin, mid-water contact lenses. ICLC 1993;20:95–101.
25. Refojo MF. Rigid Contact Lens Materials and Oxygen Permeability. In HD Cavanagh (ed), The Cornea: Transactions of the World Congress on the Cornea III. New York: Raven Press, 1987;267–271.
26. Ang JHB, Efron N. Carbon dioxide permeability of contact lens materials. ICLC 1989;16:48–58.

27. Ang JHB, Efron N. Corneal hypoxia and hypercapnia during contact lens wear. Optom Vis Sci 1990;67:512–521.

28. Holden BA, Mertz GW. Critical oxygen levels to avoid corneal edema for daily and extended wear contact lenses. Invest Ophthalmol Vis Sci 1984;25:1161–1167.

29. Hoekel JR, Maydew TO, Bassi CJ, et al. An evaluation of the 8.4-mm and 8.8-mm base curve radii in the CIBA NewVue vs the Vistakon Acuvue. ICLC 1994;21:14–18.

30. La Hood D. Daytime edema levels with plus powered low and high water content hydrogel contact lenses. Optom Vis Sci 1991;68(11):877–880.

31. Brennan NA, Carney LG. Optimizing the thickness–water content relationship for hydrogel lenses. CLAO J 1987;13:264–267.

32. Little SA, Bruce AS. Role of the postlens tear film in desiccation staining. CLAO J 1995;21:175–181.

33. Little SA, Bruce AS. Osmotic influences on postlens tear film morphology and lens movement. Ophthalmic Physiol Opt 1995;15:117–124.

34. Golding TR, Harris MG, Smith RC, et al. Soft lens movement: effects of humidity and hypertonic saline on lens settling. Acta Ophthalmol Scand 1995;73:139–144.

35. Golding TR, Bruce AS, Gaterell LL, et al. Soft lens movement: effect of blink rate. Acta Ophthalmol 1995;73:506.

36. Little SA, Bruce AS. Hydrogel (Acuvue) lens movement is influenced by the postlens tear film. Optom Vis Sci 1994;71(6):364–370.

37. Brennan NA, Lindsay RG, McCraw K, et al. Soft lens movement: temporal characteristics. Optom Vis Sci 1994;71(6):359–363.

38. Bruce AS, Mainstone JC. Lens adherence and postlens tear film changes in closed-eye wear of hydrogel lenses. Optom Vis Sci 1996;73:28.

39. Little SA, Bruce AS. Environmental influences on hydrogel lens dehydration and the postlens tear film. ICLC 1995;22:148–155.

40. Fatt I. Water flow conductivity and pore diameter in extended wear gel lens materials. Am J Optom Physiol Opt 1978;55:43–47.

41. Holden BA, Sweeney DF, Cox I, et al. Water in a contact lens material of similar modulus and design prevents lens adherence. Optom Vis Sci 1994(suppl);71:79.

42. Barr J, Stepphen R. Tips to improve your contact lens inspections. CL Spectrum 1995;10(5):26.

43. Bachman WG. Measuring soft contact lens thickness on the eye using an ultrasonic pachymeter. ICLC 1993;20:113–115.

44. Efron N, Brennan NA. The soft contact lens refractometer. Optician 1987;194(5117):29–41.

45. Efron N, Holden BA. A review of some common contact lens complications. 1: The corneal epithelium and stroma. Optician 1986;192(5057):21–26.

46. Bruce AS, Brennan NA. Corneal pathophysiology with contact lens wear. Surv Ophthalmol 1990;35:25–58.

47. La Hood D, Sweeney DF, Holden BA. Overnight corneal edema with hydrogel, rigid-gas-permeable and silicone elastomer contact lenses. ICLC 1988;15:149–154.

48. Terry RL, Schnider CM, Holden BA, et al. CCLRU standards for success of daily and extended wear contact lenses. Optom Vis Sci 1993;70:234–243.

49. Sweeney DF. Corneal exhaustion syndrome with long-term wear of contact lenses. Optom Vis Sci 1992;69:601–608.

50. Lawrenson JG, Doshi S, Ruskell GL. Slit-lamp and histological observations of the normal limbal vasculature and their significance for contact lens wear. J Br CL Assoc 1991;14:169–172.

51. Bruce AS, Brennan NA. Comparison of diagnostic tests in hydrogel extended wear. Optom Vis Sci 1994;71:98–103.

52. Stark WJ, Martin NF. Extended wear contact lenses for myopic correction. Arch Ophthalmol 1981;99:1963–1966.

53. Fleiszig SMJ, Fletcher EL, Lowe R. Microbiology of Contact Lens Care. In ES Bennett, BA Weissman (eds), Clinical Contact Lens Practice. Philadelphia: Lippincott, 1992(36);1–29.

54. Cohen EJ, Gonzalez C, Leavitt KG, et al. Corneal ulcers associated with contact lenses including experience with disposable lenses. CLAO J 1991;17:173–176.

55. Sankaridurg PR, Sharma S, Gopinathan U, et al. *Haemophilus influenzae*: a causative organism in the pathogenesis of contact lens–induced acute red eye. Invest Ophthalmol Vis Sci 1995(suppl);36:S630.

56. Wilcox MDP, Sweeney DF, Sharma S, et al. Culture-negative peripheral ulcers are associated with bacterial contamination of contact lenses. Invest Ophthalmol Vis Sci 1995(suppl);36:S152.

57. Golding TR, Bruce AS, Fletcher EL. Non-ulcerative infiltrative keratitis in RGP daily wear. Clin Exp Optom 1990;73:178–183.

58. Efron N, Wohl A, Toma NG, et al. *Pseuodomonas* corneal ulcers associated with daily wear of disposable hydrogel contact lenses. ICLC 1991;18:46–52.

59. Kotow M, Holden BA, Grant T. The value of regular replacement of low water content contact lenses for extended wear. J Am Optom Assoc 1987;58:461–464.

60. Campbell R, Caroline P. Furrow staining reveals lens tightening. CL Spectrum 1993;8(11):56.

61. Seger RG, Mutti DO. Conjunctival staining and single-use CLs with unpolished edges. CL Spectrum 1988;3(9):36–37.

62. Bruce AS, Golding TR, Wai Man Au S, et al. Mechanisms of dryness in soft lens wear—role of BUT and deposits. Clin Exp Optom 1995;78:168–175.

Chapter 11

Soft Lens Materials

Milton M. Hom

I. **Soft lens polymer components,** or **monomers,** are added to lens material to give it certain properties. When two or more monomers are polymerized together, a **copolymer** is made. Copolymers may be referred to simply as **polymers.** Soft lenses are made from hydrophilic, or "water-loving," copolymers. Most monomers are designed to increase the hydrophilicity, or water contents, of the lens material.

    A. **Dk** is related to water contents. Lenses that are 38% water have a Dk of approximately 9. As water content increases, Dk increases. For a lens of 55% water content, the Dk is approximately 18. A lens of 75% water content has a Dk of approximately 36.[1]

    B. The concept of the **"washing line"** is a simple way to understand soft lens polymers. The "washing line" is a long polymer chain that has many groups—the "wash"—suspended from it. These hydrophilic groups are needed to attract water to the polymer chain. The washing lines are fastened to each other at intervals called cross-linkages. Cross-linking makes the polymer stronger and more stable.[2]

    C. **Hydroxyethylmethacrylate** (HEMA) was the first soft contact lens material. HEMA is the monomer form, and **polyHEMA** is the polymer form; however, polyHEMA can also be referred to simply as HEMA.[2] HEMA is hydrophilic because it contains a free hydroxyl group that can bond with water. The HEMA lens water content is 38%.[3] Lenses with a water content of more than 38% must have other hydrophilic monomers to increase water content above 38% and are not 100% HEMA.[4] As the polymer hydrates, or **plasticizes,** spaces called pores within the lens enlarge and fill with water, and water-soluble substances are allowed in and out of the pores. Higher-water-content lenses have larger pores. Although HEMA is a comfortable material, it has some drawbacks, including fragility, easy soilage, difficult handling when used in low minus prescriptions, low Dk, bacterial adherence, discoloration, and compromise of vision in astigmatic patients.[2,4] Many manufacturers have sought to improve HEMA by adding monomers, but most of the soft lens polymers available today still contain some form of HEMA.

D.   Methacrylic acid (MA) is an organic acid that increases water content in a soft lens polymer. An additional hydroxyl group is added when MA is used. MA is commonly seen in rigid gas-permeable materials as a wetting agent.

E.   N-vinyl pyrrolidone (NVP), sometimes referred to simply as vinyl pyrrolidone, is a hydrophilic monomer. It can be used separately or together with HEMA to form a soft lens copolymer. When combined with another hydrophilic monomer such as HEMA or MA, it increases the water content of the material. NVP has a carboxyl group that binds water with even greater attraction than MA or HEMA.[3,4]

F.   Methyl methacrylate (MMA) adds strength and rigidity to the lens. It is derived from polymethyl methacrylate, the "grandfather" of contact lens materials.[4]

G.   Acrylamide also adds water content to lenses. Like NVP, it contains a carboxyl group that attracts water.

H.   Ethylene glycol dimethacrylate is a cross-linking agent commonly used in contact lens materials.

Pearl: Interested in what the lens is made of? Read the package insert.[4]

II. HEMA-based contact lens materials are common. Many of the soft lenses available today are either 100% HEMA or HEMA copolymers.

A.   HEMA lenses are used by CIBA Vision (Duluth, Georgia) (tefilcon), Bausch & Lomb (Rochester, New York) (polymacon), Ocular Sciences/American Hydron's (South San Francisco, California) Edge and Biomedics, and Wesley-Jessen's Natural Touch (Des Plaines, Illinois).[1]

B.   HEMA lenses with **copolymers** are used to increase water content past 38%.

    1.   HEMA and **NVP** are used together in Bausch & Lomb Toric and Optima Toric (helfilcon A and helfilcon B), Unilens (Unilens, Largo, Florida), and SimulVue (Unilens).

    2.   HEMA, NVP, and **MMA** are polymerized together in CooperVision's (Fairport, New York) Vantage and Preference (tetrafilcon) and in CIBA Vision's Focus, Spectrum, and Newvue (vifilcon A).

    3.   HEMA and **MMA** are found in Wesley-Jessen's Durasoft lenses (phemfilcon A & B) Durasoft materials have a neutral rather than negative surface charge. This decreases the affinity for deposits.

    4.   HEMA and **acrylamide** are in Wesley-Jessen's Hydrocurve lenses (bufilcon A).

    5.   HEMA and **MA** are in Vistakon's (Jacksonville, Florida) 58%-water Acuvue and Surevue (etafilcon A). Sunsoft (Albuquerque, New Mexico), Ocular Sciences/American Hydron (Edge III), and CooperVision (Fairport, New York) also use these copolymers in 55%-water methafilcon. The middle level of water content of both these polymers gives the lenses adequate Dk without the fragility and deposit tendencies of higher-water lenses. Both the Sunsoft and CoastVision toric lenses use thicker prism ballast. A better Dk is required for these thicker areas.

6. **HEMA, NVP,** and **MA** are found in CooperVision's Permalens. Permalens has a very high (71%) water content. Both NVP and MA are added to maximize the water content. The high water content requires a thick lens because the material is very fragile. The material has a great affinity for deposits.

III. **Non–HEMA-based materials** are usually based on vinyl pyrrolidone.

A. **NVP** and **MMA** make up many Bausch & Lomb lenses, including Medalist and FW Toric (lidofilcon A). The NVP supplies a higher (70%) water content because of its strong attraction to water. The MMA gives the material extra strength and resistance to tearing.

B. **Glycerylmethylmethacrylate (GMA)** is used in Wesley-Jessen's CSI and Aztech lenses. Glyceryl gives the material hydrophilicity because each molecule has two hydroxyl groups.[4] MMA is included for rigidity. The MMA monomer imparts better optics than are found in HEMA lenses. GMA produces superior clarity of lensometer mires compared with other soft lens materials. GMA has a small pore size, which makes for better deposit resistance. Before the development of disposable lenses, GMA was the first choice for treating giant papillary conjunctivitis. Unfortunately, there are reports of greater dehydration and fragility with GMA. The manufacturer recommends instilling a wetting drop in the eye before removing the lens. There are also several incompatibilities when this lens is used with certain solutions (see Chapter 13). A new material that may be helpful for dry-eye patients is a combination of **GMA** and **HEMA** made by Benz Research and Development (Sarasota, Florida).[5]

IV. **Soft lens groupings** are used by the U.S. Food and Drug Administration to differentiate the lenses. The groups are based on the lens material. Lenses with less than 50% water content are considered to have low water content, whereas those with more than 50% water are considered to have high water content. All hydrogel lenses have the suffix "filcon."[1]

A. **Group I** includes lenses with low-water, nonionic polymers. Lenses in this group can be disinfected with heat, chemicals, and peroxide. Lenses of 100% **HEMA** are in this group, as are Wesley-Jessen's **CSI** (GMA) lenses.

B. **Group II** includes lenses with high-water, nonionic polymers. They should not be heat-disinfected. Heat cycles over time greatly reduce the life of high-water materials.

C. **Group III** includes lenses with low-water ionic polymers that can be disinfected with heat, chemical and peroxide.[1] Lenses in both groups III and IV contain ionic polymers. The presence of methacrylic acid makes a lens ionic.[6]

D. **Group IV** includes lenses with high-water ionic polymers. Except for the 71% Permalens (perfilcon), this group has lenses with water contents of approximately 55–58%. Most of these lenses contain middle levels of water. Many of the disposable and planned-replacement lenses are in this group, including Acuvue, Surevue, Newvue, Focus, and Spectrum.

    1. **Protein deposition** has been found with group IV materials at a much greater rate than in those of either group I or group III.[7] The presence of MA groups combined with the larger pore size gives these materials great affinity for lysozyme. The prevalence of MA attracts the protein, and the large pores allow great penetration into the lens matrix. The stannate anion used as a stabilizer in peroxide may also contribute to the protein deposition found on group IV lenses.[6]

    2. **Potassium sorbate** or **sorbic acid** preservatives have been reported to discolor this group of lenses.[1] Preservatives of these types should be avoided as a precautionary measure. Group IV lenses should not be heat disinfected, although chemical and peroxide disinfection methods can be safely prescribed.

Pearl: Protein accumulation is more material-dependent, while lipid deposition is patient-dependent.[7]

REFERENCES

1. White P, Scott C. Contact lenses and solutions summary. CL Spectrum 1994(suppl);9(12):1–24.
2. Tighe BJ. Contact Lens Materials. In AJ Phillips, J Stone (eds), Contact Lenses (3rd ed). London: Butterworth, 1989;72–124.
3. Mandell RB. Basic Principles of Rigid Lenses. In RB Mandell (ed), Contact Lens Practice. Springfield, IL: Thomas, 1988;173–202.
4. Hom MM. An inside look at soft lens materials. CL Forum 1985;15(12):38–39.
5. Businger U. GMA/HEMA: first report on a clinical trial. CL Spectrum 1995;10(8):19–25.
6. Sack RA. Harvey H, Nunes I. Disinfection associated spoilage of high water content ionic matrix hydrogels. CLAO J 1989;15(2):138–145.
7. Franklin V, Horne A, Jones L, et al. Early deposition trends on group I (polymacon and tetrafilcon A) and group III (bufilcon A) materials. CLAO J 1991;17(4):244–248.

Chapter 12

Soft Contact Lenses for Astigmatism

Milton M. Hom

I. **Indications** for soft toric lenses are numerous.[1] Toric soft lenses offer clear, comfortable vision and high patient satisfaction. Lenses have never been easier to fit than those presently used, and success rates have never been greater. Unlike with rigid lenses, there is no significant tear lens to compensate for, and complex calculations are not necessary.[2] Toric soft lenses are much easier to fit than toric rigid gas-permeable (RGP) lenses.[3] A typical patient has astigmatism equal to or more than 0.75 D and a desire to wear soft lenses.

A. A **total refractive astigmatism** of 0.75 D or more is an indication for an astigmatic soft lens.[4,5] A sizable 40% of the spectacle-wearing population are potential astigmatic lens candidates.[2]

Pearl: Patients with 0.75 D of astigmatism usually prefer a soft toric over a spherical soft lens.[5]

B. Many of the indications for **soft toric lenses** are the same as those for soft spherical lenses.[2] Common factors include rigid lens intolerance, use in dusty environments, involvement in contact sports, and occasional wear.[1]

C. **Against-the-rule astigmatism** can present physical fit problems for rigid lenses.[1,6] A rigid lens decenters nasally and temporally if the corneal toricity is high enough. Soft lenses in general have better centration than rigid lenses with against-the-rule astigmatism than rigid lenses.

D. A large degree of **internal astigmatism** (also called calculated residual astigmatism or lenticular astigmatism) is corrected well with toric soft lenses.[2,7] The first choice for near-spherical corneas with astigmatism of 0.75 D or more is soft toric lenses.

E. **RGP lenses** are the other major alternative to soft toric lenses.[1] When there are high visual demands and a need for durability and ease of care, RGP lenses may be a better choice. Some refractive errors are better managed with RGP lenses.

1. **Cylindrical errors greater than sphere power** seem to do better with a spherical rigid lens.[6] A typical example would be –0.25 –1.00 × 180. Rotational changes will be more apparent to the patient when there is a large amount of astigmatism relative to sphere power. Visual changes caused by rotation will be more annoying to a patient wearing a soft toric lens.
2. **When refractive astigmatism is less than corneal toricity,** a rigid lens is also preferred.[7] The rigid lens would mask the residual astigmatism and afford better vision. When the refractive astigmatism is greater than corneal toricity, a soft toric lens is preferred.[2] This usually means that internal astigmatism is present. Soft torics correct internal astigmatism effectively.
3. **Poor visual acuity with soft toric lenses** usually indicates a rigid lens.[1] If the soft toric cannot give the patient the desired visual quality, there is a good chance a rigid lens will. Another alternative would be a SoftPerm lens (Wesley-Jessen, Des Plaines, Illinois).

   Pearl: Although visual clarity is better with RGP lenses, most patients prefer soft toric lenses, even for video display terminal work.[8]

4. **Noncoincident axes** between the refractive astigmatism and the corneal toricity can be an indication for a rigid lens.[2] Soft toric lenses tend to align with the primary corneal meridians rather than the refractive axis. This may cause a problem with unwanted lens rotation. A rigid lens circumvents potential rotational problems by masking astigmatism with the tear lens.[7]
   F. The **"four-to-one rule"** is helpful in determining whether a toric lens should be used. The numbers refer to the ratio between spherical and cylinder power. When the spectacle cylinder power is no more than 25% of the sphere power, a spherical lens should be tried first. If spectacle cylinder is more than 25% of the sphere power, a toric is suggested.[9]
II. **Patient selection** for soft toric contact lenses is similar to that used with spherical soft lenses.
   A. **Soft toric lens patients** must possess the same qualities as good candidates for spherical soft contact lenses. Aside from optic considerations, a poor candidate for soft spherical lenses would probably be a poor candidate for soft toric lenses. The problems seen with spherical soft lens wearers (such as poor compliance and deposits) would probably continue to plague a soft toric lens wearer.
   B. **Lids** ideally should have normal lid tension and a wide aperture.[2] Blinking and closure should be complete.
   C. **Poor tear film** and dry eyes are usually the factors that prevent patients from succeeding with these lenses. In some cases, however, a prism-ballasted soft lens can help dry eyes (see Chapter 16).

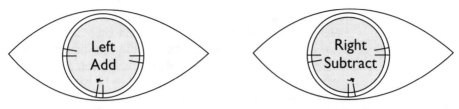

FIGURE 12.1 *LARS is the acronym for left add, right subtract. On the left, the diagnostic lens rotates to the observer's left (clockwise), requiring 10 degrees to be added for compensation. For a spectacle power of –2.00 –1.75 × 180, the ordered power would be –2.00 –1.75 × 10 (180 +10 = 10). On the right, the axis is rotated 10 degrees to the right (counterclockwise) and is subtracted. For a spectacle power of –1.75 –1.75 × 05, the ordered power should be –1.75 –1.75 × 175 (05 – 10 = 175). The new power should orient exactly the same as the diagnostic lens.*

> **Pearl:** *For a with-the-rule dry-eye patient, a prism-ballasted lens takes advantage of the effect of a prism sphere lens. The thicker prism can act to reduce lens hydration.*[10]

III. **Fitting** of toric lenses usually involves diagnostic lenses.[2] Some authors suggest **empirical fitting,** however.[11–13] A typical empirical fit consists of giving the manufacturer the spectacle refraction and K readings to determine the lens required.

   A. **Spherical soft lenses** and toric lenses follow many of the same fitting principles. Lens performance factors such as movement, centration, and lens lag are judged in the same manner.

   B. The **trial lenses** should be as close as possible to the desired power. If there are several lenses to choose from, first select the trial lenses where the cylinder axis is the closest (± 20 degrees). From these similar axis lenses, select the lenses with the cylinder power closest to the desired power, preferably lower than desired. It is better to undercorrect the cylinder power than overcorrect because the ordered cylinder power should be 80–85% of the vertexed spectacle cylinder.[2,14] Finally, the trial lens with the closest spherical power should be chosen from the remaining lenses already selected for cylinder axis and power. Trial lenses should be allowed to equilibrate on the eye for 10 minutes.[15] The extra time is needed to help stabilize the lens rotation.[2]

   C. "Left Add, Right Subtract" **(LARS)** is a method commonly used to determine the final cylinder axis of a toric lens (Figure 12.1). When the trial lens is placed on the eye, the rotation is measured. If the base of the lens rotates 10 degrees to the left, the amount of rotation, 10 degrees, is added to the **final cylinder axis** (Left Add). Rotation to the right requires subtracting the amount from the axis (Right Subtract).

      1. The **rotation** for the ordered lens should be exactly the same as that for the diagnostic lens. Sometimes, the lens will not act as ex-

pected, especially if there is a significant difference in power between the diagnostic and ordered lens. Under the LARS method, the performance of the ordered lens should be treated as another diagnostic factor and the lenses should be reordered again. Past studies have shown it takes an average of 1.4–1.8 lenses per eye to obtain a successful fit.[2,16]

2. **"Chasing the axis"** occurs when the lens orientation is different each time a new reordered lens is placed on the eye. Under these frustrating conditions, it may seem that the correct axis will never be found. This costly fitting situation happens especially with oblique-axis torics.[3] It is to be hoped that the newer, more stable lens designs have reduced the occurrences of "chasing the axis." Some manufacturers offer sample toric lenses the patient can take home for a trial period.

3. **Spherical over-refraction** determines the final spherical power. Cylinder power can also be roughly over-refracted. Setting the cylinder power at the spectacle axis works well if the axes of the diagnostic contact lens and spectacle cylinder are within 20 degrees of each other.[17]

D. **Crossed-cylinder calculations** are another method of determining final power.[18,19] After the trial lens is placed on the eye, a **spherical cylindrical over-refraction (SCO)** is performed.[20] The clinician inputs the precise over-refraction, spectacle prescription, and trial lens power into a programmable calculator to determine the final power. Before programmable calculators were easily available, cumbersome tables were used.[20-22] Many practitioners prefer SCO and a pocket calculator to using LARS. A clear over-refraction endpoint and a toric lens labeled with true specifications are essential for success with this technique. In the early 1980s, soft toric lenses were known as **snowflakes** because, like snowflakes, no two lenses were alike; in other words, reproducibility was poor.[23-25] Manufacturers today offer pocket calculators to simplify crossed-cylinder calculations. Many practitioners using this technique believe that checking lens rotation and LARS are no longer necessary. Based on their experience, they believe that the lenses will not display significant rotation and that SCO is very accurate.[18] A lensometer and trial frame can be used to determine crossed-cylinder powers if a calculator is unavailable. The trial contact lens power and SCO are both applied to a trial frame with loose lenses. The resultant power is neutralized with a lensometer.[26]

Pearl: In "target labeling," a lens vial is labeled as ordered. In "true specification labeling," the vial is labeled with the exact measured lens power.[27] Using a pocket calculator and SCO requires true specification. Make certain you know which method the manufacturer uses.

E. **Flexure effects** of soft toric lenses influence the over-refraction and subsequent lens power. Because of thickness, the front surface does not flex as much as the back surface. This incomplete flexure creates a minus tear lens that requires more plus compensation in the spherical lens power. The cylinder also needs less power and should be reduced.[24,27,28]

F. **Near vision** should be tested as well. Lenses may rotate differently on downgaze and change the vision.[2] Adjusting the cylinder axis may be necessary.

IV. **Special tests** have been developed to enhance soft toric fitting.

   A. The **Becherer twist test** is a useful screening test for soft torics.[1] It helps in determining patient tolerance for the lens rotation commonly seen with toric lenses. Rotate the best cylinder in the phoropter until blur is just noticeable. If less than 5 degrees elicits a response, there is a high level of visual sensitivity. A spherical gas-permeable lens may be a better choice than a soft toric.

   B. **Dialing** in rotation while the lens is on the eye is helpful in checking rotational velocity.[2,24] Rotational velocity is the speed at which a lens returns to the proper position when mislocated. With a finger on the lens, the lens is rotated about 45 degrees. The lens should take no more than 15 seconds to reorient itself in the proper position with blinking. Most people, especially athletes, prefer fast rotational velocities.

   C. **Retinoscopic reflex** can tell a great deal about the optic quality and fit of the lens. Distortion may indicate a steep lens, a flat lens, poor lens optics, or irregular wrapping of the lens to the cornea.[2]

   D. **Overkeratometry** can reveal a steep fit, flat fit, or irregular wrapping.

      1. **Distorted mires** appear only after blinking with a steep fit. For a flat fit, the opposite occurs. The mires clear immediately after blinking and remain distorted at all other times (Figure 12.2).

      2. **Irregular wrapping,** or **draping,** will produce a continuous distortion of the mires. The overkeratometry readings will not correspond to the known corneal toricity and axis.[2] If the diagnostic lens does not show any irregularity, the lens is defective and needs to be replaced.

   E. The **rotation** for use with LARS can be determined with many methods, including measuring with a slit lamp that has measuring reticules and a protractor, a trial frame, and "guesstimation."

      1. **Reticules** are available to place into the slit lamp eyepiece for measurement. This method is highly accurate and easy to perform.

      2. **Protractors** can be etched into the slit lamp focusing rod. The slit is rotated to match the axis mislocation, then measured on the protractor.

      3. **A marked cylindrical trial lens** can be rotated to measure mislocation. A low-power trial lens is marked along the cylinder axis. The patient wears the trial lens in a trial frame while being examined with the slit lamp. The narrow slit beam is rotated to match

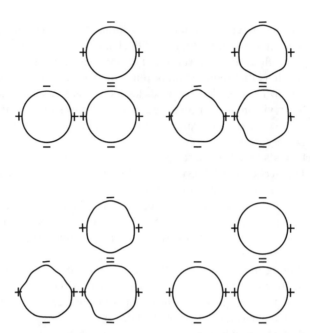

FIGURE 12.2   *Obtaining K readings while the patient is wearing his or her contact lenses (overkeratometry) is useful for diagnosing problems with soft toric lenses. In the top row are the mires for a steep fit. The bottom row are mires for a flat fit. The mires for a steep fit appear clear before blinking (upper left), then distorted after blinking (upper right). The mires for a flat fit appear distorted before blinking (lower left), then clear immediately following the blink (lower right). Mires that appear distorted at all times indicate that the lens has wrapped around the cornea in an irregular manner. A good fit should appear clear at all times, before and after blinking. (Adapted from SB Eiden. Precision management of high astigmats with toric hydrogel contact lenses. CL Spectrum 1992;7[6]:43–48.)*

the mislocation. The mislocation is measured by aligning the marked trial lens to the beam.

4. **"Guesstimation"** is the simplest and probably the most common method of measuring rotation.[2] The clock dial is visualized by the practitioner with each "hour" (space between adjacent numbers, such as 5 and 6) equaling 30 degrees (Figure 12.3). Dividing the hour into three parts produces 10-degree increments. A gross estimate is then made. In addition to being simple and easy to perform, "guesstimation" can be accurate. One study found that mean rotational estimates were within 2 degrees of actual values with no significant differences between the types of marking.[29]

F. **Crossed-cylinder calculations** can be avoided by measuring trial lenses in the lensometer. Trial lenses of the axis and powers of the toric lens

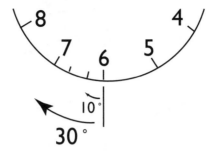

FIGURE 12.3 *"Guesstimation" can be accurate when properly done. The practitioner visualizes a clock dial, with each hour representing 30 degrees. The hour is mentally divided into thirds to produce 10-degree increments.*

and over-refraction can be stacked together and measured directly. This method works well when no programmable calculators are handy.

V. **Methods of stabilization** make toric lenses different from spherical lenses. Different designs are used to prevent rotation and aid stabilization.[30] Many of these designs are very reliable when used in combination with one another.

    A. **Rotational forces** come mainly from the lids. The lids close in a temporal-to-nasal fashion, producing the so-called zipper effect.[31] Rotational influence has been found to be greatest for oblique-axis astigmatism followed by with-the-rule then against-the-rule astigmatism.[32–34] The greatest rotation occurs because the lid meets the thickest part of the edge at an angle, as in the case of an oblique axis.[32] Ocular cyclorotation may also play a role.[35]

    B. **Prism ballast** is a very common method of stabilization. Thickness is added to the inferior lens edge. **Optima** and **Gold Medalist** (Bausch & Lomb [B&L], Rochester, New York), **CSI Toric** (Wesley-Jessen), **Hydrasoft** (CooperVision, Fairport, New York), and **Focus Toric** (CIBA Vision, Duluth, Georgia) make use of prism ballast.[15,26,36,37]

        1. The **"watermelon seed" principle** explains the effectiveness of prism ballast. When pressure is applied from the upper lid, the thickest part of the lens is expelled away. The expelling of the thickened inferior edge stabilizes the lens and helps resist rotation.[38]

        2. **Prism ballast, dynamic stabilization, or both** are commonly used by virtually all the manufacturers.[39] After blink, visual performance is better with a prism-ballasted lens than with dynamic stabilization.[40]

    C. **Truncation** is often combined with prism ballast. Lens material is removed from the lower edge, forming a nonround lens. Older designs, such as **Ocular Science's** (South San Francisco, California) **Zero T** and **Wesley-Jessen's Durasoft 2** and **Durasoft 3** toric lenses, use truncation.

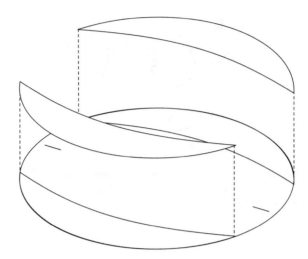

FIGURE 12.4   *Dynamic stabilization. Thin zones are shown above the Torisoft lens by CIBA Vision (Duluth, Georgia). Thin zones are located in the superior and inferior portions of the lens.*

    1.   An **anchoring effect** comes from the lobes or ends of the truncation and the conjunctiva. The truncation creates an adherence effect that helps to stabilize rotation.[2,7]

    2.   **Lower lid contact** with the truncation helps prevent the lens from rotating. The angle of the lid with respect to horizontal is known as the **lid angle** or **lid slope.**[7] If the lower lid is at an oblique angle (lid slope other than 180 degrees), truncation will create mislocation rather than stability. The lens will rotate in an undesirable direction.

D.   **Dynamic stabilization or thin zones** are incorporated into the **CIBA Vision Torisoft** lens. There are two thin zones, one inferior and one superior (Figure 12.4). **Wesley-Jessen's Optifit** and **Signature Toric** also use thin zones.

> *Pearl: Instruct patients with tight lids to apply the lenses to the eye with the markings in the correct position.*[41]

    1.   The **"watermelon seed principle"** also works in dynamic stabilization. Both the upper and lower edges are thinned, creating a biprism effect.[2,38] The lid forces expel the thick portion (along the 180-degree meridian) to hold the thin portions (upper and lower edges) in place, stabilizing lens rotation.

> *Pearl: For an against-the-rule patient, some practitioners prefer a thin-zone over a prism-ballasted design. Thin-zone lenses are*

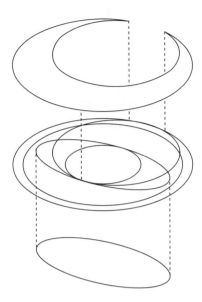

FIGURE 12.5   *The Hydrasoft Toric by CooperVision (Fairport, New York) is prism-ballasted with back surface toricity (posterior toroidal curve). The posterior toroidal curve is shown below the lens. Anterior eccentric lenticulation reduces mass and edge thickness in the Hydrasoft Toric design. The lenticulation is shown above the lens.*

> *thinned superiorly and inferiorly, which complements the thickness distribution of an against-the-rule lens.[10]*

2. **Comfort** is greatly enhanced because the edges are very thin. Comfort is often superior to that of a prism-ballasted lens.[42]
3. That there is **no induced prismatic effect** may be another advantage of dynamic stabilization. Problems due to a vertical imbalance are eliminated because of the absence of prism. One study, however, found that the induced vertical prism imbalance was only one-fourth to one-third of the actual lens prism. And symptoms due to vertical imbalance are rarely reported.[43]

E. **Eccentric lenticulation, chamfer,** and **slab off** on the front lens surface act to thin the edges.[7] The effect of lenticulation reduces lens mass and increases comfort. Lenticulation allows a more uniform edge thickness around the entire lens to effectively decrease lid influence and add stability. In eccentric lenticulation, the zone is decentered **superiorly. Hydrasoft Toric** (CooperVision), **Kontur 55 Toric** (Kontur Kontact Lens, Richmond, California), **Classic Toric** (Sunsoft, Albuquerque, New Mexico), **Preference Toric** (CooperVision), and **Eclipse Toric** (Sunsoft) all use eccentric lenticulation and prism ballast (Figure 12.5). **Optima** (B&L) uses regular lenticulation along with prism ballast.[15]

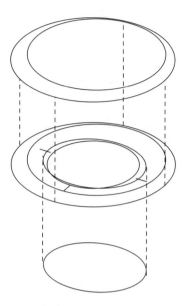

FIGURE 12.6   *The Focus Toric by CIBA Vision (Duluth, Georgia) is pictured in the middle. The lens is stabilized with prism ballast and back surface toricity (posterior toric optic zone). The posterior toric optic zone is shown at the bottom. Because prism ballast adds thickness to the inferior edge of the lens, a circumferential comfort bevel reduces inferior edge thickness and allows a uniform thickness around the lens. The circumferential comfort bevel is pictured at the top.*

    F. **Back surface toricity** allows a more aligned fit and may increase stabilization. Some studies, however, question the effectiveness of back surface toricity for stability.[15,44] Most of the newer designs use back surface toricity in concert with other stabilization methods, most notably prism ballast. **Kontur 55, Metrosoft Toric** (MetroOptics, Austin, Texas), **Ocuflex 55 Toric** (Ocu-Ease, Pinole, California), **Hydrocurve II** (Wesley-Jessen), **Accugel Custom Toric** (Accu-Lens, Carmichael, California), **Optifit Toric** (Wesley-Jessen), **Hydrasoft Toric XW** (CooperVision), **Preference Toric** (CooperVision), and **Focus Toric** (CIBA Vision) have back surface toricity (Figures 12.6 and 12.7).

    G. **Periballast** has prism in the periphery but no prism in the optic zone. The superior portion of a high-minus lenticular carrier is removed, leaving a peripheral ballast. The result is thinner edges all around and reduced mass.

  VI. **Different modalities** and **features** are available in soft toric lenses. Daily wear lenses include **Durasoft 2 Optifit** and **Signature** (both by Wesley-Jessen), **Torisoft** (CIBA Vision), **Optima** (B&L), **Hydrasoft** (CooperVision), **Toric** (Sunsoft), and **Westhin** (Westcon, Grand Junction, Colorado). Extended- or flexible-wear lenses include **Durasoft 3 Optifit** (Wesley-Jessen),

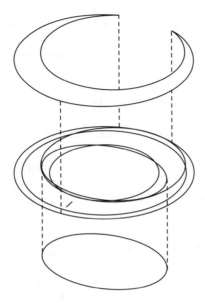

FIGURE 12.7 *Preference Toric by CooperVision (Fairport, New York). The Preference Toric is stabilized with prism ballast and back surface toricity. Below the lens is the toric optic zone located on the back surface. Above the lens is the eccentric lenticular zone on the front surface. It helps to provide a uniform edge thickness.*

Hydrasoft XW and **Hydrocurve series** (both by CooperVision), **Eclipse** and **Toric** (both by Sunsoft), and **Spectrum Toric** (CIBA Vision). Planned replacement torics include **Focus** (CIBA Vision), **Preference** (CooperVision), and **Medalist** series (B&L). Tinted torics include **Durasoft Optifit Toric Colors** (Wesley-Jessen), and **Torisoft SoftColors** (CIBA Vision).

VII. **Troubleshooting soft torics** has become easier in recent years with improved designs and the availability of pocket calculators.

    A. **Stable blurred vision** is a common complaint. It can be due to several factors. One study found that the three leading causes of toric lens reorders were mislocation of axis, power change, and poor visual quality (when over-refraction is not helpful).[11] All three leading causes were related to blurred vision.

        1. **Axis mislocation** occurs for a variety of reasons. Usually the lens rotation is not the same as that of the diagnostic lens. For these cases, think of the mislocating lens as the new diagnostic. LARS or SCO and a calculator can be used to determine the reorder powers.

        2. **Power changes** are best determined with an SCO and calculator.[6] LARS can also be used. The format of the over-refraction should be with cylinder power twice that of the spherical power and with an opposite sign.[31,32,45] The SCO axis is usually between 30 and

60 degrees different from the original axis for lens rotation of less than 30 degrees. Any deviation from this format probably means the lens is mislabeled. The power should be verified. If the SCO does not yield a good endpoint, the fit or quality of the lens should be questioned.[22]

3. Following is an **example** of SCO:

> Contact lens power = −2.00 −1.75 × 175
> SCO = +0.25 −0.50 × 35
> **Crossed-cylinder new power = −2.00 −2.00 × 03**

The SCO follows the proper format. Cylinder power (−0.50) is twice that of the sphere power (+0.25) and of opposite sign.[31,45] The lens should be reordered in the new power.[45]

4. **Verification of lens power** should be performed if there is a deviation from the proper over-refraction format. The lens is blotted, preferably with a coffee filter, and held base-down in the lensometer with the convex side up.[7] A small aperture of 3–4 mm is recommended.[2] The **Tori-Check** (General Ophthalmics, Park Ridge, Illinois) is another helpful device used to hold the lens in place while neutralizing the power.[46]

5. **SCO** and **LARS** can be used together. The result is a very powerful diagnostic tool.[45] Using the information in the earlier example:

> Contact lens power = −2.00 −1.75 × 175
> Lens rotation = 10 degrees left (clockwise)
> Visual acuity = 20/25
> SCO = +0.25 −0.50 × 35
> Visual acuity = 20/20
> **Crossed-cylinder new power = −2.00 −2.00 × 03**

With LARS, the 10 degrees of rotation would be added to the original contact lens power (Left Add), yielding **−2.00 −1.75 × 05.** This result is close to the crossed-cylinder new power of −2.00 −2.00 × 03. Both methods are in approximate agreement and confirm the need to reorder a new power.

Pearl: Axis may need to be rounded to the nearest 5–10 degrees, depending on the manufacturer.[26]

6. **Poor visual quality** that cannot be improved by over-refraction that is due to the nature of soft toric lenses themselves, a steep fit, or a defective lens.[22] If the lens is defective, a replacement is needed. The optics of a prism-ballasted lens degrades vision, and

some patients reject the visual quality of soft lenses.[47] An RGP lens may be a better option. If the lenses are not fitting properly, the base curve should be adjusted.

B. **Unstable blurred vision** can be caused by a steep or flat lens. Both a steep and flat lens can be diagnosed with overkeratometry.

    1. **A steep lens** may show an irregular flexure. The vision will improve immediately after the blink, then be followed by blur. Another indication of steepness is creeping rotation.[2,48] The lens rotates slowly in one direction.

    2. **A flat lens** may rotate erratically, again causing unstable vision, especially with blinking.[10,49]

    3. **For a good fit** with unstable blurred vision, a different design with a different type of stabilization should be tried. The present method of stabilization is probably ineffective.

C. **Edema** and **neovascularization** are a concern because of the thickness of soft toric lenses.[2,50] New vessel growth has been reported in the corneal periphery due to soft toric lenses. A thinner lens or smaller diameter should be used. A double thin-zoned CIBA Vision Torisoft is an excellent option.[50]

REFERENCES

1. Quinn TG. Choosing between soft torics and RGPs. CL Spectrum 1995;10(3):15.
2. Remba MJ, Blaze P. Toric Hydrogel Lens Correction. In ES Bennett, BA Weissman (eds), Clinical Contact Lens Practice. Philadelphia: Lippincott, 1991(41);1–12.
3. Mandell RB. Hydrogel Lenses for Astigmatism. In RB Mandell (ed), Contact Lens Practice (4th ed). Springfield, IL: Thomas, 1988;659–680.
4. Gerber PC. Prescribing soft toric lenses for the low astigmat. CL Forum 1990;11(11):50–53.
5. Dabkowski JA, Roach MP, Begley CG. Soft toric versus spherical contact lenses in myopes with low astigmatism. ICLC 1992;19:252–256.
6. Andrasko G. Are you going soft on astigmats? CL Spectrum 1995;10(3):19.
7. Remba MJ. Clinical evaluation of toric hydrophilic contact lenses. J Am Optom Assoc 1981;52(3):211–221.
8. Snyder C, Wiggins NP, Daum KM. Visual performance in the correction of astigmatism with contact lenses: spherical RGPs versus toric hydrogels. ICLC 1994;21:127–131.
9. Hanks AJ, Weisbarth RE. Troubleshooting soft toric contact lenses. ICLC 1983;10(5):305–317.
10. Quinn TG. Sorting through soft torics. CL Spectrum 1995;10(5):16.
11. Remba MJ. Evaluating the Hydrasoft Toric. CL Forum 1987;12(3):45–51.
12. Lieblein JS, Wells MM. To trial fit torics or not. CL Spectrum 1991;6(4):35–37.
13. Kleinstein RN. Simplified fitting procedures for toric soft contact lenses. J Am Optom Assoc 1984;55(10):777–778.
14. Ewell D. Clinical application of toric soft lenses. CL Forum 1980;5(10):23–29.
15. Ames KS, Erickson P, Medici L. Factors influencing hydrogel toric lens rotation. ICLC 1989;16:221–225.

16. Remba MJ. Clinical evaluation of contemporary soft toric lenses. ICLC 1985;12(5):294–300.

17. Myers RI, Jones DH. Meinell P. Using overrefraction for problem solving in soft toric fitting. ICLC 1990;17:232–235.

18. Purcell H, Teig D, Eiden B, et al. How to fit true specification labeled torics. CL Spectrum 1993;8(8):21–25.

19. Edrington TB, Ackley KD. Evaluation of the Toric Tamer. CL Spectrum 1989;4(3):77–80.

20. Myers R, Castellano C, Becherer D, et al. Lens rotation and spherocylindrical overrefraction as predictors for soft toric evaluation. Optom Vis Sci 1989;66(9):573–578.

21. Myers RI. Off-axis fitting of soft toric contact lenses. Int Eyecare 1985;1(7):486–488.

22. Hallack J. Standard soft toric lenses: a problem of orientation. ICLC 1982;9(4):250–255.

23. Becherer PD, Becherer PF. The expanding role of soft toric CLs. CL Forum 1989;10(5):54–58.

24. Blaze PA, Downs SF. Fitting toric soft lenses in high astigmats. J Am Optom Assoc 1984;55(12):902–904.

25. Payor RE, Robirds SR, Zhang X, et al. Soft toric lens power accuracy and reproducibility. CLAO J 1995;21(3):163–168.

26. Jurkus JM. Toric Soft Lenses. In CA Schwartz (ed), Specialty Contact Lenses: A Fitter's Guide. Philadelphia: Saunders, 1996;42–48.

27. Eiden SB. Precision management of high astigmats with toric hydrogel contact lenses. CL Spectrum 1992;7(6):43–48.

28. McCarey BE, Amos CF. Topographic evaluation of toric soft contact lens correction. CLAO J 1994;20(4):261–265.

29. Snyder C, Daum KM. Rotational position of toric soft contact lenses on the eye—clinical judgments. ICLC 1989;16:146–151.

30. Jurkus JM, Furman DW, Colip MK. Stability characteristics of toric soft lenses. ICLC 1993;20:65–68.

31. Blaze P. Refining toric soft lens correction. CL Forum 1988;13(11):53–58.

32. Holden BA. The principles and practice of correcting astigmatism with soft contact lenses. Aust J Optom 1975;58:279–299.

33. Gundel R. Effect of cylinder axis on rotation for a double thin zone design toric hydrogel. ICLC 1989;16:141–145.

34. Castellano CF, Myers RI, Becherer PD, et al. Rotational characteristics and stability of soft toric lenses. J Am Optom Assoc 1990;61(30):167–170.

35. Baron WS. Cyclorotation impacts on toric contact lens fitting and performance. Optom Vis Sci 1994;71(5):350–352.

36. Ghormley NR. The CSI toric soft lens—a winner. ICLC 1993;20:5–6.

37. Ghormley NR. Gold Medalist toric—a new planned lens replacement soft toric lens. ICLC 1994;21:125–126.

38. Hanks AJ. The watermelon seed principle. CL Forum 1983;8(9):31–35.

39. Lowther GE. Progress with hydrogel toric contact lenses. ICLC 1989;16:159.

40. Tomlinson A, Ridder WH, Watanabe R. Blink-induced variations in visual performance with toric soft contact lenses. Optom Vis Sci 1994;71(9):545–549.

41. Rakow PL. Problem solving with toric hydrogels. CL Forum 1990;11(11):29–36.

42. Hanks AJ, Weisbarth RE, McNally JJ. Clinical performance comparisons of toric soft contact lens designs. ICLC 1987;14(1):16–21.
43. Staarmann T, Andrasko G. Vertical imbalance induced by a unilateral prism-ballasted contact lens. Int Eyecare 1985;1(4):310–314.
44. Tomlinson A, Chang F, Hitchcock J. A comparison of the stability of front and back surface toric soft lenses. Int Eyecare 1986;2(4):218–222.
45. Dishman A, Akerman D, Barron C, et al. Using crossed-cylinders resolution to solve toric soft lens acuity problems. CL Spectrum 1992;7(4):29.
46. Wodis M. Tori-Check—simple method for checking soft toric power. CL Forum 1987;12(3):52–54.
47. Kienast EJ, Malin AH. A clinical study of two toric lenses: the SBH Signature vs. B&L Optima. CL Spectrum 1991;6(10):21–24.
48. Jurkus J, Tomlinson A, Gilbault D, et al. The effect of fit and parameter changes on soft lens rotation. Am J Optom Phys Opt 1979;56(12):734–736.
49. Quinn TG. Troubleshooting with soft toric contact lenses. CL Spectrum 1995;10(7):17.
50. Westin EJ, McDaid K, Benjamin WJ. Inferior corneal vascularization associated with extended wear of prism-ballasted toric hydrogel lenses (a case report). ICLC 1989;16:20–23.

Chapter 13

Soft Contact Lens Care and Patient Education

Milton M. Hom

I. **Soft contact lenses** require cleaning and disinfection. As far back as 1888, Fick boiled glass shells (early contact lenses) before applying them to the eye. Presently, 1-day disposable lenses have brought us closer to the ultimate goal of making cleaning and disinfection obsolete.[1]

A. **Selection** of a care system depends on the past **history** of the patient. Ask what solutions are currently used and why changes, if any, were made in the past.[2] Knowledge of past problems is helpful in choosing a care system.

*Pearl: Having solutions on display is a helpful reminder for patients. The patient can **"point and shoot"** at the brands he or she is using.[3,4]*

B. **Simplifying the number of care systems** prescribed by the practitioner is helpful. Some practitioners use only two systems.[5] One multipurpose solution (**MPS**) regimen and one peroxide system will cover most cases.

C. **Trial lens disinfection** should be done on a regular basis. Lenses can be placed in unpreserved saline, sealed, and heat disinfected. Even high-water-content lenses can withstand an occasional heat cycle.[6,7] ReNu Multi-Purpose Solution (Bausch & Lomb [B&L], Rochester, New York) stored in **inverted** vials can be effective for in-office storage. Digitally cleaning the lens and stopper combined with storage in an inverted position helps ensure an environment free of bacterial growth.[8] The continual antimicrobial effect of a solution such as Softwear saline (CIBA Vision, Duluth, Georgia) may be the best option for storage presently available.

D. **Long-term storage** is best done after heat disinfection. Part of the storage method is allowing the lens to completely air dry. Patients need to carefully rehydrate dried lenses before applying them.[6]

Pearl: A lens that is too old to wear is too old as a spare.[9]

E. **Packaging solutions** in large 3- to 6-month supplies helps reduce purchase confusion.[5] Many practitioners ship the solutions to patients for convenience.

F. **Sterilization** has occurred when all viable microbes have been eliminated. **Disinfection** is substantially reducing the level of microbial contamination. Most lens care systems, with the exception of heat, disinfect rather than sterilize.

G. **Food and Drug Administration (FDA) testing** subjects lens care systems to six challenge organisms: *Pseudomonas aeruginosa, Staphylococcus epidermis, Serratia marcescens, Candida albicans, Aspergillus fumigatus,* and Herpes simplex.

1. A **multi-item microbial challenge test** cultures 20 lenses subjected to microbes after disinfection by the test system. Tested systems must show no growth after a 14-day incubation period.

2. A **contribution-of-elements test** evaluates each step in the disinfection process for its contribution to the overall efficacy of the system.[1] The FDA requires that the entire cleaning system be evaluated as a whole, not just one step at a time.[10] Low-toxicity MPSs rely heavily on the contributions of different elements for complete and effective disinfection.[11] Successful disinfection depends on performing all the cleaning steps in the proper order. Skipping cleaning steps results in incomplete disinfection and can lead to infection.[12]

3. A **D-value test** produces an index of disinfection rate, the time required to reduce a population of organisms by 90%. The lower D values are better.[1,10]

II. **Solution components** serve different functions to make the solution as safe and effective as possible.

A. **Preservatives** are necessary to ensure that a solution remains safe for use after air contact. Preservatives are agents that prevent contamination or decompensation by microorganisms. Weaker components are used in salines, although polyquad (polyquaternium-1) and polyamino propyl biguanide (DYMED) are used in both salines and disinfectants.[13]

1. **Benzalkonium chloride (BAK)** solutions rarely cause problems with rigid lenses. Soft lenses absorb BAK and gradually release it to cause epithelial toxicity, however.[14,15] BAK increases the permeability of epithelial cells because of toxicity. BAK can also disrupt bacterial cell membranes and interfere with intracellular enzymes. Patients who wear soft lenses should avoid solutions containing BAK.[16]

2. **Thimerosal** is a slow-acting, effective disinfecting agent that contains mercury.[17] It kills cells by inhibiting bacterial enzymes and cell membrane functions. Thimerosal is not absorbed by the matrix, but it does adhere to protein deposits.[16] The disinfection effect is enhanced by the presence of disodium ethylenediaminetetraacetic acid **(EDTA)**.[15] Thimerosal is also combined with chlorhexidine for

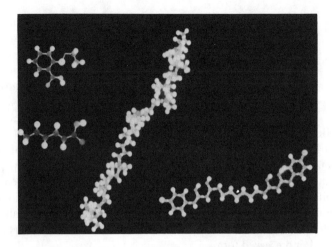

FIGURE 13.1 *Different relative sizes of preservative molecules. Thimerosal is on the upper left, sorbic acid on the left, alkyl trienthanol ammonium chloride on the lower right, and polyquad in the center. As shown, polyquad is a much larger molecule. Neither thimerosal nor alkyl trienthanol ammonium chloride is commonly used as a preservative at the present time. (Reprinted with permission from GE Lowther. Contact Lens Solutions and Care Systems. In JD Bartlett, SD Jaanus [eds], Clinical Ocular Pharmacology [3rd ed]. Boston: Butterworth–Heinemann, 1995;413.)*

disinfection.[18] Because of the high incidence of hypersensitivity, thimerosal has all but disappeared from soft lens solutions.[19]

3. **Sorbic acid** in 0.1% concentration is a bacteriostatic agent that produces a low incidence of hypersensitive reactions.[15] There have been reports that it causes lens discoloration when combined with hydrogen peroxide, however. Sorbic acid is an unstable compound that breaks down into an aldehyde, and it is this that causes discoloration.[20]

4. **DYMED** is a high-molecular-weight preservative that alters the phospholipid groups found in bacterial cell walls.[18] There is some absorption into the soft lens matrix.[16]

5. **Polyquad** is another preservative whose high molecular weight prevents it from being absorbed into the contact lens matrix (Figure 13.1). It resembles BAK in composition and action, but it does not cause adverse effects.[18,21]

B. **Buffers** are necessary to keep the pH within a normal range of 6–8. Tears have a natural phosphate buffer to maintain pH. Buffering chemicals can be identified by the suffix "-ate" on the label.[22] A weak acid or base and its corresponding salt make up the buffer in a solution. The borate buffer commonly found in some solutions consists of boric acid and sodium borate. Borate also has some antimicrobial benefits. Other buffers used are bicarbonate and citrate.[18,23] A low pH causes lenses (especially high-water-content, ionic lenses) to lose hydration and change shape.[21,22]

Pearl: If lenses cause discomfort or lens properties change, check for outdated or long-opened solutions. Solutions commonly have an acidic drift over time.[24-26]

III. **Salines** are used for wetting, rinsing, storage, and application of the soft contact lens. Salines are made to resemble tears. They are **isotonic** with tears, containing 0.9% NaCl, and have a pH between 7.0 and 7.4. Low-pH (acidic) salines can cause stinging when applied to the eye.[27] They were originally available in salt tablet form, and the patient had to prepare the homemade solution with distilled water. Although economical, homemade saline carries a high risk of ***Acanthamoeba*** infection. Present salines are available in unpreserved or preserved forms.

   A. **Nonpreserved saline** is available as unit doses or in aerosol cans. Aerosol offers the best preservation of sterility. Sensitized patients benefit the most from unpreserved salines.

   B. **Preserved saline** is available in multidose containers.[28] Preserved salines last much longer than nonpreserved salines when exposed to air.

      1. **Common preservatives** currently in use are polyquad (Opti-Soft by Alcon, Fort Worth, Texas) and DYMED (ReNu and Sensitive Eyes Plus by B&L). Sorbic acid is used in Alcon's Saline Solution Especially for Sensitive Eyes and B&L's Sensitive Eyes. Potassium sorbate is used in SOFT-MATE Saline by Allergan (Irvine, California).[29]

      2. **SoftWear Saline** by CIBA Vision relies on an antimicrobial buffer system that provides natural protection from contamination without sensitizing the patient.[30,31] The carbon dioxide from the atmosphere causes formation of trace amounts of hydrogen peroxide from the borate buffers in the solution. The trace amounts provide antimicrobial action while being nontoxic to the eye. Sensitivities have not been a significant problem. There have been recent anecdotal reports to the contrary, however.[30,32]

IV. **Daily cleaning** and **surfactant cleaning** are important to remove grime and bacteria adhering to the lens.[10] They have been called the most important step in the care system because it significantly reduces the microbial hazards of contact lenses.[1,33] Daily cleaning greatly enhances the disinfection step. Surfactant cleaning is designed to be used on a daily prophylactic basis.[34]

   A. **Surfactants** in the cleaner emulsify lens debris, allowing the contaminants to be rinsed away.[28] Active rubbing with a daily cleaner for 20 seconds followed by rinsing is recommended. **Rubbing and rinsing** reduces the bioburden by about 3 log units.[35,36] In investigating cases of *Pseudomonas* with daily disposable lenses, Efron found evidence that elimination of the rub-and-rinse step is a pervasive factor in cases of ulcerative keratitis.[37]

Pearl: If foaming is present during hydrogen peroxide disinfection or enzyme cleaning, the lens was not thoroughly rinsed after daily cleaning.[38]

B. **Cleaning solutions** contain detergents (ionic and nonionic), wetting agents, chelating agents, buffers, and preservatives.
C. The **recommended procedure** for cleaning is to place the lens in the palm of the hand, rinse with saline, apply the daily cleaner, rub, then rinse thoroughly with saline.[38] Remembering to place the lens in the palm of the hand is important, as rubbing between fingers can cause lens damage.[28]

Pearl: Use simple instructions when teaching the patient: Rub the lens thoroughly as you would rub a casserole dish, rinse the lens as you would rinse a glass just washed with detergent, and soak in totally fresh solution.[14]

D. **Opti-Clean** by Alcon has polymeric beads that provide abrasive action when the lens is rubbed. The cleaner must be shaken prior to use because the beads usually settle at the bottom of the container. **Opti-Clean II** and **Opti-Free Daily Cleaner** are both preserved with polyquad.[15,38] The newer Opti-Free Daily Cleaner has fewer beads for easier rinsing because Opti-Clean required large amounts of saline for removal.[5,30]
E. **MiraFlow Extra-Strength Cleaner** by CIBA Vision contains isopropyl alcohol (20%). The alcohol makes the cleaner very effective, especially for lipid depositors.[38] Lenses should be rinsed quickly because the cleaner may induce parameter changes.[30]
F. **Sorbic acid** is found in Alcon's PreFlex and Pliagel, B&L Sensitive Eyes Daily Cleaner, and CIBA Vision Cleaner.[29]

*Pearl: **Insufficient rubbing and insufficient rinsing** are two significant errors in lens care.[39]*

V. **Disinfectants** inactivate the microorganisms present in contact lenses. There are basically three types of disinfection: heat, chemical, and chemical hydrogen peroxide.
A. **Heat disinfection** is a simple and highly effective method of disinfection.[38] A heat unit disinfects the lenses for the proper amount of time and temperature (10 minutes at 80°C). Continual heating of the polymer, however, shortens lens life and bakes on deposits. High-water-content lenses especially do not withstand repeated heat disinfection very well. Other drawbacks are power requirements and nonfunctioning units. Despite these disadvantages, some practitioners still prefer heat disinfection because of its superior effectiveness against microbes.[11]

B. Chemical disinfection is convenient and widely available. Four-hour soak times after daily cleaning are usually recommended. Chemical disinfection is more costly than heat. Some patients practice "topping off" the lens case each day to save solution. Unfortunately, this diminishes the disinfection effect. Used solution must be replaced with fresh solution during each cleaning cycle. Other than cost, the major disadvantages of chemical disinfection are solution reactions.

Pearl: A bottle of saline should last the patient 1 month. A patient who uses a new bottle every 2 to 3 months may be "topping off."

   1. **Fewer reactions** occur with large-molecule chemical disinfectants such as **DYMED** and **polyquad.** These disinfectants are present in lower concentrations and consequently avoid the risk of toxicity. **Toxicity** occurs when the preservative cannot differentiate between the microbes and epithelial cells.[1] Both DYMED and polyquad are not very effective against fungi and *Acanthamoeba*.[40]

   Pearl: A major goal for solutions is that they not be harmful or cause sensitization while promoting good disinfection.[41]

      a. **DYMED** is the disinfectant found in **ReNu Multi-Purpose Disinfection Solution** by B&L.[15,38]
      b. **Polyquad** is the main preservative in **Opti-Soft** and **Opti-Free** by Alcon.[15,38] At one time, use of CSI lenses (Wesley-Jessen, Des Plaines, Illinois) with Opti-Soft would cause keratitis. Opti-Soft was reformulated to solve this incompatibility. The reformulated solution is Opti-Free.[14]
   2. **Chlorhexidine** disrupts bacterial cell membranes. It binds to protein deposits, is absorbed by the lens matrix, and has little effect on fungi.[16] When used alone, the kill time is slow, with a minimum soak of 10 hours.[18] **SOFT-MATE Disinfecting Solution** (Allergan) containing chlorhexidine, when directly compared with DYMED and polyquad, was the only solution effective against *Serratia marcescens* within 4 hours, however.[42] It is not commonly used for soft lenses anymore because of past hypersensitivity reactions.[15] Presently, it is commonly seen in rigid gas-permeable (RGP) lens solutions. Alcon's **Flex-Care** once contained chlorhexidine.[38]
   3. **Quaternary ammonias** and thimerosal are used in **Allergan Hydrocare Cleaning and Disinfecting solution.** [18,43] There were reports of incompatibilities when used with CSI lenses.[14]
C. Chemical hydrogen peroxide is an **oxidative system** that has none of the sensitizing elements seen with other chemical disinfection systems.[44] Hydrogen peroxide has been shown to be the most effective system in regi-

men challenge studies.[17] The decompensation of hydrogen peroxide produces a highly reactive and chemically promiscuous free radical that produces rapid and effective bactericidal action. The free radicals convert to water and oxygen.[45,46] Daily cleaning and rinsing are necessary prerequisites to ensure that lens debris does not interfere with the disinfection.[45] Although sometimes complicated to use, it is the system of choice for hypersensitive patients.[18] Soaking times are commonly 10 minutes to overnight. Hydrogen peroxide, in itself, is highly irritating to the eye and needs to be neutralized after disinfection. Residual amounts after neutralization are 1 ppm for catalase, 1.8–15 ppm for platinum, and 200 ppm by dilution.[13] Peroxide is effective against **human immunodeficiency virus (HIV)**, but can not disinfect cystic *Acanthamoeba*.[12] Soaking for about 2.4 hours is effective against **fungi,** but the shorter soak times seen in systems such as the **AOsept Disinfection System** (CIBA Vision) showed poor performance.[47] Available peroxide systems vary in the their methods, type of neutralization, and level of convenience.[45]

1.   **ULTRACARE** by Allergan uses a coated catalase-neutralizing tablet that time-releases over a 2-hour period.[38] The disinfection solution turns into a pink indicator color when the tablet is added. An older Allergan system is **OXYSEPT,** which is neutralized with the **Oxytab.**[30]

2.   The **AOsept Disinfection System** neutralizes the peroxide with a platinum catalyst disc. The disc needs replacement every 3 months or 90 uses.[38,45] The previous **Septicon** system was a two-step process. The lenses were first soaked in Lensept (peroxide) (CIBA Vision) and then transferred to saline and platinum disc for the second neutralization step. AOsept uses a simpler one-step process. The platinum disc and lenses are placed in AOsept (peroxide and salt) and neutralized into saline. Neutralization by disc is also found in CIBA Vision's new peroxide system, **PureEyes.**

3.   The **CONSEPT system** by Allergan has an additional surfactant cleaner combined with 3% hydrogen peroxide (CONSEPT 1). After disinfection in CONSEPT 1, the lenses are neutralized by CONSEPT 2. CONSEPT 2 contains sodium thiosulfate. The lenses are disinfected in the Hydramat II (Allergan), a handy "hands-off" cleaning device that enhances cleaning activity by agitation of the lenses in solution.[48]

4.   **MiraSept** by Alcon uses chemical neutralization with sodium pyruvate. MiraSept Disinfecting Solution (Step 1) contains peroxide. MiraSept Rinsing and Neutralizing Solution (Step 2) contains sodium pyruvate.[29,38]

5.   **Temporary disinfection** rather than continuous action is a drawback of peroxide. Chemical disinfectants maintain bacteria populations during storage of the lenses. Neutralized hydrogen peroxide

systems show extremely large increases in bacteria during storage of the lenses.[49] Lenses need redisinfection if stored for more than 7 days with peroxide.[13] For **long-term storage,** the complete sterilization effect of heat is the best.[50]

   D.   **Chlorine tablets** are convenient, but there are problems with bleaching tinted lenses, and they are ineffective against fungi.[11]

VI.   **Wetting agents** are used for the dryness associated with contact lens wear. Preservatives commonly used are thimerosal (Allergan's LENS WET and B&L's Lens Lubricant), polyquad (Alcon's Opti-Tears, Opti-One and Opti-Free Rewetting drops), and sorbic acid (B&L's ReNu Rewetting and Sensitive Eyes).[15,29]

   A.   **LENS PLUS Rewetting Drops** by Allergan is available in unit dose form and has no preservatives. It is packaged in several single-use vials.

   B.   **Poloxamer 407** is used as a viscosity builder and wetting agent for artificial tears. It has mucomimetic (mucuslike) properties and is found preserved with sorbic acid in Alcon's Clerz 2 and CIBA Vision's Lens Drops.[15,38]

   C.   **Polyvinyl alcohol** helps the solution spread across the corneal surface.[18] It is commonly used in RGP lens solutions.

VII.   **Enzyme cleaners** hydrolyze the proteins left behind by daily cleaning.[1] Enzymes in tablet form are dissolved into saline or hydrogen peroxide. Hydrogen peroxide, heat, or rinsing deactivates the enzyme.[34] Enzyme cleaning is normally done on a weekly basis. Chlorhexidine can be problematic when used with enzyme cleaners.[14]

   A.   **Papain** was the first enzymatic cleaner for contact lenses. The papain in **ALLERGAN ENYMATIC Contact Lens Cleaner** is from papaya. Papain has been shown to remove heavy deposits more effectively than pancreatin.[51,52] Despite better effectivity against protein, papain produced significantly more ocular discomfort than pancreatin.[52] Shorter soaking times are recommended for high-water-content lenses because of reported adverse reactions.[2,18] The enzyme is neutralized by rinsing or heat disinfection (if utilized).

   B.   **Pancreatin** is found in Alcon's **Opti-Free Enzymatic Cleaner** series. It comes from the pancreas of hogs or oxen. Pancreatin has additional lipase and amylase for better efficacy against lipid and mucoid deposits.[34] Enzymatic cleaning can be combined into a one-step process with simultaneous disinfection in Opti-Free.[30]

   C.   **Subtilisin-A** is an enzyme made from the controlled fermentation of *Bacillus lichenformis*.[15] **ReNu Enzymatic** series by B&L, **ULTRAZYME** by Allergan, and **Enzyme Plus Surfactant Cleaner** by Allergan are all made of subtilisin-A.[53,54] ULTRAZYME can be used for a variety of lenses and is optimized for use in 3% hydrogen peroxide.[34,55] Enzyme Plus Surfactant Cleaner has a surfactant poloxamer 338 added for better cleaning.[54]

VIII.   Patients prefer an **MPS** because of ease and convenience.[56,57] One solution is used for rubbing, rinsing, and disinfection. It has been shown that use of an

MPS does not completely guarantee compliance in itself, however. Careful patient training and frequent reinforcement of proper lens-handling techniques are still necessary.[58]

A. **ReNu Multi-Purpose Solution** by B&L uses DYMED (polyamino-propyl biguanide) and has poloxamine for deposit resistance. The solution has an effective surfactant and is nonirritating.[59]

B. **Opti-One Multi-Purpose Solution** by Alcon contains polyquad citrate. The citrate buffer competes with proteins for lens binding sites. It also chelates and sequesters calcium.[14,60] Comparative studies have shown citrate to enhance cleaning efficacy. The cleaning effect of the citrate buffer continues even during the passive disinfection soak.[60] Other MPSs with polyquad are Opti-Free and Opti-Soft (both by Alcon Laboratories).

C. **QuickCARE** by CIBA Vision is actually two solutions, a starter solution followed by a finishing solution. The starter solution is hypertonic, with surfactants and isopropyl alcohol. Ten drops of the starter solution are rubbed onto the lens for 30 seconds. The lens is then rinsed with the finishing solution and placed into the case for at least 1 minute. The finishing solution is a saline solution not unlike CIBA Vision's SoftWear saline. The entire cycle should take about 5 minutes.[61] The QuickCARE starter solution (CIBA Vision) has a decided speed advantage over other MPSs. Eighty percent of the challenge organisms were killed in 1 minute during one study. This compares with 2–24 hours for other MPSs.[62] QuickCARE is also effective against *Acanthamoeba*.[14] One drawback, however, is the reluctance of patients to rub the lenses with the starter solution.

D. **COMPLETE Brand Multi-Purpose Solution** by Allergan contains the preservative polyhexamethylene biguanide (TrisChem). COMPLETE also contains tromethamine and tyloxapol, a surfactant. Patient response is similar to that for ReNu, although COMPLETE contains slightly more of the same preservative as ReNu.[14]

E. **SOLO-CARE** is a new MPS by CIBA Vision. It is preserved with polyhexanide with poloxamer 407 as the surfactant.

IX. **Microwave irradiation** has been studied as a form of disinfection. Five minutes of microwave irradiation in vented saline-filled cases were sufficient to kill microorganisms. Lens parameters were not clinically affected over an equivalent of 6 months of time.[63]

X. **Purilens** (American Vision, New Jersey) uses ultraviolet light and subsonic turbulence to clean and disinfect.[64] Ultraviolet light is an effective germicidal agent.[65] The lenses are placed in preservative-free saline for a 15-minute cycle. A 3-month study showed no severe eye complications and high patient satisfaction.[66]

XI. **Standing waves** apply strong, vertically directed vibrational energy to clean lenses. Allergan's Hydramat II device and lenses are placed into the SOFT-MATE Automatic Cleaning Unit for a 12-minute cycle. Standing waves are effective for daily cleaning but not for disinfection.[67,68]

XII. **Cycling lenses** is a method of prolonged (7-day) cleaning to extend the life of the lens instead of replacing it. Two sets of lenses are ideal for this system. One set is worn; the other is soaked in a Hydramat with Allergan's SOFT-MATE Protein Remover for 5 days. Prior to and following the soak, the lenses are agitated for 30 seconds. Lenses are then disinfected for 24 hours with Allergan's CONSEPT system, followed by a fresh overnight soak in CONSEPT 2. The cleaning cycle lasts for 7 days and is alternated between the two pairs of lenses.[69]

XIII. **Contraindications** and **reactions** related to care systems include toxicity, sensitivity, allergy, lens-solution interaction, solution-solution interaction, parameter changes, and compliance issues.[1]

    A. **Solution reactions** result in red, irritated eyes when the patient wears the contact lenses. Reactions are often accompanied by conjunctival chemosis, injection, infiltration, a follicular or papillary response, and staining.[1]

        1. **Thimerosal** hypersensitivity has been reported in up to 50% of patients.[16]

            a. **Superficial punctate keratopathy (SPK)** and an injected eye usually results from a solution reaction. There can be **corneal infiltrates,** usually sterile in nature, located at the limbal area.[28,70] **Pseudodendritic lesions, neovacularization,** and **epithelial opacification** are sometimes present.[70]

            b. **Switching** to preservative-free solutions and hydrogen peroxide disinfection is the best treatment. Replacing with fresh lenses is ideal but not necessary. The lenses can be **purged** of sensitizing chemicals by several cycles of heat disinfection in distilled water or hydrogen peroxide followed by a final cycle in unpreserved saline.

        2. **Chlorhexidine** is more likely to cause reactions when lenses are protein-coated and poorly rinsed.[14]

    B. **Deposits** are the most important reason for lens replacements.[28] Deposits from tears commonly bind to the lens surface. The components of the tear film adhere and begin to impregnate into the polymer as soon as the lens is applied to the eye.[71]

        1. **Pellicle** is the mucoprotein coating on the lens surface. The pellicle begins to form 1 minute after lens application. Despite regular cleaning, the pellicle continues to form as new layers are laid down over old layers. Unfortunately, not only lens performance is compromised, but there is also a risk of bacteria adherence to the pellicle.[28] Ionic polymers have greater pellicle formation than nonionic polymers. Extended wear produces more pellicle formation than daily wear, making frequent replacement desirable.[71]

        2. **Rudko classification** is used to evaluate lens deposits. A lens removed from the eye is held against a dark background. A beam of light illuminates the lens edge from the side. The lens is typed as I,

II, III, or IV depending on the amount of visible deposits. Type I
has no visible deposit with 15× magnification. Type II indicates a
visible deposit on a wet lens with 15× magnification. Type III
shows a visible deposit on a dry lens without magnification. Type
IV shows a visible deposit on a wet lens without magnification.[71]

3. **Lipid deposits,** also called **jelly bumps** or **lens calculi,** are commonly seen with high-water extended-wear lenses. Lipid deposits
   often involve the lens matrix and leave a hole or dent when removed.[72] The lipid forms first and is sometimes followed by a secondary **calcium deposit.** Patients with lipid deposits usually have a
   tear film potassium deficiency. Other risk factors for lipid deposits
   include dry eyes, meibomian gland dysfunction, high-fat diets,
   medications affecting tear film, and alcohol consumption.[71] Disposable lenses, dry-eye therapy, and potassium-containing solutions are effective treatment strategies.

4. **Protein coatings** affect visual acuity and comfort. The proteins in
   tears are normally clear, but they denature and adhere to lenses.
   The denatured proteins are no longer clear and can obscure vision.
   An familiar example occurs during heating of an egg; when heated,
   the clear part of the raw egg becomes opaque because the protein
   denatures. Coatings consist of denatured proteins loosely adherent
   to the lens surface and appear hazy.[71]

   a. **Lens haze** has been reported in group IV lenses and peroxide
      disinfection. The sodium stannate found in peroxide is a con-
      tributing factor. Stannate is used to remove trace contaminants
      in peroxide to prevent decomposition.[73]

   b. Giant papillary conjunctivitis (GPC) is associated with lens
      soilage. The altered proteins can be a primary cause of an anti-
      genic response such as GPC.[74] Lenses with heavy coatings
      should be replaced.[71]

5. **Rust spots** appearing as a circular orange-red deposits usually result from use of tap water to clean lenses.[30]

6. **Infection** may be a higher risk when lenses have deposits because
   bacteria may adhere to deposits.[10]

7. **Mascara** appears as an iridescent filmy or greasy deposit on lens
   surfaces. Reminding patients to wash their hands before handling
   lenses is very helpful.[30] Mascara in the form of lash thickeners is
   especially troublesome because of their fiber content. Make-up containers can also harbor infectious bacteria colonies and should not
   be shared.[75] Cosmetics are best applied after application of lenses.
   Lenses should be removed before any removal of make-up.[76]

8. **Intensive cleaning** can be performed by heating the lens in a solution containing demineralized water, alcohol (ethanol), citric acid,
   acetic acid, hydrogen peroxide, and hydrochloric acid. For lenses

of more than 45% water, the alcohol and hydrochloric acid are omitted.[72] Keep in mind that these are in-office techniques.

C. **Lens discoloration** has been described in a number of lens and solution combinations.[14] Sorbic acid or potassium sorbate causes discoloration as the solution ages and after absorbing protein. It is not a good idea to store group IV lenses in these salines.[16] Thimerosal with heat can cause lenses and cases to blacken. Hydrogen peroxide (brown-bottle type) can turn lenses pink or other colors. Benzyl peroxide and chlorine from a pool can cause fading of tinted lenses. Accidental instillation of fluorescein while the patient is wearing lenses will cause discoloration, but it can sometimes be removed by soaking the lenses in hydrogen peroxide.[14]

D. **Lens precipitates** occur when preservatives of opposite charge are mixed together. Cationic disinfectant preservatives such as chlorhexidine, polyquad, and DYMED should not be mixed with anionic preservatives such as sorbic acid surfactant cleaners.[23,77]

   1. **Gel precipitates** are sometimes produced when polyvinyl alcohol interacts with borate buffer solutions.[14]
   2. **Chlorhexidine** has been known to cause a fine black precipitate when placed into 3% hydrogen peroxide.[38,77]
   3. **Catalase** can gum up the platinum disc if placed into the case.
   4. **Phosphate-buffered peroxides** (AOsept, OXYSEPT) can form calcium phosphate precipitates.
   5. **Poloxamer 407** (MiraFlow and Pliagel) and Allergan SOFT-MATE Cleaner can cause cloudy precipitates when mixed together.[77]

E. **Lens parameter changes** can occur when AOsept patients use Lensept or OXYSEPT. After disinfection with these solutions, their lenses are shaped like a taco. The lens changes shape because it has been soaking in water, not saline. Resoaking the lens in saline will help it resume its normal shape.[14] Group IV lenses with methacrylic acid will also change parameters when soaked in peroxide for long periods.[38] Soaking lenses in cleaners containing alcohol also changes parameters.[30,38]

F. **Lens clouding** has been seen when ReNu Thermal Enzymatic cleaner (B&L) is heat disinfected with CSI and Aztech lenses (both by Wesley-Jessen). Reformulation of the enzyme has since cleared up the problem. Surface haziness has been shown when group IV lenses disinfected with a one-step system (AOsept) are switched to a two-step system.[77]

G. **Staining** has been reported when Allergan's **ACDS** and Alcon's **Opti-Soft** was used with CSI (crofilcon) lenses.[14] Irritation has been reported when protein-coated lenses are used with chlorhexidine-preserved solutions.

   1. **Keratitis** can develop when enzyme cleaners are switched. One case involved the use of Allergan Enzymatic tablets in AOsept instead of ULTRAZYME (also by Allergan). A chemical keratitis was the result.[78]

2. **Switching chemical disinfectants** can result in undesirable combinations and increase penetration into the cornea.[77] One example is filling a case with chlorhexidine and topping it off with Allergan's ACDS.[23]

3. **Hydrogen peroxide disinfection** can cause keratitis. The keratitis appears as a wide horizontal formation of small punctate lesions that stain in the inferior paracentral cornea. Switching patients to a peroxide system that uses a catalase neutralization step from a catalytic disc solves the problem. The keratitis takes about 7–10 days to resolve.[46]

H. *Acanthamoeba* cause a severe infection that can result in necrotizing stromal melt and corneal perforations. Corneal transplants are needed if the disease is not treated early.[28] Acanthamoeba comes in two forms: the vegetative (trophozoite) and cyst form. The cyst form is more resistant to disinfection than the trophozoite. Thorough rubbing and rinsing can remove both the trophozites and cysts.[12]

1. **Ionic, high-water-content lenses** (group IV) lenses showed the greatest *Acanthamoeba* adherence. Low-water-content, nonionic lenses had significantly lower adherence.[79]

2. **Low-tonicity environments,** such as fresh or pool water, break down the epithelial fluid barrier with edema. This may be the crucial factor in increasing the risk of *Acanthamoeba* keratitis. There is a connection with fresh water exposure such as **tap** or **hot tub water** with this infection.[80]

Pearl: Tap water alone should never be used with soft lenses.[1]

3. **Heat disinfection** is completely effective against the cysts. Heat is not compatible with many lenses, however.

4. **MiraFlow,** with 20% isopropyl alcohol, is highly effective. Because the **QuickCARE** starter solution (CIBA Vision) is similar to Miraflow, it is also effective. Solutions containing **thimerosal** are effective as well. **ReNu** and **Opti-Free** show poor antiacanthamoebal activity.[40] **Hydrogen peroxide** is not very effective.[81]

I. **HIV** collects in contact lenses. Patients should be cautioned against using lenses worn by HIV-infected individuals. For acquired immunodeficiency syndrome patients, contact lens wear may not be appropriate because the lenses themselves can act as a highly desirable medium for bacteria.[28]

J. **Soft contact lens toxic occlusion phenomenon** is a rare reaction appearing as central deep stromal edema, epithelial edema, or both. Type I cases experience foggy vision. Type II cases may have foggy vision with moderate discomfort and photophobia. The causes are unknown, but it may be related to eucalyptus spray exposure in steam baths.[82]

   K. Discomfort from solutions can occur when the solution pH is acidic,
       when the lens cleaner or enzyme has not been rinsed off, when too much
       residual peroxide remains, or when solution tonicity is not right.[38]
XIV. Patient education is necessary to ensure compliance with proper lens care
       procedures.[48] Compliance in itself is a problem. According to a B&L study,
       35% of contact lens wearers think saline is for disinfection, 37% do not clean
       and disinfect as they should, and 47% use products not recommended by the
       practitioner.[83] Continual patient education is the key to combating noncom-
       pliance. Over time, even an enthusiastic patient can become bored, compla-
       cent, and forgetful about proper lens care.[29,84,85]

*Pearl: Even in life-and-death situations, noncompliance is a problem. Half
of all patients taking medications have been found to be noncompliant.[4]*

   A. Factors that reduce compliance are complicated regimens, cost, patient
       misunderstanding, and poor patient-clinician relationship.[39] Practition-
       ers are legally liable and should provide every reasonable means for pa-
       tients to follow appropriate care procedures.[86] Writing down the names
       of the solutions patients should use is imperative.[4] Printed materials,
       videotapes, and constant review are helpful.[87] Alternative solutions for
       use when the first choices are unavailable can be listed for the patient
       on a printed handout.[4,88–90] Unfortunately, the longer a patient wears
       lenses comfortably without proper care, the more he or she feels the doc-
       tor overemphasizes it needlessly.[85]

*Pearl: Have the patient **tell you how** he or she is disinfecting lenses during follow-up. Don't simply ask if the patient has been disinfecting.[84,85,89]*

   B. Proper application and removal are important for successful contact
       lens wear.
       1. Hands must be washed before handling the lenses. Hand washing
           with an antibacterial soap significantly reduces bacterial contamina-
           tion of lenses.[91] Patients should be told to avoid soaps that contain
           lanolin or oil. The lens should first be **visually inspected** for nicks,
           cracks, and tears. The lens is then placed on the tip of the **index finger**
           with adequate moisture.[34] Too much moisture, however, will cause the
           lens to adhere to the finger and make application more difficult. The
           patient should make certain the lens is not **inside-out.** The edges of
           an inside-out lens will appear flared out. An inside-out lens can pro-
           duce discomfort, slightly reduced vision, and excessive movement.[30]

*Pearl: Patients follow the practitioner's example. If you do not fol-
low proper procedure (hand washing, for example), do not expect
the patient to follow your instructions.[4]*

2. **Application** of the soft lens can be done with the scleral or corneal method. The normal procedure is to always apply and remove the **right lens first.** This avoids reversal of lenses. A mirror can be helpful.[92]

   a. In the **corneal method,** the patient looks directly at the lens (centrally) during application. Usually, the upper lashes (not the lids) are held open with one hand. On the other hand, the middle finger holds the lower lashes and the index finger holds the lens. The lens is placed onto the cornea.

   b. **The scleral method** is preferred by practitioners. The method is similar to the corneal method with the exception that the patient fixates up or down while placing the lens on the sclera.[34,92]

   c. **Lightly massage** the lids to help center the lens and remove bubbles after placement.

   Pearl: Patients should demonstrate successful application and removal at least four times before they are allowed to take the lenses with them.

   Pearl: If a lens is dried out, the patient should soak the lens in saline for at least an hour before applying.[2]

3. **Removal** is usually easier than application. After washing the hands, the lens is gently pinched off the cornea or pulled down first onto the sclera and then pinched off.[34,92]

   a. **Sliding** the lenses off the eye is effective for patients with long nails. While looking down over a flat surface, the patient touches the lens with the index finger and slides it off the cornea toward the ear. The lens will flick out when it comes in contact with the lateral canthus. Unfortunately, lenses can easily be lost if the patient is not careful.

   b. **Squeezing** the lens out like removing a rigid lens is another method. The finger of one hand is placed on the edge of the top lid. The finger of the other hand is placed on the edge of the bottom lid.[92] While looking at the nose, the patient pulls the lids toward the ear.

   Pearl: For a patient who has problems with damaging lenses, use of a soft-tipped tweezer while removing lenses will greatly reduce damage rate.[93]

C. **Cleaning and disinfection** should be performed each time the lens is worn. The daily wear lenses need cleaning and disinfection every day. Enzymes are usually prescribed for use once a week. Wetting drops can be used as needed. Remind the patient to use wetting drops before lens removal.

D. Lens cases should be cleaned and rinsed. Some practitioners recommend cleaning with a **surfactant cleaner.** The most effective is a hydrogen peroxide rinse, but this can result in significant amounts of residual peroxide. A hot water rinse followed by air drying has also been found effective against *Pseudomonas* case contamination. There may be a risk of *Acanthamoeba* contamination if tap water is used, however.[94] Cases should be replaced regularly (every 3–6 months) because 40–60% of the contact lens cases are contaminated.[11,84,95–97] For patients with corneal ulcers, the offending microorganism is usually colonizing in their contact lens cases. There is probably less risk of infection, however, with heat disinfection.[4]

Pearl: Cleaning lenses is like washing dishes in a dishwasher. The dishes are cleaned (surfactant cleaner), rinsed off (saline rinse), and then run through the dishwasher (disinfection). If you put them in the dishwasher without cleaning or rinsing, your dishes (lenses) will be caked with sterile dirt. If you let the dirty dishes (lenses) sit until the next day and then run them through the dishwasher, it is more difficult to remove the debris.[98]

E. Patients should be given specific instructions: Do not overwear the lenses, do not wear lenses in the hot tub, do not wet the lenses with saliva, remove the lenses if the eyes are red, and have regular follow-ups.[39]

F. Wearing schedules can vary. One guideline is to commence with 4 hours the first day and increasing 1 hour every day after until 8–10 hours are reached. The first day is 4 hours, the second day is 5 hours, the third day is 6 hours, and so on for the first week. Lenses can be worn up to 12–15 hours per day after the first week if needed.

*Pearl: Fitting the contact lens is the easy part. Taking care of it over time is the difficult part. Remember, **"don't quit the fit."**[39]*

REFERENCES

1. Efron N, Henriques A, Merkz JTM, et al. Contact lens maintenance systems. ICLC 1992;19:153–156.
2. Fontana FD. Every lens care dilemma has its solution. CL Forum 1989;14(9):43–53.
3. Schnider CM. When the solution is the problem. CL Spectrum 1990;5(12):25.
4. Focus group on compliance. CL Spectrum 1989;4(12):39–43.
5. Snyder C, West WD, Jameson M, et al. Patient control and lens care systems—the vital link. CL Spectrum 1992;7(6):49–54.
6. Campbell RC, Caroline PJ. Between the lines: long-term lens storage dilemma. CL Forum 1989;14(11):56.

7. Campbell RC, Caroline PJ. Do your in-office disinfection procedures measure up? CL Spectrum 1992;7(12):63.

8. Dramen GE, Dramen GD, Schnider CM. Evaluation of an enhanced cleaning and storage method for in-office disinfection of hydrogel contact lenses. ICLC 1992;19:240–245.

9. Davis LJ, Auker TA. Should a worn hydrogel lenses be saved? A case report. ICLC 1989;16:176–177.

10. Fleiszig SM, Fletcher EL, Lowe R. Microbiology of Contact Lens Care. In ES Bennett, BA Weissman (eds), Clinical Contact Lens Practice. Philadelphia: Lippincott, 1992(36);1–29.

11. The changing face of disinfection and care. CL Spectrum 1990;5(4):51–64.

12. Shovlin JP. Resistant pathogens following disinfection: the significance of "contribution of elements." ICLC 1989;16:126–128.

13. Rosenthal RA, McNamee LS, Schlech BA. Continuous anti-microbial activity of CL disinfectants. CL Forum 1988;13(11):72–75.

14. Barr JT. What you need to know about solution interactions. CL Spectrum 1994;9(8):15–21.

15. Carney LG, Barr JT, Hill RM. Lens Solution Chemistry. In ES Bennett, BA Weissman (eds), Clinical Contact Lens Practice. Philadelphia: Lippincott, 1991(35);1–7.

16. Townsend W. The preservative problem. CL Spectrum 1994;9(11):49.

17. Reinhardt DJ, Kaylor B, Prescott D, et al. Rapid and simplified comparative evaluations of contact lens disinfecting solutions. ICLC 1990;17:9–13.

18. Gasson A, Morris J. Care Systems. In A Gasson, J Morris (eds), The Contact Lens Manual. Oxford, England: Butterworth–Heinemann, 1992;234–244.

19. Janoff L. The relative toxicity of five common disinfecting/preserving agents as determined by a modified neutral red dye release assay and the agar overlay technique (clinical implications). ICLC 1992;19:134–135.

20. Epstein AB. Contact Lens Complications. In CA Schwartz (ed), Specialty Contact Lenses: A Fitter's Guide. Philadelphia: Saunders, 1996;251–311.

21. Krezanoski JZ. Chemical buffering of contact lens solutions. CL Forum 1988;13(12):60.

22. Hill RM, Carney LG, Barr JT, et al. Soft lens solutions: a look at what's not on the label. CL Spectrum 1988;3(10):43–46.

23. Rakow PL. Solution incompatibilities and confusion: observations and caveats. CL Forum 1989;14(9):60–64.

24. Hill RM. Salines and their pH problems. ICLC 1991;18:203–204.

25. Hill RM. Soothing solutions: acidity. ICLC 1991;18:75–76.

26. Carney LG, Hill RM, Barr JT, et al. Do contact lens solutions stand the test of time? CL Spectrum 1990;5(8):53–56.

27. Edwards G. Saline pH value: a critical key to soft CL comfort. CL Forum 1989;14(4):40–42.

28. Mandell RB. Symptomatology and refitting. In RB Mandell (ed), Contact Lens Practice (4th ed). Springfield, IL: Thomas, 1988;598–643.

29. Schwartz CA. Seeking better compliance through education, new products. CL Forum 1988;13(9):29–65.

30. Henry VA. Lens Care and Patient Education. In ES Bennett, VA Henry (eds), Clinical Manual of Contact Lenses. Philadelphia: Lippincott, 1994(10);230–259.

31. Christensen B, Janes JA. Clinical investigation of the new SoftWear saline. CL Spectrum 1990;5(11):37–40.

32. Ziglar L. SoftWear saline and the sensitive patient. CL Spectrum 1990;5(12):50–51.

33. Shih KL, Hu J, Sibley MJ. The microbiological benefit of cleaning and rinsing contact lenses. ICLC 1985;12:235–242.

34. Mandell RB. Lens Handling, Care and Storage. In RB Mandell (ed), Contact Lens Practice (4th ed). Springfield, IL: Thomas, 1988;568–597.

35. Leach N. Contamination of soft lens storage solutions in private practice. Clin Eye Vis Care 1993;5(2):65–69.

36. Shih KL, Hu J, Sibley MJ. The microbial benefit of cleaning and rinsing contact lenses. ICLC 1985;12:235–242.

37. Efron N, Wohl A, Toma NG, et al. *Pseudomonas* corneal ulcers associated with daily wear of disposable hydrogel contact lenses. ICLC 1991;18:46–51.

38. Weisbarth RE. Hydrogel Lens Care Regimens and Patient Education. In ES Bennett, BA Weissman (eds), Clinical Contact Lens Practice. Philadelphia: Lippincott, 1993(34);1–27.

39. Shannon BJ. Problems in Compliance. In JA Silbert (ed), Anterior Segment Complications of Contact Lens Wear. New York: Churchill Livingstone 1994;337–349.

40. Davies DJG, Anthony Y, Meakin BJ, et al. Evaluation of the anti-acanthamoebal activity of five contact lens disinfectants. ICLC 1990;17:14–21.

41. Lubricating and rewetting solutions: a roundtable discussion. Part II. CL Spectrum 1989;4(5):47–52.

42. Shih KL, Raad MK, Hu JC, et al. Disinfecting activities of non-peroxide soft contact lens cold disinfection solutions. CLAO J 1991;17(3):165–168.

43. Piccolo MG, Boltz RL, Rice RW, et al. Hydrogen peroxide and quaternary ammonium care systems for extended wear lenses. ICLC 1985;12(4):212–226.

44. Stokes DJ, Morton DJ. Antimicrobial activity of hydrogen peroxide. ICLC 1987;14:146–149.

45. Sibley MJ. Hydrogen peroxide systems. CL Forum 1987;12(7):57–63.

46. Epstein AB, Freedman JM. Keratitis associated with hydrogen peroxide disinfection in soft contact lens wearers. ICLC 1990;17:74–81.

47. Lowe R, Vallas V, Brennan NA. Comparative efficacy of contact lens disinfection solutions. CLAO J 1992;18(1):34–40.

48. Lowther GE. Do your contact lens patients adhere to your prescribed procedures? ICLC 1989;16:312–313.

49. Rosenthal RA, Stein JM, McAnally CL, et al. A comparative study of the microbiologic effectiveness of chemical disinfectants and peroxide-neutralizer systems. CLAO J 1995;21(2):99–110.

50. Schnider CM. Part-time lens wear, full time lens care. CL Spectrum 1994;9(1):17.

51. Kurashige LT, Kataoka JE, Edrington T, et al. Protein deposition on hydrogel contact lenses: a comparison study of enzymatic cleaners. ICLC 1987;14:150–158.

52. Lasswell LA, Tarantino N, Kono D. Enzymatic cleaning of extended wear lenses: papain vs. pancreatin. Int Eyecare 1986;2(2):101–104.

53. Ghormley NR. Ultrazyme and ReNu Enzyme cleaners—a difference? (continued) ICLC 1989;16:80.

54. LaPierre M, St-Arnauld F, Doyon J, et al. Efficiency comparison: Enzyme Plus versus Ultrazyme. CL Spectrum 1991;6(11):37–41.
55. Ghormley NR. Ultrazyme and ReNu Enzyme cleaners—a difference? ICLC 1988;15:6.
56. New solutions flood market CL Spectrum 1994;9(7):5.
57. West W, Gallia M. Concept testing. CL Spectrum 1993;8(8):49–53.
58. Turner FD, Gower LA, Stein JM, et al. Compliance and contact lens care: a new assessment method. Optom Vis Sci 1993;70(12):998–1004.
59. House HO, Leach NE, Edrington TB, et al. Contact lens daily cleaner efficacy: multipurpose versus single purpose products. ICLC 1991;18:238–243.
60. Hong BS, Bilbault TJ, Chowhan MA, et al. Cleaning capability of citrate-containing vs. non-citrate contact lens cleaning solutions: an in vitro comparative study. ICLC 1994;21:237–240.
61. Ghormley NR. Quick Care—a new soft lens disinfection system. ICLC 1994;21:77–78.
62. Ajello L, Ajello M. A comparison of the antimicrobial spectra and kill rates of three contact lens care solutions: QuickCARE starting solution, ReNu multi-purpose solution, and Opti-Free rinsing, disinfecting, and storage solution. ICLC 1995;22:156–163.
63. Harris MG, Can CM, Grant T, et al. Microwave irradiation and soft contact lens parameters. Optom Vis Sci 1993;70(10):843–848.
64. Admoni M, Bartolomei A, Qureshi MN, et al. Disinfection efficacy in an integrated ultraviolet light contact lens care system. CLAO J 1994;20(4):246–248.
65. Gritz DC, Lee TY, McDonnell PJ, et al. Ultraviolet radiation for the sterilization of contact lenses. CLAO J 1990;16(4):294–298.
66. Bartolomei A, Alcaraz L, Bottone E, et al. Clinical evaluation of Purilens, an ultraviolet light contact lens care system. CLAO J 1994;20(1):23.
67. Efron N, Lowe R, Vallas V, et al. Clinical efficacy of standing waves and ultrasound for cleaning and disinfecting contact lenses. ICLC 1991;18:24–29.
68. Sibley MJ. Use of vibrating standing waves to clean contact lenses. CL Forum 1987;12(5):60–61.
69. Malin AH. Cycling lenses for longer life. Part II. CL Spectrum 1989;4(2):52–56.
70. Arentsen J. Noninfectious medical complications induced by soft contact lenses. CL Forum 1987;12(11):21–26.
71. Hart DE. Deposits and Coatings: Hydrogel Lens/Tear-Film Interactions. In ES Bennett, BA Weissman (eds), Clinical Contact Lens Practice. Philadelphia: Lippincott, 1992(33);1–32.
72. Jacob R. Principles of cleaning soft contact lenses. ICLC 1988;15:317–325.
73. Sack RA. Harvey H, Nunes I. Disinfection associated spoilage of high water content ionic matrix hydrogels. CLAO J 1989;15(2):138–145.
74. Minno GE, Eckel L, Groemminger S, et al. Quantitative analysis of protein deposits on hydrophilic soft contact lenses. I. Comparison to visual methods of analysis. II. Deposit variation among FDA lens material groups. Optom Vis Sci 1991;68(11):865–872.
75. Ng A, Mostardi B, Mandell RB. Adherence of mascaras to soft contact lenses. ICLC 1988;15:64–68.
76. Baldwin JS. Cosmetics: too long concealed as culprit in eye problems. CL Forum 1986;11(6):38–41.

77. Rakow PL. Solution incompatibilities. CL Forum 1988;13(6):41–46.
78. Campbell RC, Caroline PJ. Do your in-office disinfection procedures measure up? CL Spectrum 1992;7(12):63–64.
79. Seal DV, Bennett ES, McFadyen AK, et al. Differential adherence of *Acanthamoeba* to contact lenses: effects of material characteristics. Optom Vis Sci 1995;72(1):23–28.
80. Bergmanson JPG. An expert guide to contact lenses and the corneal epithelium. CL Spectrum 1994;9(7):34–41.
81. Conner CG, Hopkins SL, Salisbury RD. Effectivity of contact lens disinfection systems against *Acanthamoeba culbertsoni*. Optom Vis Sci 1991;68(2):138–141.
82. Williams CE. Soft contact lens toxic occlusion phenomenon. CL Spectrum 1986;1(11):14–18.
83. Optimize your lens care options. CL Spectrum 1995;10(3):27.
84. CL problems start when patient motivation wanes. CL Forum 1986;11(6):42–47.
85. Marren SE. Negotiating compliance with contact lens care. ICLC 1990;17:63–66.
86. Harris MG. Are you legally vulnerable when prescribing contact lens care products? CL Spectrum 1990;5(6):63–66.
87. Shannon BJ. Patient training prevents noncompliance. CL Forum 1988;13(7):39–43.
88. Wish list for solutions. CL Forum 1985;10(9):44–51.
89. Berenblatt AJ. Lens care systems: a practitioner's wish list. CL Forum 1988;13(3):37–38.
90. McGeehon M. Guidelines to handling problem patients. CL Forum 1988;13(4):23–28.
91. Barlow M, Plank D, Stroud S, et al. The effectiveness of typical hand-cleaning methods on hydrogel contact lenses. ICLC 1994;21:232–235.
92. Atkinson KW, Port MJA. Patient Management and Instruction. In AJ Phillips, J Stone (eds), Contact Lenses (3rd ed). London: Butterworth Publishers, 1989;299–332.
93. Attridge JG. Monitoring the effectiveness of soft-tipped tweezers to reduce hydrogel lens damage. ICLC 1993;20:76–79.
94. Larragoiti ND, Diamos ME, Simmons PA, et al. A comparative study of techniques for decreasing contact lens storage case contamination. J Am Optom Assoc 1994;65(3):161–163.
95. Siwoff R, Haupt EJ. Bacterial growth on contact lens cases: do solutions make a difference? CL Forum 1986;11(9):47–52.
96. Lowther GE. How safe are hydrogel disinfection systems? ICLC 1991;18:124.
97. Ghormley NR. A disposable contact lens case? ICLC 1991;18:45.
98. Connelly S. CL care: you wash your dirty dishes nightly, don't you? CL Forum 1989;14(9):77–79.

PART IV

Disposable and Extended Wear

Chapter 14

Rigid Extended Wear and Complications

Milton M. Hom

I. **Rigid gas-permeable (RGP) extended wear** is healthier than soft extended wear and has high success rates.[1–4] During overnight wear, corneal coverage is less, tear exchange is greater (due to **rapid eye movement**), and materials are more permeable than those of soft lenses.[5–9] Although materials are less than optimal, normal tear pumping reduces overnight swelling more rapidly than soft extended wear.[6,10] Complications are fewer and less severe than soft lenses.[11] Rigid lenses require less replacement, cost less, produce more stable vision, are easier to care for, are available in custom lens designs, and can be modified.[12,13] In the past, much of the early work was performed with aphakes. Currently, most rigid extended-wear lenses are fitted for myopes and hyperopes.[14–16]

II. A number of issues pertaining to **lens design and fitting** must be taken into account.

    A. **Patient selection** for rigid extended wear is similar to that for daily wear, with some special concerns. Astigmatic patients who fail with soft lenses because of visual acuity are ideal candidates. Aphakic patients are also good candidates.[17] Patients with poor compliance and hygiene are not desirable candidates. When examination and history reveal the presence of coalesced staining areas, giant papillary conjunctivitis (GPC); chronic injection; or use of antihistamines, diuretics, or tranquilizers, the patient is a poor candidate for rigid extended wear.[12] Systemic conditions related to poor wound healing **(diabetes)** and immunosuppression should be also ruled out.[18] Special attention should be paid to dry-eye concerns because of adhesion risk. Conditions related to staphylococcal keratitis **(blepharitis, meibomian gland dysfunction)** should be treated prior to rigid extended contact lens wear.[18] Other conditions affecting topography **(pterygia** and **pinguecula)** may predispose the patient to peripheral complications of rigid extended wear such as **peripheral corneal desiccation.**[18]

257

Pearl: Daily wear rigid lens success is a necessary prerequisite for RGP extended wear.[18]

B. Fitting of rigid extended wear lenses follows many of the same guidelines as are used for daily wear. A successful daily wear design may cause problems as an extended-wear lens, however.[19] Close attention must be paid to edge lift and peripheral systems.

   1. The **recommended diameter** and **base curve relationship** vary with authors.[5,12,20–23] Diameters of approximately 9 mm with alignment to slight apical clearance (flat K to 0.50 D steeper than K) are effective.[20,21] Overly **large diameters** and **flat lens fitting** should be avoided because of adhesion.[1] There should be 1–2 mm of blink-induced movement.[24]

   2. **Edge lift** is an important feature because of peripheral corneal desiccation. An ideal 0.4- to 0.5-mm wide band of fluorescein at the edge should be seen when fitting. Width is more critical than depth in rigid extended wear.[20]

   Pearl: Do not duplicate a successful daily wear design for extended wear without close evaluation of the peripheral system and diameter. Lens adhesion problems occur because of large diameter, narrow edge width, and reduced edge clearance.[19] Redesign the lens for extended wear.

   3. **Flexure** is common with the higher-Dk materials. Fitting sets made of the same material as the ordered lens are recommended because of property differences.[12,25,26]

C. Material selection is largely influenced by oxygen permeability. The highest level of permeability is desirable. Fluorosilicone acrylates are currently the most widely used for rigid extended wear (see Chapter 5).

   1. The **boundary layer effect** makes the effective Dk on the eye around half of the nominal Dk[5,12,27] (see Chapter 5). Since a Dk of 75 is needed as the ideal minimum for manageable overnight swelling, an absolute minimum Dk/t of 30 is necessary for extended wear.[5,12,28]

   2. A **general guideline** for rigid extended wear is to have Dks of 60–100 for resolving overnight swelling within 1–2 hours of eye opening (a higher Dk is required to resolve overnight swelling faster but lenses with these Dks are not made with satisfactory performance).[5,18,27] Dks of 50–60 may be adequate for occasional overnight wear. Extended wear on a regular basis requires a Dk of more than 90.[18]

   Pearl: There is a higher patient dropout rate with lower-Dk lenses.[12] Strive to fit the highest-Dk materials.[1]

III. **Patient education and management** to ensure safe and comfortable wear is important.

    A. **The wearing schedule recommended by the Food and Drug Administration** is a maximum of 7 days and 6 nights. The lenses should be removed at least 1 night. Before commencing extended wear, the patient should be on a daily-wear schedule. One month of daily-wear success is strongly advised before the patient proceeds with overnight wear.[20,29]

    B. The **follow-up schedule** when extended wear is initiated includes an early morning visit within 2 hours of awakening during the first week of overnight wear.[19] Conditions such as lens adhesion and edema are best viewed shortly after awakening.[29] Other follow-ups are at 1 week, 1 month, and 3 months for nonproblematic patients. Subsequent visits at 3-month intervals are advised on a regular basis.[18,30]

    Pearl: *Expect to see keratometric flattening during follow-up.*[27,31,32]

    C. **Care systems** are similar to those used with rigid daily wear (see Chapter 9). Lenses should be disinfected and cleaned the evenings they are not worn.

        1. **High-viscosity** solutions can cause prolonged blurring in the morning, producing a so-called ointmentlike effect, and they are not recommended.[12]

        2. **Rewetting drops** are important to use before sleep and on awakening. The drops rinse away trapped debris and enhance lens movement.[5,12]

        Pearl: *Instruct your patients to instill a wetting drop before sleep to help prevent adhesion.*[19]

IV. **Complications** of rigid extended wear are usually related to corneal hypoxia or mechanical trauma.[33] Many of the complications are the same as those seen in soft extended wear, although they usually occur at a reduced rate.[1,5,27,34] There is an especially low occurrence of infiltrates with RGP extended wear. The better tear flushing, smaller corneal coverage, and reduced lens contamination contribute to a healthier extended-wear lens.[12]

    A. **Vascularized limbal keratitis (VLK)** is a rare inflammatory condition related to rigid extended wear lenses. The typical patient is a female who formerly wore polymethyl methacrylate lenses with a large diameter, steep fit, and low-edge lift.[35]

        1. The **progression of VLK** is described in stages (I–IV). Elevations or heaping of the limbal epithelium with staining first appear. A peripheral corneal infiltrate forms adjacent to the elevation. The cornea becomes inflamed with conjunctival hyperemia. Superficial and deep vascularization emanates from the limbus and encircles

the infiltrate in a leashlike manner. Untreated, the elevation will break down into a painful erosion.

2. **Treatment** entails discontinuation of lens wear and use of topical steroids to treat the infiltrate and regress the vascularization. Topical antibiotics with cessation of lens wear also help produce rapid regression. The patient should be refitted with an alignment lens of smaller diameter and with moderate edge lift.[36]

B. **Ptosis** is a benign complication of rigid extended wear that resolves with discontinuation of lens wear. The mechanical trauma of the lens is believed to cause edema or hypertrophy of the upper lid.[18,37]

C. **Fluorescein staining of the cornea** usually indicates a break in the protective corneal barrier. Infection is more likely with large amounts of staining. Dellen formation, new vessel growth, and peripheral corneal ulcers can be the end results of staining.[5,23,38] Because overnight (8 hours) lens removal does not completely resolve light staining, only minimal levels of staining should be acceptable.[19,38] Strategies must be used to eliminate staining.[39]

1. **Peripheral corneal dessication (PCD), or 3 and 9 o'clock staining,** is related to numerous patient and fit factors. It is best assessed in an afternoon visit after 1–2 weeks of extended wear. Three-and-9-o'clock staining is punctate staining at the outside edge of the lens along the horizontal meridian. It often appears as an inverted (base-up) triangle and extends above and below the horizontal meridian.[40] PCD is a common finding in rigid extended wear.[18,27,41]

2. The **causes** of PCD are usually a poor tear film, inadequate peripheral lens design, or decentering lenses. Patients prone to staining have higher levels of conjunctival hyperemia, poor tear film integrity, poor lens centration, and insufficient edge clearance.

3. **Dry eyes** are often associated with staining. An eye with hyperemia and unstable tear film should be treated with lubricating drops in mild cases. Correcting poor blinking is also effective[39] (see Chapter 16). Often, the patient also has an associated deposit problem.[42]

Pearl: A thin, uneven tear film with debris and injection may indicate a predisposition to PCD.[29]

4. **Modifications** and **design changes** are necessary to remedy an inadequate peripheral system. Increasing the edge lift usually decreases peripheral staining.[42] A thorough blend, widening or flattening the peripheral system, and tapering the edge are effective modifications for insufficient edge lift.[43] If the edge lift is too excessive, the lens should be reordered in most cases.[18]

5. **Against-the-rule corneas** or a **laterally displaced corneal apex** can cause a chafing effect with a horizontally displaced lens. Ep-

ithelial staining and compression of the lens edge result from lateral decentration.[36] Design changes, such as a bitoric lens for toric corneas, are sometimes necessary.

6. **Inferiorly fitted lenses** are correlated with desiccation staining.[5,27,44] Seventy-three percent of low-riding lenses have 3 o'clock and 9 o'clock staining.[12,27] Minus lenticular designs for all plus and low minus can help to raise the lens and decrease staining.[40,44] Plus lenticulars are used for higher (more than 6 D) minus lenses[45] (see Chapter 4).

D. **Lens adhesion,** or "early morning lens adherence," is a significant complication for rigid extended wear.[16,24] It is usually associated with peripheral corneal staining, vascularization, ulceration, and significant corneal distortion. A typical adhesion patient would wake up in the morning with the lens "stuck" in his or her dry eye.[39] Lens adhesion is the leading reported cause of cessation of rigid extended wear.[46] Most studies find adherence in at least 10–50% of participants.[18,30,47–49] Lens binding has been reported for daily wear as well[50] (CD-ROM: RGP Cases: Case 5).

1. **Exact causes** are not known. Several theories are proposed.
   a. **Mucus adhesion** of the lens to the eye is currently the most accepted theory. A loss of aqueous creates a highly viscous, mucus-rich tear layer that acts as an adhesive between the lens and eye.[24,51,52]
   b. **Intraocular pressure (IOP)** may be another cause. The estimated time of adherence (after 5 hours) approximately correlates with the higher diurnal pressure in the morning. The increased IOP induces lateral stresses that cause lens surface deformation, indentation, and subsequent adherence.[53]
   c. **Negative pressure,** or a suction effect of the lens against the eye, may be another cause.[27,52] The flexible materials required for extended wear are prone to creating a suction effect on the eye.[12] Because lens adhesion still occurs with fenestrated lenses, however, this theory is questionable.[51]

2. **Symptoms** are dryness, blurred vision, spectacle blur, and injection.[18] Patients often report that the lens feels as though it needs **more cleaning.**[54] Symptoms are typically minimal.

3. **Signs** are distorted mires; central and peripheral **compression ring,** or **corneal indentation ring;** and a poorly centering (usually inferior) nonmoving lens.[5,49] The signs can disappear within 2 hours of awakening.[18]
   a. **Corneal distortion** is probably due to the compression ring. When one side of the keratometric mires appears wavy, distortion is present.
   b. **Compression rings** are caused by the lens edge leaving a circular indentation on the cornea.[5,31,51,55,56] Many times, the

tears break up in a arcuate pattern within the compression ring, and there is pooling of fluorescein on either side of the ring.

c. **Superficial punctate keratitis (SPK)** can appear as an elongated arcuate shape or a broader circular shape within the indentation ring. Central SPK can be accompanied by peripheral fluorescein staining adjacent to or at a point opposite to the curve of the ring.[57]

d. **Silicone acrylate surface hazing** is a protein film on the lens surface that may also lead to adhesion.[12] Scrupulous cleaning is necessary.

4. **Treatment** includes lens design changes, patient education, and solution changes.

a. **Reduction of lens diameter** and use of **wide and flat peripheral curves** are highly recommended.[18,49] Lens adhesion is exacerbated by an edge lift that is too narrow or too shallow.[1] Fitting philosophies that advocate large-diameter, alignment lenses with small edge lift may work well with daily wear, but in reality, they set the patient up for lens adhesion.[12,29,51] Unfortunately, there may be some confusion because lower edge clearances have been recommended in the past for extended-wear rigid lenses.[23]

b. **Steepening the base curve** is effective.[54] The contact area for the adhesive mucin to bind the lens to the eye is reduced when the lens is steepened. Preventative measures can be taken by not fitting the lenses flat.

c. **Self-assessment** by the patient is effective for diagnosis and management.[5,29] It is not unusual for lens binding to go unnoticed by the practitioner. Subjective lens-binding assessment is a very reliable method of monitoring.[50] When the patient awakens, the patient should experience free lens movement. If not, the patient should use rewetting or digital manipulation to free the lens. If dislodging the lens becomes a difficult or chronic problem, cessation of extended wear should be considered.

d. A **change of solutions** may be needed. It is reported that switching patients from Boston Advance conditioning solution to the original Boston Conditioning solution (Bausch & Lomb, Rochester, New York) has solved some problems of adhesion.[18] For patients who have silicone acrylate surface hazing, changing to an abrasive cleaner and enzymatic cleaners is recommended.[12,58]

e. **Regular replacement** has been shown to reduce the incidence of lens binding. Replacement brings new, clean lens surfaces on a regular basis. A 3- or 6-month replacement schedule is recommended.[50]

E. **Hypoxia** and **acidosis** have been reported in 90% of patients who wear these lenses.[33] Edema is a normal response in extended wear because current materials have insufficient oxygen transmission.[59] It often appears to the patient as morning blur on awakening, without any other clinical signs. A patient reporting fogginess that persists for more than 15–20 minutes indicates very high levels of residual edema.[18]

   1. **Microcysts** are irregular refractile lesions of 15–50 μm that usually exhibit **reversed illumination.** Microcysts originate at the basement membrane and migrate forward to the epithelium, sometimes breaking through and staining. They take 3–4 months to clear and can temporarily increase after discontinuation of lens wear.[46] Negative staining sometimes appears at elevated areas where microcysts are preparing to break through. Microcysts numbering 50 or more indicate cessation of extended wear or a material change.[1] **Vacuoles** are often present, showing **unreversed illumination** (see Chapter 3).

   2. **Striae** and **folds** appear when there is corneal swelling due to edema. Striae are fine, gray-white vertical lines in the stroma seen at 5–6% corneal swelling.[18,60] Folds appear at 10–12% swelling and appear as dark lines in the posterior stroma. Striae have been noted less frequently with rigid lenses than soft lenses despite similar amounts of swelling. If striae or folds appear, overnight wear should be reduced and a change in material made.[1]

   3. **Polymegethism** and pleomorphism in minimal increases have been reported with high-Dk RGP lenses.[16,18] The consequences of polymegethism and pleomorphism are unclear.[1]

F. **GPC** and **contact lens papillary conjunctivitis (CLPC)** result from the mechanical irritation of a rigid lens and deposit formation.[19] The incidence is lower for rigid lenses than for soft lenses. The papillary response differs from that seen with soft lenses in location and appearance. The response begins closest to the lid margins (area 3) and progresses toward the fold (areas 2 and 1). The lid inflammation seen in CLPC precedes the papillary response.[18] Deposits usually cause the lid inflammation, and enzymatic cleaning is highly recommended.[61]

G. **Discomfort** is a major reason for discontinuance of lens wear.[31,33,62] Some patients are not able to adjust to rigid lenses because of scratchiness, burning, and tearing.[19] Soft lenses should be considered.

H. **Contact lens acute red eye (CLARE)** is often referred to as a soft extended-wear complication (see Chapter 15). CLARE is seen with rigid extended wear when associated with lens adhesion.[2,6,18] The patient typically awakens in the middle of the night with severe pain in one eye.

Infiltrates and severe redness are seen during examination. Treatment of the associated lens adhesion usually resolves the condition.[18]

I.   Corneal ulceration has been reported with rigid extended-wear lenses. It is usually in the peripheral cornea and is caused by lens adherence.[29,33,58] Treatment consists of antibiotics if the ulcer is infectious.[18,63]

J.   A mosaic pattern, also known as **an anterior corneal mosaic** or a **Fischer-Schweitzer pattern,** has been observed on the corneal surface. The polygonal staining pattern is caused by lens compression and resolves several hours after awakening.[5,12,64,65]

K.   Parameter changes such as warpage have been reported because of the softer nature of higher-Dk materials.[7,12,27,61,66] With the use of fluorosilicone acrylates, however, warpage is less of a problem.[47] Some authors have also reported surface changes in the form of **crazing** for silicone acrylates after several months of wear.[12,61,67] Both of these changes may require a new lens.

REFERENCES

1.   Schnider CM. Rigid gas-permeable extended wear. CL Spectrum 1990;5(9):101–106.
2.   Weiss L. Clinical study of extended wear lenses: hydrogel vs. gas-permeable. CL Forum 1987;13(9):41–46.
3.   Koetting RA, Castellano CF, Nelson DW. Extended wear with low-Dk hard gas-permeables. CL Forum 1985;11(2):77–78.
4.   Rengstorff RH, Odby A. Adaptation to Paraperm extended wear lenses: a clinical study in Sweden. J Am Optom Assoc 1986;57(8):600–603.
5.   Bennett ES. RGP extended wear: a modality for the future? CL Forum 1987;13(5):27–41.
6.   Bridgewater BA. Extended wear: rigid gas-permeable versus disposable. CL Spectrum 1991;6(2):56–62.
7.   Mandell RB. Rigid lens occasional extended wear. CL Spectrum 1990;5(10):49–53.
8.   Koetting RA, Castellano CF, Nelson DW. A hard lens with extended wear possibilities. J Am Optom Assoc 1985;56(3):208–211.
9.   Mandell RB. Extended Wear. In RB Mandell (ed), Contact Lens Practice (4th ed). Springfield, IL: Thomas, 1988;683–717.
10.   Young G, Port M. Rigid gas-permeable extended wear: a comparative clinical study. Optom Vis Sci 1992;69(3):214–226.
11.   Schnider CM, Terry RL. Evaluation of success for RGP EW contact lenses: survival versus clinical criteria. Invest Opthalmol Vis Sci 1989(suppl);30:258.
12.   Bennett ES, Ghormley NR. Rigid extended wear: an overview. ICLC 1987;14(8):319–331.
13.   Soloman J, Snyder R, Klein P. A clinical experience with extended wear RGP lenses. CL Spectrum 1986;1(7):49–51.
14.   Benjamin WJ, Simons MH. Extended wear of rigid contact lenses in aphakia: a preliminary report. ICLC 1984;11(1):44–54.

15. Benjamin WJ, Simons MH. Extended wear of oxygen-permeable rigid lenses in aphakia. ICLC 1984;11(9):547–561.

16. Bennett ES, Grohe RM. Extended Wear. In ES Bennett, RM Grohe (eds), Rigid Gas-Permeable Contact Lenses. New York: Professional Press, 1986;431–445.

17. Ghormley NR. Rigid extended wear: patient selection. ICLC 1987;14:10.

18. Schnider CM. Rigid Gas-Permeable Extended Wear Lenses. In JA Silbert (ed), Anterior Segment Complications of Contact Lens Wear. New York: Churchill Livingstone, 1994;317–336.

19. Terry R, Schnider CM, Holden BA. Maximizing success with rigid gas-permeable extended wear lenses. ICLC 1989;16(6):169–175.

20. Schnider CM. An option overlooked: make room in your practice for RGP extended wear. Rev Optom 1995;132(4):51–59.

21. Benjamin WJ. RGP extended wear: fit 'em small or fit 'em large? ICLC 1987;16(9–10):307–308.

22. Ghormley NR. Rigid EW lenses: lens design and fitting procedures. ICLC 1987;14(4):175–176.

23. Andrasko G. Commonly asked questions concerning hard gas-permeable EW lenses. CL Spectrum 1987;2(6):30–32.

24. Greco A. Avoiding complications with rigid extended wear. ICLC 1987;14(1):38.

25. Lowther GE. High- versus low-Dk RGP materials for daily wear. ICLC 1987;14(5):174.

26. Yamane SJ. Fitting RGP lenses for extended wear. CL Forum 1988;14(8):24–28.

27. Henry VA, Bennett ES, Forrest JF. Clinical investigation of the Paraperm EW rigid gas-permeable contact lens. Optom Vis Sci 1987;64(5):313–320.

28. Holden BA, Mertz GW. Critical oxygen levels to avoid corneal edema for daily and extended wear contact lenses. Invest Ophthalmol Vis Sci 1984;25:1161–1167.

29. Terry R, Holden BA, Schnider CM. Peripheral corneal ulceration in rigid gas-permeable extended wear: a case report. ICLC 1989;16(11–12):323–326.

30. Polse KA, Rivera RK, Bonnano J. Ocular effects of hard gas-permeable-lens extended wear. Optom Vis Sci 1988;65(5):358–364.

31. Young G, Port M. Rigid gas-permeable extended wear: a comparative clinical study. Optom Vis Sci 1992;69(3):214–226.

32. Kamiya C. Cosmetic extended wear of oxygen-permeable hard contact lenses: one year follow-up. J Am Optom Assoc 1986;57(3):182–184.

33. Levy B. Rigid gas-permeable lenses for extended wear—a 1-year clinical evaluation. Optom Vis Sci 1985;62(12):889–894.

34. Gullion M. Rigid gas-permeable extended wear today. Int Eyecare 1985;1(3):213.

35. Grohe RM, Lebow KA. Vascularized limbal keratitis. ICLC 1989;16(7–8):197–209.

36. Grohe RM. A complete guide to detecting and managing limbal complications. CL Spectrum 1994;9(6):26.

37. Fonn D, Holden BA. Extended wear of hard gas-permeable contact lenses can induce ptosis. CLAO J 1986;12:93.

38. Andrasko G. Peripheral corneal staining: incidence and time course. CL Spectrum 1990;5(7):59–62.

39. Bailey NJ. Favorable forecast for extended wear RGPs. CL Forum 1985;11(6):27–35.

40. Ghormley NR. Corneal desiccation—clinical management. ICLC 1990;17:5–8.

41. Lowther GE. Trends in RGP lenses. ICLC 1988;15(10):301.
42. Andrasko G. Peripheral corneal staining: edge lift and extended wear. CL Spectrum 1990;5(8):33–35.
43. Khorassani AA, Peterson JE. Effects of peripheral curve width and radius changes on retention forces measured for PMMA and Boston IV rigid lenses. ICLC 1988;15(10):311–315.
44. Lebow KA. Reduce three-and-nine corneal staining with moderate edge-lift profiles. CL Spectrum 1990;5(7):29–33.
45. Jones DH, Bennett ES, Davis LJ. How to manage peripheral corneal desiccation. CL Spectrum 1989;4(5):63–66.
46. Levy B. Complications of rigid gas-permeable lenses for extended wear. Optom Vis Sci 1991;68(8):624–628.
47. Maehara JR, Kastl PR. Rigid gas-permeable extended wear. CLAO J 1994;20(2):139–143.
48. Swarbrick HA, Holden BA. Rigid gas-permeable lens adherence: a patient-dependent phenomenon. Optom Vis Sci 1989;66(5):269–275.
49. Swarbrick HA, Holden BA. Rigid gas-permeable lens binding: significance and contributing factors. Optom Vis Sci 1987;64(11):815–823.
50. Woods CA, Efron N. Regular replacement of rigid contact lenses alleviates binding to the cornea. ICLC 1996;23:13–19.
51. Swarbrick HA. A possible etiology for RGP lens binding (adherence). ICLC 1988;15(1):13–19.
52. Goldberg JB. RGP contact lens adherence: flexure or tear film thinning—can we define the cause? ICLC 1994;21:26–28.
53. Kwok LS. Is intraocular pressure a risk factor in contact lens wear? Optom Vis Sci 1992;69(6):489–491.
54. McLaughlin R. How to handle RGP lens adhesion. CL Spectrum 1993;8(10):15.
55. Benjamin WJ, Boltz RL. RGP lens adhesion is not a benign phenomenon. ICLC 1989;16(2):60–62.
56. Dougal J. Abrasions Secondary to Contact Lens Wear. In A Tomlinson (ed), Complications of Contact Lens Wear. St. Louis: Mosby, 1992;123–156.
57. Kenyon E, Polse KA, Mandell RB. Rigid contact lens adherence: incidence, severity, and recovery. J Am Optom Assoc 1988;59(3):168–174.
58. Schnider CM, Zabiewicz K, Holden BA. Unusual complications associated with RGP extended wear. ICLC 1988;15(4):124–129.
59. Holden BA, Mertz GW. Critical oxygen levels to avoid corneal edema for daily and extended wear contact lenses. Invest Ophthalmol Vis Sci 1984;25:1161–1167.
60. Josephson JE, Caffrey BE. Evanescent corneal striae in a rigid g/p extended wear patient. Am J Optom Physiol Opt 1987;64(4):298.
61. Ghormley NR. Rigid EW lenses: complications. ICLC 1987;14(6):219.
62. Sigband DJ, Bridgewater BA. Fluoroperm 151 extended wear: a clinical study. CLAO J 1994;20(1):37.
63. Ehrlich M, Weissman BA, Mondino BJ. *Pseudomonas* corneal ulcer after use of extended wear rigid gas-permeable contact lens. Cornea 1989;8(3):225–228.
64. Zantos SG, Zantos PO. Extended wear feasibility of gas-permeable hard lenses for myopes. Int Eyecare 1985;1(1):66–76.

65. Osborn GN, Andrasko GJ, Barr JT. RGP lenses daily wear vs. extended wear. CL Spectrum 1986;1(4):32–49.
66. Quinn TG, Comstock TL, Badowski L. Clinical experience with 92-Dk fluorosilicone-acrylate contact lens. CL Spectrum 1989;4(5):57–60.
67. Ghormley NR. The Fluoroperm family—part I. ICLC 1988;15(8):239–240.

Chapter 15

Soft Extended Wear and Complications

Milton M. Hom and Joseph P. Shovlin

I. **Extended-wear** lenses are those that are worn while sleeping overnight. Soft extended-wear lenses can be worn as conventional lenses, as disposable or planned-replacement (PRP) lenses, or as flexible-wear lenses.
   A. **Conventional soft extended wear** is more convenient than daily-wear.
      1. The **advantages of conventional soft extended wear** are that this approach entails less handling and maintenance and therefore fewer lens solutions and lower costs. Patients can wake up in the morning and see clearly the instant they awake.[1] People who travel frequently also enjoy the convenience of extended wear.[2]
      2. **Thirty days** of continuous wear has been approved by the U.S. Food and Drug Administration in the past.[3] Presently, a 6-night maximum of overnight wear followed by cleaning and disinfection is recommended by the FDA.[1]
      3. The **disadvantages of conventional soft extended wear** are the complications associated with extended wear. There is increased risk of corneal edema, ulceration, and other conditions compared with daily wear.[4,5]
   B. **Disposable** or **PRP** lenses for extended wear are the choices for healthier, easier maintenance.[6] **Disposable** lenses are worn once or twice by the patient and thrown away. **PRP** lenses are replaced on a regular, scheduled basis.[7] Disposable cycles are usually shorter (2 weeks); PRP cycles are longer (1 month or more). Eighty-seven percent of patients preferred disposable lenses over conventional lenses when directly compared.[8] **Acuvue** (Vistakon, Jacksonville, Florida) is the most documented lens of this modality and is often perceived as the standard. Both PRP and disposable lenses are supplied in **multipacks** and are designed for replacement at regular intervals.[9] Most are meant for both daily wear or extended wear. **Focus** (CIBA Vision, Duluth, Georgia), **CooperVision Preference** (CooperVision, Fairport, New York), **See-**

Quence 2 and **Medalist** (both by Bausch & Lomb, Rochester, New York), and **Edge III Proactive** and **Biomedics 55 lenses** (both by Ocular Sciences, South San Francisco, California) are approved for either daily or extended wear.[9,10]

1. **Disposable and PRP lenses have reduced lens spoilage** and related complications compared with conventional extended wear.[9]

   a. **Clear vision** from fresh clean lenses is an advantage of reduced lens spoilage.[11] Problems stemming from deposits are virtually eliminated. Comfort is often better.[9]

   b. **Enhanced compliance** is also possible with disposable lenses.[11] Disposable and PRP lenses have the potential for better compliance because care procedures are simplified.

   c. **Complications** such as giant papillary conjunctivitis (GPC), contact lens papillary conjunctivitis (CLPC), contact lens acute red eye (CLARE), and solution sensitivity are all reduced with disposable lenses.[6]

2. **The major disadvantage of disposable soft extended wear** is that all the problems associated with extended wear are not solved.

   a. **Corneal infections** and **ulcers** still occur at the same rate with disposable soft extended wear as with conventional extended wear,[9,12] although sometimes overall complications are less with disposable lenses.[12]

   b. **Cost** is sometimes perceived as a disadvantage. Although each lens is lower in cost, total lens cost is higher because many more lenses are needed. Some practitioners argue, however, that the need for fewer solutions more than offsets the additional expense.[11,13]

   c. **Lens abuse** does occur with PRP and disposable lenses.[13] Replacement less frequently than prescribed constitutes lens abuse. Many patients view disposable lenses as cheaper, longer-term lenses that don't need replacement as prescribed.[14] A telling example is a patient who buys a 6-month supply and returns 12 months later.[13] Unfortunately, lens abuse eliminates any advantages disposable lenses offer.

C. **Flexible wear** lenses are worn overnight on an occasional basis, perhaps one or two nights a week.[15] Practitioners are moving toward flexible wear with PRP and disposable lenses.[16]

II. **Lens design and fitting** is similar to daily-wear soft contact lenses.

A. **Patient selection** is critical for success. Superior hygiene is a must.[1] Many of the qualities of a successfully compliant daily wear patient are also important for extended wear.

   Pearl: Korb summed up successful contact lens wear as a "clean wet lens on a clean wet eye."[9]

Patients with lid infections or recurring conjunctivitis and patients who do not follow directions are not very good candidates.[17] Tear film problems, corneal thinning (keratoconus), chronic allergies, and poor general health may be contraindications.[18]

Pearl: Extended wear is not recommended for symptomatic daily lens wearers.[19] For such patients, extended wear creates more problems than it solves.

B. **Fitting** is very similar to that used with daily wear soft lenses. Use of diagnostic lenses is recommended. Usually the median base curve is selected as the initial lens, and adequate movement is necessary.[1,3] Lenses should be allowed to equilibrate on the eye for 20 minutes before checking lens performance.[9]

Pearl: Most manufacturers offer free trial lenses. A 1- to 2-week trial period with diagnostic lenses is very helpful in determining any potential problems with disposable lenses.[9]

1. The **initial lens** can be a medium-water-content, medium-thickness (group IV), loosely fitting lens. If there are edematous signs or new vessel growth develops, a high-water-content, looser-fitting lens can be chosen.[3]

Pearl: Acuvue produces significantly better visual acuity than other disposable lenses.[20–22]

2. **Base curve** choices for lens selection are an Acuvue 8.8-mm base curve or a NewVue (CIBA Vision) 8.4-mm base curve. These base curves fit 80–90% of patients.[23]

C. **Types of lenses** can be classified by material and water content.

1. **FDA** classification is by material groups (see Chapter 11). Disposable or frequent-replacement lenses such as **Vistakon's Acuvue** and **Surevue** (etafilcon 58%), and **CIBA Vision's NewVues** and **Focus** (vifilcon 55%) are group IV lenses. **Bausch & Lomb's SeeQuence, SeeQuence 2,** and **Medalist,** and **Ocular Sciences' Edge II** and **Proactive** lenses are all made from polymacon 38% and are group I lenses. **CooperVision's Preference** (polymacon 38%) is also group I.

2. **Water content** is another method of classification. Lenses are grouped into low (up to 43%), medium (55–58%), and high (70% or more).

3. **Major manufacturers** use the same materials for both disposable and PRP lenses.

   a. **Acuvue** and **Surevue** are made of the same material but have
      different designs. Acuvue is the disposable lens for extended
      wear, whereas Surevue is the daily wear PRP lens. **NewVue**
      and **Focus** lenses are also similar, with the same materials but
      different designs and different modalities. NewVue is a dis-
      posable extended-wear lens; Focus is a PRP daily-wear lens
      that can be also used for extended wear.
   b. **SeeQuence 2** and **Medalist** (both 38% water polymacon) can
      be fit with the same set of trial lenses. They are both front-
      surface spin-cast and lathe-cut on the back surface. See-
      Quence 2 is meant for 1- to 2-week replacement. Medalist is
      designated for daily wear with a 1- to 3-month replacement
      cycle. The lenses have a visibility tint. The significant advan-
      tage of these lenses over other midwater-content lenses is
      much greater protein resistance.[24,25]

III. **Patient education and management** should be highly structured to minimize the likelihood of complications.[3]
   A. **"Six on, one off"** is the maximum wearing schedule recommended by
      FDA guidelines. Every six nights of overnight wear are followed by one
      night with no lenses.[9] Cleaning and disinfection are usually done on the
      "off" night. A common maintenance schedule is disposal of the lenses
      after 1–2 weeks.[11]

   Pearl: *If the patient doesn't feel a significant difference between wearing the new lenses and the old lenses, you are probably replacing them at
   a right time in the cycle.*[26]

   B. The **follow-up schedule** is normally 1 day after sleeping in the
      lenses, then 1 week, 1 month, and every 3–4 months thereafter. New
      patients can wear lenses on a daily-wear basis for adaptation pur-
      poses before commencing extended wear.[1] A wearing cycle of ex-
      tended wear can be recommended at the 1-week visit. Immediate
      removal of the lenses is advised if there is any pain, redness, or de-
      creased vision.[1]
      1. The **Yamane triad** is a three-point safety check the patient should
         perform every morning.[27]
         a. **Feel good.** After blinking six to eight times, the patient should
            ask, "Do my lenses feel good?"
         b. **Look good.** The eyes must look clear and white in the mirror.
         c. **See well.** Vision should be checked by alternately covering
            each eye.
      2. **Special attention** must be paid to limbal areas for neovasculariza-
         tion, to endothelium for buckling, to stroma for striae, and to ep-
         ithelium for microcysts or staining during follow-up.[3]

C. **Care systems** are almost identical to those used for daily-wear soft lenses (see Chapter 13). Some manufacturers bundle solution packages for PRP lenses. Many patients prefer one-step multipurpose solutions for convenience.[9]

D. **Risk factors** must be explained to the patient for liability reasons. Videotapes and written material are particularly useful when training the patient.[27]

Pearl: The best defense against extended-wear complications is continual patient education.[17]

IV. **Complications** from overnight wear are well documented. Fitting by physiology is a comprehensive method that considers the management of complications for both daily and extended wear. Many of the following conditions are also covered in Chapter 10.

A. **Hypoxia** and **acidosis** are significant challenges for extended wear lenses. Under closed-eye conditions, only 55 mm Hg of oxygen is available. This is a considerable decrease from 155 mm Hg of oxygen available under open-eye conditions. Decreased oxygen availability due to closed-eye conditions and impeded oxygen flow by the contact lens (barrier effect) impose great stresses on the cornea during extended wear.[2,19,28] Acidosis results from **hypercapnia** (increase of carbon dioxide) and is often associated with hypoxia. Acidity increases because of the barrier effect of the contact lens. The release of carbon dioxide waste products is impeded by the lens. Soft lenses show three times the carbon dioxide transmissibility as rigid gas-permeable (RGP) lenses of the same Dk.[29] Some individuals with low oxygen needs may tolerate current extended-wear lenses with minimal adverse effects.[19]

1. **Corneal edema** is almost always expected with current lenses.[15] Under hypoxic stress, water enters the cornea, and swelling results.

    a. A **Dk/t** of 24 is needed for successful daily wear. For extended wear, a Dk/t of 87 is needed to limit overnight swelling to 4%.[30,31] A Dk/t of 34 is sufficient to limit the swelling to 8%. The cornea can recover to normal thickness (**deswelling**) shortly after eye opening if the swelling is limited to 8%.[31] Because the Dk/t of current lenses is too low, overnight swelling is 10–15%, usually leaving residual corneal edema.[15]

    b. **Striae** and **folds** result because of corneal swelling. Striae are vertical, grayish-white, wispy lines in the stroma seen with a parallelepiped.[15,32] Folds appear as buckling in Descemet's membrane and are seen as black, deep grooves with direct focal illumination. Striae appear when edema exceeds 5%, while the more severe folds appear at 10% or more.[15,32] Extended wear should be discontinued when striae and folds still remain after 1 hour of open-eye wear.

    c. **Symptoms** of edema are decreased vision, glare, halos, and photophobia. These appear when swelling levels are 8% or higher.[15]

    d. **Swelling** and **ulcers** are distinctly correlated. When *Pseudomonas* was applied to rabbit corneas, 20% swelling resulted in corneal ulcers for half of the corneas tested. Swelling of 43% resulted in all of the corneas developing ulcers.[33]

  2. **Epithelial edema** associated with rigid lenses is referred to as **central corneal clouding** or **Sattler's veil.**[34] With soft lenses, the edema covers a much larger area and is more difficult to detect. Patients may complain of hazy vision, and staining is often present. Mild epithelial edema appears as surface mottling or waffling. More severe edema results in staining.[35]

  3. **Loss of transparency** in the stroma is indicative of edema of 20–25%. The cornea appears hazy or milky against the black pupil.[32]

B. **Corneal microcysts** are asymptomatic, small (15–50 μm) inclusions or dots located in the epithelial midperiphery, appearing after 3 months of extended wear.[15,28] They usually show as **reversed illumination** with a biomicroscope.[2] Reversed illumination occurs only when the contents of the cyst have high-index material, however. Basement membrane debris and basal cell breakdown material have high indices. Fluid-filled cysts are not high index and will show unreversed rather than reversed illumination. Sometimes, microcysts appear as both reversed and unreversed illuminations, depending on their contents[36] (see Chapter 3). The presence of microcysts prior to lens wear may indicate **epithelial basement membrane dystrophy.**[37]

Pearl: *Microcysts can look like salt on a jellyfish.*[38]

  1. The **cause** of microcysts is not known, but it is definitely linked to hypoxia.[39,40] The number of microcysts has been used as a clinical index of hypoxic corneal stress.[28] Microcysts can appear in non-lens wearers, however.[15]

  2. Patients are usually **asymptomatic.** The normal course for the microcyst is to originate in the deeper layers and migrate anteriorly. If the cysts reach the surface, they break, causing staining and subsequent interference in vision.[40] Microcysts that elevate above the surface before breaking can show as dry spots or negative staining. Staining may be misinterpreted as a surface problem and not as a problem caused by edema.[41]

  3. **Treatment** is discontinuance of lens wear. More than 50 microcysts indicate too much interference with corneal metabolism and lenses should be discontinued until the number is reduced, ideally to zero.[2,15] Recovery takes 6–8 weeks, and

more microcysts (**daughter cells**) typically appear 1–2 weeks after lens discontinuation.[15]

C. **Epithelial vacuoles** are larger than microcysts and can be differentiated with unreversed illumination. Virtually all extended-wear patients have vacuoles if lenses are worn for 1 year. Patients are usually **asymptomatic,** and only monitoring is needed. Temporary discontinuation is indicated if the vacuoles coalesce and stain.[15]

D. **Corneal staining,** also called **superficial punctate staining (SPS)** or **superficial punctate keratitis (SPK),** can vary from small punctate spots to large, dense, confluent patches.[15,42] It is important to monitor staining because it represents a break in the epithelial barrier. There is a standing army of bacterial troops waiting to breach the barrier.[43] Causes of staining include dehydration, solution toxicity, exposure, mechanical causes, and hypoxia.[15] Dehydration and exposure staining are further discussed in Chapter 16. Toxic staining is discussed in Chapter 13. Mechanical staining is discussed in Chapter 10.

1. **Hypoxia** adversely affects the epithelial structure. Epithelial adhesion is reduced with extended wear.[44] Cell mitosis, hemidesmosome density, and epithelial sensitivity are also reduced.[45] Increased fragility results in greater susceptibility to damage and microbial infection.[43]

2. **Epithelial integrity loss** commonly results in SPS, or SPK.[34] The fragile epithelium is easily broken. This explains why staining and epithelial edema are commonly seen together. Hypoxic SPK usually occurs in the superior cornea.[46]

3. **Symptoms** can range from none to severe pain and are usually coincident with the amount and depth of staining.[15]

4. **Treatment** entails removing lenses for periods from 24 hours to over 7 days, depending on the severity of staining.[15] Because there are numerous reasons for staining, the underlying causes must be diagnosed and treated accordingly.

E. **Follicular conjunctivitis** associated with extended wear may be a precursor to keratitis and subsequent corneal ulceration. The causative organisms in one study were *Penicillium, Pseudomonas, Staphylococcus aureus,* and those that cause epidermitis. Extended-wear patients experienced hyperemia, mild to moderate discomfort, and tearing, all of which are related to follicular conjunctivitis. Conjunctival follicles were found without corneal involvement.[47]

F. **Ulcerative keratitis,** or **microbial keratitis,** is the most serious complication of extended wear.[48] The major population at risk is the approximately 24 million contact lens wearers we have today. Severe stromal scarring or loss of eye can occur within 24 hours with a *Pseudomonas* ulcer.[6] There is an overwhelming increased risk for overnight wear and extended wear compared with daily wear. Patients with conventional and

PRP or disposable extended wear are 5–15 times as likely to develop ulcerative keratitis as those who use daily wear.[12]

1. **Compromised epithelium, bacterial adherence,** and **contamination** increase the chances of microbial infection. Epithelial cells are larger and more fragile during extended wear.[44] Some experts believe the larger cells with fewer microvilli reduce mucus protection against bacterial adherence.[49,50] Evidence shows that extended-wear lenses have enhanced ***Pseudomonas* adherence.**[51] *Pseudomonas* attachment is greater in new Acuvue lenses than in those previously worn.[52] Any time the epithelial membrane becomes compromised, there is an increased risk of corneal infection. The microorganisms adhere to the corneal surface and then invade the compromised tissue. The microorganisms then spread and multiply, inducing a host of inflammatory responses. The host's immune factors encounter the microorganisms that first cause tissue damage, which is followed by tissue repair and recovery.[53,54] Contact lenses can be common vectors for microbial **contamination** through lens care products, the contact lens case, and adherence of bacteria to the lens. Other sources of contamination are the natural skin flora and cosmetics.

2. **Risk factors** for corneal infection related to contact lenses include poor compliance, diabetes, blepharitis, epithelial trauma, corticosteroid use, smoking, trichiasis, neuroparalytic keratitis, keratitis sicca, Bell's palsy, lagophthalmos, patching, steroids, compromised immunocompetence, rheumatoid arthritis, malnutrition, alcoholism, hospitalization in an intensive care unit, mental illness, dacryocystitis, and perhaps hypoxia and warm climate.[6,55]

3. **Characteristics** of infected and sterile ulcers were identified by Stein et al.[48] Infected ulcers produced moderate to severe **pain** and unilateral **photophobia, discharge, larger infiltrates, epithelial defects,** and **anterior chamber reactions** (**hypopyon** in severe cases).[15] Sterile ulcers produced smaller infiltrates; no discharge; a likelihood of no epithelial defect; and absent or mild pain, photophobia, and anterior chamber response.[48]

4. **Documentation** is very important; the clinician should note the size and shape of the epithelial defect, the depth and location of the infiltrate and surrounding stromal inflammation, and the presence or absence of anterior chamber and scleral involvement. The ulcer must be graded. It can be classified as mild, moderate, or severe.

   a. A **mild** ulcer is less then 2 mm in size with a corneal depth no greater than 20%. The infiltrate is superficial with no scleral involvement.

b. A **moderate** ulcer is about 2–5 mm in size with a 20–50% corneal depth involvement. The infiltrate is dense and mid-stromal with no scleral involvement.

c. A **severe** ulcer is more then 5 mm in diameter with a corneal depth of more than 50%. The infiltrate is dense with deep stromal involvement, and the sclera may be involved.

5. **Perilimbal redness** is sometimes present in an adjacent conjunctival quadrant.[56] For large central ulcers, there can be **extreme hyperemia** 360 degrees around the limbus.[15] **Lid swelling** is a common finding with microbial keratitis.[44] **Corneal edema** is often seen surrounding the affected area.[15] *Pseudomonas* ulcers produce extremely severe edema, giving the entire cornea a **soupy appearance.**[43] *Staphylococcus* ulcers are usually concentrated in the affected area, whereas the rest of the cornea retains transparency. The affected area has a edematous **ground-glass appearance.** Full-thickness epithelial loss with underlying stromal infiltrates can be seen.[41] Both the epithelium and stroma stain rapidly.[15]

6. The **leading causative organism** is *Pseudomonas,* followed by *Staphylococcus*, gram-negative and gram-positive bacteria, fungi, and amebas.[42,56] Most of these organisms are part of the normal bacterial flora of the eye. The normal healthy bacterial flora can prevent or inhibit the growth of unhealthy unwanted bacteria; however, the normal flora can sometimes be harmful and cause a microbial keratitis.

7. **Cultures** are mandatory for corneal ulcers, neonatal conjunctivitis, hyperacute conjunctivitis, and dacryocystitis. Cultures are recommended for chronic conjunctivitis, chronic blepharitis, hospital-acquired infections, ulcerative conjunctivitis, epidemic conjunctivitis, atypical external disease, and follicular conjunctivitis. Cultures are rarely helpful in diagnosing ulcers, acute blepharitis, papillary conjunctivitis, hordeolum or chalazion, corneal abrasion, and allergic conjunctivitis.

8. **Treatment** should be a broad-spectrum antibiotic, which should be chosen for initial coverage.[6] Multiple-agent therapy is recommended over use of a single agent. There should be a rapid and intensive topical therapy with daily evaluation; the antibiotic choice can be tailored by culture results and clinical response. Hydrogen peroxide systems are prescribed for these patients if lens wear is resumed.[57]

a. **Mild** to **moderate keratitis**, or **nonsuppurative** ulcers, have a subacute onset with a chronic, slow progression. The virulence of infection is uncertain, and laboratory studies may be delayed because they require special laboratory materials. Initial treatment of antibiotics should be based on smears and a biopsy.

Table 15.1   Initial therapy of infectious keratitis

Organism	Antimicrobial	Topical Dose	Subconjunctival
Gram-positive cocci	Cefazolin	50 mg/ml every 15–30 min	100 mg in ⅓ ml
Gram-negative rods	Tobramycin or gentamicin	13.6 mg/ml every 15–30 min	20 mg in ½ ml
No organism or multiple organisms	Cefazolin and tobramycin	See above for dosages of each agent	
Gram-positive rods	Penicillin and gentamicin	100,000 units/ml, every 15–30 min; see above for gentamicin	
Gram-negative cocci	Ceftriaxone or ceftazidime	50 mg/ml every 15–30 min	
Acid-fast bacilli	Amikacin	20 mg/ml every 15–30 min	20 mg in ½ ml

Source: Adapted from AY Matoba. Infectious keratitis. Focal Points: Clinical Modules for Ophthalmologists. 1992;10(8):1–10.

    b.   **Severe,** or **suppurative,** ulcers have an acute, rapid onset and progression. Virulence is highly likely, and immediate, urgent laboratory studies using standard materials are needed. The initial, immediate antibiotic should be a broad-spectrum antimicrobial agent, which can be changed later once the smears are cultured.

9.   Several **methods of drug delivery** are available. The most common method is topical every 15 minutes to 1 hour for the initial 24–48 hours. A collagen shield reconstituted in water-soluble, fortified antibiotic can be used for 12 hours. Antibiotics can also be delivered subconjunctivally by injection once or twice daily for 1–2 days or intravenously if there is an impending perforation or scleral suppuration.

10.   **Initial therapy of infectious keratitis** (Table 15.1) entails frequent dosages.

11.   **Modification of therapy** is sometimes needed. The objectives in antibiotic therapy are to eliminate replicating bacteria, avoid adverse reactions to the medication, and control the destructive components of the inflammatory process.[58] To avoid unnecessary abrupt changes in therapy, the patient's response must be adequately assessed, and sensitivity tests should be completed at the laboratory.

12. **Certain responses** may be expected when a proper and effective therapy has been applied.[59]
    a. *S. aureus* and *Streptococcus pneumoniae* may be relatively unchanged then improve rapidly after 24–48 hours. Organisms are generally eliminated in 7–10 days.
    b. *P. aeruginosa* generally appears worse at 24 hours, and the organism may persist for 14 days or longer.

    Pearl: Be patient; don't bail out of an appropriate treatment too soon.

    c. **Infection with bacteria of low virulence** (e.g., *S. epidermidis*) generally improves rapidly in 24–48 hours. The organisms are eliminated in 5–7 days.
    d. *Mycobacterium* **and filamentous fungi** respond slowly and may persist for weeks.
13. **Resistant bacteria** include methicillin-resistant *S. aureus, Enterococcus fecalis*, aminoglycoside-resistant *P. aeruginosa,* beta-lactamase-producing *Neisseria,* and atypical *Mycobacterium.* The current antibiotic recommendation for resistant bacteria is vancomycin (Vancocin), 20–30 mg/ml, and ceftazidime (Fortaz), 50 mg/ml.
14. Various kinds of **adjuvant therapy** may be provided.
    a. **Cycloplegia** is used for comfort and to prevent synechiae.
    b. **Collagenase inhibitors** (e.g., ethylenediaminetetraacetic acid [EDTA], tetracycline,) are used to minimize stromal destruction.
    c. **Steroids** may be hazardous early in treatment, and their safety and efficacy are not well established in most forms of microbial keratitis. They may be helpful in reducing harmful destruction due to host response.
    d. **Nonsteroidal anti-inflammatory drugs** help reduce inflammation and pain.
    e. **Tissue adhesives** may be used for small impending and actual perforations.
    f. **Glaucoma medication** may be used if needed; beta blockers are the drug of choice.
    g. **Debridement** may improve antibiotic penetration.
    h. **Cryotherapy** has a possible role in sclerokeratitis.
    i. A **bandage lens and collagen shield** may promote re-epithelialization and allow for slow, concentrated release of antibiotic.
    j. **Continuous antibiotic infusion devices** may produce a possible benefit in extensive sclerokeratitis.
    k. **Therapeutic keratoplasty** can be used for large perforations and central or deep medically recalcitrant keratitis.

15. **Hospitalization** is indicated when a patient or family members are unable to deliver high-frequency treatment or return for daily follow-up, or if there is threatening perforation or scleral involvement.

16. **Preventative** steps can reduce the risk of infection. Lens care contamination can be minimized by washing the hands before handling contact lenses. The contact lenses should be removed at predetermined intervals and cleaned and disinfected by using FDA-approved regimens. Solution bottles should be kept small to avoid contamination, and lens cases should be occasionally replaced. Overnight wear of contact lenses should be minimized, and when it is used, patients should be selected carefully. **Warning signs** for corneal ulcers are the appearance of infiltrates, reduced vision, and patient discomfort. These patients should be seen immediately, within 2 hours of the patient's complaint.

17. **The closed eye** is a hostile environment and is in a subclinical inflammation state for protection. Because of the harsh climate, increasing oxygen permeability and decreasing microbial adherence to lenses may not be enough to make overnight wear completely safe.[60]

G. A **culture-negative peripheral ulcer (CNPU)** is a peripheral ulcer that is clinically diagnosed based on loss of epithelium, stromal involvement, and underlying infiltrative response. CNPU affects 2% of all lens wearers per year and is associated almost exclusively with soft extended wear, although it can occur with overnight wear of RGP lenses.[61] It can be caused by a hypersensitive reaction to *Staphylococcus* exotoxins; such ulcers are referred to as a **"sterile ulcers."**[43]

1. A **CNPU** is a small (less than 2 mm diameter), circumscribed, full-thickness peripheral ulcer without raised edges. Severe pain, discharge, and an anterior chamber reaction are absent. CNPU often goes undetected by the patient.

2. **Conservative treatment** is to assume that the ulcer is caused by infection. If medical intervention is not pursued, careful diagnosis and close patient follow-up are necessary. Discontinuance of lens wear is advisable. Resolution occurs within 2 weeks without medical intervention.[6]

H. **Corneal infiltrates** are whitish-gray spots and patches composed of inflammatory tissue cells (such as lymphocytes). Infiltrates can be focal (well-defined) or diffuse (hazy borders). They are usually located within 2–3 mm of the limbus in the epithelial, subepithelial, or stromal layers. Diffuse infiltrates can easily be mistaken for arcus senilis because of location. If the patient is asymptomatic, the infiltrates are usually under the upper lid in the superior cornea. **Causes** can be mechanical, toxic, microbiological, or chemical. Infiltrates alone represent an inflammatory response. There are many underlying causes, such as CLARE, keratoconjunctivitis, trauma, solution sensitivity, and hypoxia.[15] Loss of epithelial integrity is evidence of an ulcer, which must be treated immediately. **Opti-Free solution** (Alcon Laboratories, Fort Worth, Texas) was once thought to cause infiltrates, but studies found a low incidence of 0.7% among users of this solution. Ruling out other causes such as allergic reactions and low-grade infections is recommended when dealing with infiltrates.[13]

Pearl: Look for infiltrates in the corneal quadrant adjacent to the redness. Many times, hard-to-find infiltrates appear there.[38]

1. **Marginal** or **sterile infiltrates** are frequently mistaken for marginal ulcers. An ulcer is an actual loss of corneal tissue and can be sterile. Infiltrates are an accumulation of cells and debris. Ulcers appear depressed, whereas infiltrates appear raised.[61] Most marginal ulcers are actually sterile infiltrates. **Sterile infiltrates** or **infiltrative keratitis** can be caused by *Staphylococcus* exotoxins or related to solution hypersensitivity (an allergic reaction).[62] They are usually located in the peripheral cornea. Other conditions that must be ruled out are chlamydial keratitis, adenoviral epidemic keratoconjunctivitis, and contact lens superior limbic keratoconjunctivitis (CLSLK). **Infectious infiltrates** are usually bacterial in nature and are seen in microbial keratitis.

   Pearl: There are three questions to ask to aid in the diagnosis of infiltrates: (1) Is it an infiltrate or ulcer? (2) Is it allergic? and (3) Is it viral?[63]

2. **Symptoms** include foreign body sensation, irritation, photophobia, lacrimation, and localized hyperemia.[15]
3. **Resolution** is in 2 weeks, by which time infiltrates disappear. Lenses should not be worn if the patient has infiltrates. The color of the infiltrates changes to a whitish brown and becomes more granular looking. Patient should be restricted to daily wear for 2 weeks before resuming extended wear.[15]

I. **Post-tear lens debris** can indicate potential problems with extended wear.[41] It is usually associated with a nonmoving lens. **Lens adherence** with extended wear is common. Virtually all soft lenses will adhere to the eye after 45 minutes of eye closure. The impaired circulation of the tear film under closed-eye conditions probably contributes to the compromised extended-wear eye.[64] The debris that accumulates may be sloughed epithelial cells and metabolic waste products.[41,65] Conjunctivitis, staining, and infiltrative keratitis can result from the presence of debris. Lenses must be cleaned, lubricated, and loosened.[41,66]

J. **CLARE,** also known as **tight lens syndrome,** is an alarming event to the patient.[6,28] The patient awakens in the early morning, often between two and four o'clock, with severe pain, redness, tearing, and extreme photophobia in one eye.[15,38] Marked hyperemia and infiltrates are seen at the limbus, indicating an inflammatory response.[28]

1. The **cause** is usually a tight lens, although there are reported cases involving flat lenses.[2,6] Other causes may include bacterial contamination, solution reaction, lens protein, hypoxia, and general physical stress.[15]

2. **Treatment** is discontinuation of lens wear until infiltrates resolve. This normally takes 2–3 weeks but can take up to 3 months. New lenses are refitted, and daily wear is prescribed for 2 weeks before extended wear is resumed. Using new lenses and reducing the number of nights sleeping in lenses will decrease recurrence.[15] If a microbial cause for the infiltrates is suspected, therapeutic treatment must be started as soon as possible.

K. **Limbal hypertrophy (LH)** and **furrow staining** are similar conditions. Both are bunching of the limbal and perilimbal areas caused by a **tight lens.**

1. **LH** is actually a pooling of fluorescein in a ringlike pattern in heaped-up areas just within the limbus.[67] It can appear in one quadrant of the peripheral cornea and ultimately form a narrow band that encircles the cornea.[68]

2. **Furrow staining,** often without symptoms, appears as groovelike furrows perpendicular to the limbus. It is a more severe form of LH and is often combined with epithelial splitting. Fluorescein cannot be irrigated from furrow staining. Appearing most frequently in extended-wear patients, it occurs when the epithelium corrugates from a tight translimbal fit.[68]

3. **Treatment** of both conditions is refitting with a loose midwater soft lens.[67,69] Resolution usually occurs in 7–10 days.[69]

L. **Epithelial splitting,** also called **superior epithelial arcuate lesion** or **soft lens arcuate keratopathy,** appears in the superior limbal area and is usually asymptomatic.[15,69]

1. A **linear crack** approximately 0.5 mm wide and 2–5 mm in length appears along the superior limbus when stained.[15,70] Edges are irregular and appear slightly roughened or thickened. There is usually normal epithelium separating the area from the limbus.[70] It may be mistaken for a dendrite, except that it does not have bulbs or staining. Epithelial splitting is unilateral and asymptomatic, although dry-eyed patients may complain of a mild foreign body sensation after lens removal.[69]

2. **Three stages** typify epithelial splitting: (1) arcuate punctate staining, (2) coalesced punctate patches, and (3) epithelial splitting.[15]

3. **Treatment** entails refitting into different soft or rigid lens material or design. Resolution usually occurs in 1 week.[69] Epithelial splitting may be the result of upper eyelid pressure on the lens causing trauma as a consequence of inadequate lens flexure.[71]

M. **Superior limbal epithelial staining** appears similar to epithelial splitting but is less defined. The lesion is caused by the superior cornea being sealed off by the lens and upper lid in extended-wear patients. Treatment is the same as for epithelial splitting.[69]

N. **Corneal blotting** has been seen in extended-wear patients, immediately after eye opening and for 2 hours. Larger and more diffuse than punctate stain, the bilateral blots come in a variety of shapes: round, with tails, crescent-shaped, and so forth. Factors such as debris under the lens or tear chemistry may be causes. Patients should be refitted with daily-wear soft or rigid lenses.[69]

O. **Endothelial blebs** are seen in the midperiphery within minutes of applying a soft lens to the eye. Blebs appear as dark areas with specular reflection of the endothelium. The cause is probably related to acidosis.[6] The patient is asymptomatic. The bleb response is not clinically significant, and it disappears within minutes of lens removal.[15]

P. **Endothelial bedewing** consists of clusters of droplets on the inferior endothelium. The cluster is usually seen on the inferior endothelium and consists of 20–50 droplets. A past history of inflammation is usually present. There is no treatment unless there are symptoms, in which case wearing time can be reduced.[15]

Q. **Corneal wrinkling,** or **anterior corneal mosaic,** causes rippling in the epithelium that allows fluorescein to pool. Upper lid pressure causes a lens that has a thick periphery and thin center to ripple. The force is transferred to the underlying epithelium, and wrinkling results. Rapid loss of vision can occur. The effects of the wrinkling subside when the lens is removed. Refitting the patient to another lens design is advisable.[15,69]

R. **CLPC** occurs in both soft and RGP lenses, daily and extended wear.[3] CLPC progresses to the more severe GPC if left untreated. GPC and CLPC are the most common causes of people discontinuing extended wear of soft contact lenses.[15]

    1. The **causes** of CLPC are similar to those of GPC. These include lens spoilage, solution sensitivity, and mechanical trauma.

    2. The **symptoms** at the early stages are itching and mucus discharge after sleep. Later, patients complain of stringy mucus discharge, tearing during the day, blurring, excessive lens movement and displacement, intense itching, and lens awareness.

    3. **Signs** are slight palpebral conjunctival redness and edema. The symptoms are often much more severe than the signs. In later stages, uniform, elevated, small papillae appear that progress to GPC.[6]

    4. **Treatment** consists of cessation of lens wear, which relieves symptoms. Patients should discontinue contact lens wear for up to 2 months until symptoms are resolved. Return to extended wear is not recommended.[15] Daily disposable lenses have been successfully refitted.

S. **Polymegethism** was first described among contact lens wearers in 1981, when a reduced number of normally hexagon-shaped cells and variations in cell size (**pleomorphism**) was observed in the endothelium of polymethyl methacrylate wearers. The altered cell morphology was thought to be due to compromised endothelial function. It has been hypothesized that corneal problems are likely in the future for these patients.[72] Rather than positing an actual loss of cells, newer theories characterize polymegethism as an oblique reorientation of the lateral walls of the endothelial cells. Polymegethous cells may not necessarily vary in cell volume and subsequently cause damage as previously thought.[73]

    1. Patients are initially asymptomatic. Since it has been associated with **corneal exhaustion syndrome,** patients can experience related symptoms of decreased tolerance and corneal edema.

    2. **Discontinuation** of lens wear has not been effective in reducing polymegethism.[15]

T. When related to contact lenses, **corneal neovascularization** is usually due to hypoxia.

    1. **Vascularization** is defined as the formation and extension of capillaries into an avascular cornea. **Neovascularization** is formation and extension of capillaries into a previously vascularized cornea.

    2. **Limbal hyperemia,** or limbal injection, is distention of limbal blood vessels.[74] Low-grade limbal hyperemia is commonly seen on awakening. Associated mild symptoms are irritation, grittiness, dryness, and a sensation of heat.[19] If the level of hyperemia becomes clinically significant, bulbar conjunctival trauma should be suspected.

    3. Blood vessels are usually asymptomatic in **appearance.** Vessels look like spikes, branches, or loops and extend 1.5–2.0 mm beyond the translucent limbal zone. Sometimes ghost vessels without blood remain after the neovascularization subsides. The ghost vessels, however, can fill rapidly if stimulated again.[15]

    4. **Documentation** of new vessel formation can include a description of location, depth, degree of penetration, and overall severity (based on amount of penetration and depth of vessels).[75]

    5. **Perilimbal stromal edema** seems to set the stage for new vessel formation.[34] This accounts for the fact that neovascularization is uncommon for rigid lenses. Other causes are trauma, solution sensitivity, inflammatory response, or damaged lenses.

    6. **Resumption** of extended wear is not recommended unless the underlying causes are diagnosed and eliminated.

U. **Bulbar conjunctival trauma** reveals itself as hyperemia. A hyperemic conjunctiva caused by trauma must be differentiated from CLARE and ulcerative keratitis.

    1. **Causes** are usually mild abrasion or excessive pressure from the lens. A tight-fitting lens or bad edge can cause trauma.

2. A **mild foreign body sensation** is sometimes present and accompanied by staining in the bulbar conjunctiva.
3. **Discontinuation** of lens wear is recommended until the conjunctiva heals.[15]

V. **Lens defects** associated with disposable lenses were studied by Efron and Veys. After examining 150 lenses each of Acuvue, NewVues and SeeQuence lenses, several defects were found. Acuvue had 75% lenses with defects. NewVues and SeeQuence had 5% and 9% defects, respectively.

   1. **Types of defects** include nicks, tears, roughness, excess material, splits, blemishes, eccentric optic zones, and multiple pieces.[76,77]

   2. **Ocular responses** to defects included increased microcysts and corneal and conjunctival staining.[76,78] Whether these biomicroscopic findings and ocular responses are clinically significant is controversial.[20,79]

> *Pearl: Have your patients do a visual inspection of disposable lenses prior to application, looking closely for edge nicks, tears, and roughness.[80]*

W. **CLSLK** is not a common condition related to soft lenses. The appearance is superior corneal, limbal, and conjunctival hyperemia and staining. The affected area can extend to the insertion point of the superior rectus muscle. Epithelial haze, infiltrates, and micropannus have been reported. There are reports of permanent vision loss in extreme cases.[81] It is similar to **Theodore's superficial limbic keratoconjunctivitis.**

   1. **Causes** are hypoxia under the upper lid, mechanical lens irritation, lens deposits, and solution preservatives (thimerosal). The response is thought to be inflammatory in nature.

   2. **Symptoms** are lens awareness, burning, itching, photophobia, slight reduction of vision, and lens intolerance.

   3. **Removal of lenses** for several weeks may be necessary for all signs to resolve. Lubricants can be prescribed to help the affected areas under the upper lid heal. Wear can be resumed with solutions meant for hypersensitive patients. Refitting with RGP lenses is recommended if there is recurrence.[15]

V. **Spiral of problems** can occur with soft contact lenses. As long as a contact lens remains on the eye, it may produce a spiral of increasing immunologic problems. A contact lens insults the ocular surface, which increases mucus production and leads to more deposits. More deposits produce a greater insult, more mucus, and even more deposits. The problems get larger and larger until they eventually lead to pain for the patient. Properly used disposable and PRP lenses are meant to break the spiral of increasing immunologic problems[82] (Figure 15.1).

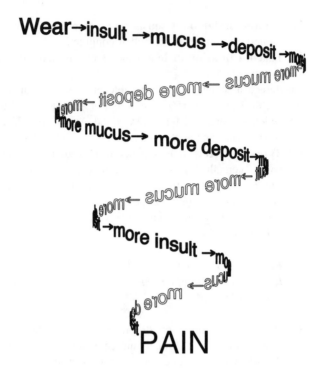

FIGURE 15.1   *Spiral of increasing problems with contact lens wear. When a contact lens is on the eye, the insult to the ocular surface induces more mucus production. More mucus induces more deposits and more insult, creating a spiral of increasing problems that eventually leads to pain. Disposable and planned-replacement lenses are designed to break this spiral. (Adapted from MR Allansmith. Immunologic effects of extended wear contact lenses. Ann Ophthalmol 1989;21:465–474.)*

REFERENCES

1. McLaughlin R. Hydrogel Extended Wear Contact Lenses. In ES Bennett, BA Weissman (eds), Clinical Contact Lens Practice. Philadelphia: Lippincott, 1991(55);1–2.
2. Mandell RB. Extended Wear. In RB Mandell (ed), Contact Lens Practice. Springfield, IL: Thomas, 1988;683–717.
3. Molinari JF. Extended wear contact lenses: a philosophy for fitting and management. Optom-Clin 1991;1(3):1–11.
4. Weissman BA, Modino BJ, Pettit TH, et al. Corneal ulcers associated with extended-wear soft contact lenses. Am J Ophthalmol 1984;97:476–481.
5. Schein OD, Glynn RJ, Poggio EC, et al. The relative risk of ulcerative keratitis among users of daily-wear and extended-wear soft contact lenses. N Engl J Med 1989;321:773–778.
6. Swarbrick HA, Holden BA. Complications of Hydrogel Extended Wear Lenses. In JA Silbert (ed), Anterior Segment Complications of Contact Lens Wear. New York: Churchill Livingstone, 1994;289–316.
7. Ghormley NR. Disposable or planned-replacement lenses? ICLC 1993;20:214.

8. Josephson JE, Caffrey BE, Campbell I, et al. Disposable contact lenses vs. contact lenses maintenance for extended wear. CLAO J 1990;16:184–188.

9. Barnhart LA, Chun MW. Disposable Hydrogel Contact Lens Systems. In ES Bennett, BA Weissman (eds), Clinical Contact Lens Practice. Philadelphia: Lippincott, 1991(57);1–8.

10. Daniels K. Evaluating a new molded disposable lens. CL Spectrum 1995;10(12):42–47.

11. Ghormley NR. Disposable contact lenses—the answer to extended wear complications? ICLC 1989;16(1):8–10.

12. Poggio EC, Abelson M. Complications and symptoms in disposable extended wear lenses compared with conventional soft daily wear and soft extended wear lenses. CLAO J 1993;19(1):31–39.

13. 10 practice-building ways to use disposable lenses. CL Spectrum 1994;9(9):44–48.

14. Lowther GE. Disposable extended wear, disposable daily wear, or disposable lenses which are not disposed? ICLC 1988;15:365.

15. Grant T, Terry R, Holden BA. Extended Wear of Hydrogel Lenses. In MG Harris (ed), Problems in Optometry. Philadelphia: Lippincott, 1990;599–622.

16. Schnider CM. Extended wear-extended care. CL Spectrum 1994;9(5):15.

17. Lowther GE. Complications. Int Eyecare 1986;2(1):6.

18. Tomlinson A. Selection of patients for contact lens extended wear. ICLC 1987;14:437–440.

19. Guillon M, Ruben M. Extended or Continuous Wear Lenses. In M Ruben, M Guillon (eds), Contact Lens Practice. London: Chapman & Hall, 1994;991–1033.

20. Guillon M. Schock SE. Soft contact lens visual performance: a multicenter study. Optom Vis Sci 1991;68(2):96–103.

21. Guillon M, Guillon J, Shah D. Visual performance stability of disposable contact lenses. ICLC 1993;20:7–17.

22. Watanabe RK, Ridder WH, Tomlinson A. Visual performance of three disposable soft contact lenses. ICLC 1993;20:106–112.

23. Hoekel JR, Maydew TO, Bassi CJ, et al. An evaluation of the 8.4-mm and the 8.8-mm base curve radii in the CIBA NewVue vs. the Vistakon Acuvue. ICLC 1994;21:14–18.

24. Ghormley NR. SeeQuence 2 and Medalist—a new planned-replacement system. ICLC 1992;19:53–54.

25. Lin ST, Mandell RB, Leahy CD, et al. Protein accumulation on disposable extended wear lenses. CLAO J 1991;17:44–50.

26. Norman C, Wood W, Rigel L, et al. Seven steps to success with disposables. CL Spectrum 1995;10(2):33–40.

27. Yamane SJ, Paragina S. Patient Education. In ES Bennett, BA Weissman (eds), Clinical Contact Lens Practice. Philadelphia: Lippincott, 1991(59);1–9.

28. Holden BA, Swarbrick HA. Extended Wear: Physiologic Considerations. In ES Bennett, BA Weissman (eds), Clinical Contact Lens Practice. Philadelphia: Lippincott, 1991(58);1–15.

29. Ang JHB, Efron N. Carbon dioxide permeability of contact lens materials. ICLC 1989;16:48–57.

30. Gruber E. Material vs. design: expand your fitting philosophy. CL Spectrum 1994;9(9):32–34.

31. Holden BA, Mertz GW. Critical oxygen levels to avoid corneal edema for daily and extended wear contact lenses. Invest Ophthalmol Vis Sci 1984;25:1161–1167.

32. Efron N. Clinical management of corneal edema. CL Spectrum 1986;1(12):13–23.

33. Soloman OD, Loff H, Perla B, et al. Testing hypotheses for risk factors for contact lens-associated infectious keratitis in an animal model. CLAO J 1994;20(2):109–113.

34. Bonnano JA. Corneal Edema. In JA Silbert (ed), Anterior Segment Complications of Contact Lens Wear. New York: Churchill Livingstone, 1994;15–27.

35. Epstein AB. Contact Lens Complications. In CA Schwartz (ed), Specialty Contact Lenses: A Fitter's Guide. Philadelphia: Saunders, 1996;251–311.

36. Lowther GE. Microcystic edema versus microcysts. ICLC 1992;19:5.

37. Schnider CM. Rigid Gas-Permeable Extended Wear Lenses. In JA Silbert (ed), Anterior Segment Complications of Contact Lens Wear. New York: Churchill Livingstone, 1994;317–336.

38. Zantos SG. Management of corneal infiltrates in extended wear contact lens patients. ICLC 1984;11(10):604-612.

39. Catania LJ. Diagnoses of the Cornea. In LJ Catania (eds), Primary Care of the Anterior Segment (2nd ed). Norwalk, CT: Appleton and Lange, 1995;203–351.

40. Bonnano JA, Polse KA. Hypoxic Changes in the Corneal Epithelium and Stroma. In A Tomlinson (ed), Complications of Contact Lens Wear. St. Louis: Mosby, 1992;21–36.

41. Silbert JA. Complications of extended wear. Optom Clin 1991;1(3):95–122.

42. Weissman BA, Mondino BJ. Ulcerative Bacterial Keratitis. In JA Silbert (ed), Anterior Segment Complications of Contact Lens Wear. New York: Churchill Livingstone, 1994;247–269.

43. Silbert JA. Microbial disease and the contact lens patient. ICLC 1988;15:221–229.

44. Lowther GE. Epithelial lesions with hydrogel extended wear: will disposable lenses prevent the problem? ICLC 1988;15:237–238.

45. Madigan MC, Holden BA. Reduced epithelial adhesion after extended wear contact lens wear correlated with reduced hemidesmosome density. Invest Ophthalmol 1992;33:314–323.

46. Onofrey B. Keep corneal insults from getting nasty. Rev Optom 1993;130(4):53–58.

47. Maguen E, Nesburn AB, Martinez, MR, et al. A long-term evaluation of myopic extended wear lenses in a primary care, nonreferral population. CL Spectrum 1992;7(10):45–50.

48. Stein RM, Clinch TE, Cohen EJ, et al. Infected vs sterile corneal infiltrates in contact lens wear. Am J Ophthalmol 1988;105:632.

49. Tsubota K, Yamada M. Corneal epithelial alterations induced by disposable contact lens wear. Ophthalmology 1992;99(8):1193–1196.

50. Tsubota K, Toda I, Fujishima H, et al. Extended wear soft contact lenses induce corneal epithelial changes. Br J Ophthalmol 1994;78:907–911.

51. Fleiszig SM, Efron N, Pier GB. Extended contact lens wear enhances *Pseudomonas aeruginosa* adherence to human corneal epithelium. Invest Ophthalmol Vis Sci 1992;33(10):2908–2916.

52. Boles SF, Refojo MF, Leong F. Attachment of *Pseudomonas* to human worn etafilcon-A contact lenses. Cornea 1992;11:47–52.

53. Smolin G. Dystrophies and Degenerations. In G Smolin, RA Thoft (eds), The Cornea: Scientific Foundations and Clinical Practice. Boston: Little, Brown, 1983;329–354.

54. Waring GO, Rodrigues MM, Laibson PR. Corneal Dystrophies. In HM Leibowitz (ed), Corneal Disorders: Clinical Diagnosis and Management. Philadelphia: Saunders, 1984:57–99.

55. Weissman BA, Mondino BJ. Corneal Infection Secondary to Contact Lens Wear. In A Tomlinson (ed), Complications of Contact Lens Wear. St. Louis: Mosby, 1992;255–274.

56. Miller D, White P. Infectious and inflammatory contact lens complications. CL Spectrum 1995;10(5):40–46.

57. Efron N, Wohl A, Toma NG, et al. *Pseudomonas* corneal ulcers associated with daily wear of disposable hydrogel contact lenses. ICLC 1991;18:46–51.

58. Matoba AY. Infectious keratitis. Focal Points: Clinical Modules for Ophthalmologists, 1992;10(8):1–10.

59. Shovlin JP. What to expect the morning after. Optom Manage 1992;24:73.

60. Sack RA, Tan KO, Tan A. Diurnal tear cycle: evidence for a nocturnal inflammatory constitutive tear fluid. Invest Ophthalmol Vis Sci 1992;33(3):626–640.

61. Schnider C. The not-so-routine visit. CL Spectrum 1994;9(12):11.

62. Catania LJ. Sterile infiltrates vs. infectious keratitis: world apart. ICLC 1987;14:412–415.

63. Townsend W. 3 questions to ask when you see infiltrates. CL Spectrum 1994;9(1):53.

64. Bruce A, Mainstone JC. Lens adherence and postlens tear film changes in closed-eye wear of hydrogel lenses. Optom Vis Sci 1996;73(1):28–34.

65. Weissman BA, Mondino BJ. Complications of extended-wear contact lenses. Int Eyecare 1985;1(3):230–240.

66. Shovlin JP. Sterile infiltrates associated with extended wear disposable contact lenses. ICLC 1989;16:239–240.

67. Grohe RM. A complete guide to detecting and managing limbal complications. CL Spectrum 1994;9(6):26.

68. Campbell R, Caroline P. Furrow staining reveals lens tightening. CL Spectrum 1993;8(11):56.

69. Dougal J. Abrasions Secondary to Contact Lens Wear. In A Tomlinson (ed), Complications of Contact Lens Wear. St. Louis: Mosby, 1992;123–156.

70. Malinovsky V, Pole JJ, Pence NA, et al. Epithelial splits of the superior cornea in hydrogel contact lens patients. ICLC 1989;16:252–255.

71. Young G, Mirejovsky D. A hypothesis for the aetiology of soft contact lens-induced superior arcuate keratopathy. ICLC 1993;20:177–180.

72. Schloessler JP Woloschak MJ. Corneal endothelium in veteran PMMA contact lens wearers. ICLC 1981;8(6):19–25.

73. Bergmanson J. Histopathological analysis of corneal endothelial polymegethism. Cornea 1992;11:133–142.

74. Efron N. Vascular response of the cornea to contact lens wear. J Am Optom Assoc 1987;58:836–846.

75. Josephson JE, Caffrey BE. Corneal Vascularization. In JA Silbert (ed), Anterior Segment Complications of Contact Lens Wear. New York: Churchill Livingstone, 1994;29–39.

76. Efron N, Veys J. Defects in disposable contact lenses can compromise ocular integrity. ICLC 1992;19:8–18.

77. Lowther GE. Evaluation of disposable lens edges. CL Spectrum 1991;6(1):41–43.

78. Seger RG, Mutti DO. Conjunctival staining and single-use contact lenses with unpolished edges. CL Spectrum 1988;3(9):36–37.

79. Efron N. A response to Professor Holden's "personal perspective." CL Spectrum 1992;7(11):37–40.

80. Barr J, Stepphen R. Tips to improve your contact lens inspections. CL Spectrum 1995;10(5):26.

81. McMahon TT. Comments on the incidence of ocular complications from contact lens wear. Int Eyecare 1985;1(4):304–306.

82. Allansmith MR. Immunologic effects of extended wear contact lenses. Ann Ophthalmol 1989;21:465–474.

PART V

Special Topics

Chapter 16

Dry Eyes and Contact Lenses

Milton M. Hom and Joseph P. Shovlin

I. **Dry-eye** problems related to contact lenses are also known as contact lens–induced dry eye (CLIDE).[1] Some practitioners believe that CLIDE is the major contributor to contact lens failure.[2] An estimated **one-fifth** of visits to eye-care practitioners are related to ocular complaints secondary to dry eye.

   A. **Preocular tear film (POTF)** is necessary for clear and comfortable vision. It serves as the primary refracting surface of the eye. Depending on the severity of decreased POTF, individuals may be limited in their ability to see clearly and comfortably. The POTF is the primary route of oxygen supply to the anterior cornea; it allows white blood cells to reach the avascular cornea and provides the eye's antibacterial properties. The POTF also lubricates the lids and flushes away corneal metabolic waste products and other debris. With a decreased POTF, the risk of developing secondary infection or chronic inflammation may be increased. Not only are lid infections commonly associated with dry eye, but there is also a higher likelihood of secondary conjunctivitis and dermatitis. Dry eye can adversely affect an individual's quality of life.

   B. **Pathologic dry eyes** may be related to any of a host of underlying medical conditions and are treated accordingly. Many times, bandage contact lenses are prescribed for the relief of pathologic dry eyes.

   C. **Marginal dry eyes** are related to contact lenses.[2] Lenses normally put a stress on the tear film. A stable tear film is necessary to accommodate a contact lens. A marginal dry eye cannot comfortably keep the lens and eye sufficiently wet. There can be innumerable reasons why contact lenses induce dry eyes in symptomatic patients. Suggested solutions themselves are often as complicated and confusing as the causes.

   D. **Ocular surface disease** is present when there is an unhealthy conjunctival and corneal epithelium. Damage to the cornea and conjunctival tissues can occur because of an abnormal tear film. Biomicroscopic signs are irregular specular reflection and staining.

293

    E. The **National Eye Institute (NEI) definition** of dry eyes is "a disorder of the tear film due to tear deficiency or excessive tear evaporation that causes damage to the intrapalpebral ocular surface and is associated with symptoms of discomfort."[3]

II. **Tear film abnormalities** have been categorized by Holly and Lemp.[4,5]

    A. **Aqueous deficiency** is usually referred to as **keratoconjunctivitis sicca (KCS).** Many times, KCS is related to medical conditions. It is usually bilateral and produces a foreign body sensation and lacrimation. This most common tear film abnormality usually results from a decrease in aqueous production by the lacrimal glands. It is commonly associated with primary **Sjögren's syndrome,** the sicca complex, and is thought to be autoimmune in origin. Sjögren's syndrome is associated with collagen-vascular and connective tissue disease, most often rheumatoid arthritis. It is more common in women who are menopausal, pregnant, or taking birth control pills, all of whom have elevated levels of estrogen and prolactin. Ocular symptoms are often the first manifestation of Sjögren's syndrome. Wetting drops are normally prescribed for KCS as initial treatment.[4]

    B. **Mucin abnormality** results from altered goblet cell function, resulting in a decrease in mucin production. The function of mucin is to enable the proper spreading of tears across the cornea surface. Dry spots occur because of abnormal or inadequate mucin.[4,6] Conditions that alter goblet cell function are ocular pemphigoid, Stevens-Johnson syndrome (SJS), allergic conjunctivitis, severe trachoma, contact lens wear, and chemical burns. Impaired goblet cell function can also result from marked vitamin A deficiency, although this is rare in developed countries. In ocular cicatricial pemphigoid (OCP) and SJS, goblet cell loss results in immunoglobulin deposits at the basement membrane zone of the conjunctiva. Bullae appear at the conjunctival subepithelial level. Continued progression of this process results in shortening of the conjunctiva and **symblepharon** formation. Goblet cell density may also increase secondary to thermal and chemical injuries. The resulting ocular surface disorders differ from OCP or SJS at the cellular level, although clinically they appear similar.

    C. A **lipid abnormality** is associated with meibomian gland dysfunction (MGD), blepharitis, and acne rosacea. A lipid-deficient dry eye can also be associated with lid disorders caused by inflammation, trauma, or scarring after eyelid surgery. The lipid layer inhibits tear evaporation. Abnormalities in the lipid layer result in increased evaporation and insufficient tears.[6] Contact lenses also increase the **tear evaporation** rate. The lipid layer on the contact lens surface is abnormal because it is either very thin or not present.[2,7,8]

    D. A **lid abnormality,** or **blink abnormality,** can predispose the eye to dryness.[5] Any structural defect of the lid can interfere with tear film distribution. Poor lid apposition, scar tissue formation, exophthalmos, and lid retraction can lead to ocular surface disease. Restricted lid movement can result in **exposure keratitis.**[4] Incomplete closure of the lids while sleeping constitutes **lagophthalmos.** Lid abnormality, or blink abnormality, can be caused by Bell's palsy, thyroid-related eye disease, foreign body (including contact lenses), or lid trauma. Other lid abnormalities that prevent efficient resurfacing of the tear layer include ptosis, lid lag, lid retraction, and madarosis.

E. **Epitheliopathy,** or **tear base abnormality,** are alterations in epithelial morphology that can affect tear film stability. When the microvilli on the epithelial surface are compromised, nonwetting areas can result.[4,6] Unhealthy microvilli, poor glycocalyx, or squamous metaplasia can result in ocular surface disease. Causes can be poor nutrition, chemical burn, Sjögren's syndrome, OCP, SJS, recurrent corneal erosions, contact lens complications, trauma from entropion, or lash abnormalities such as trichiasis.[9]

F. **"LAMBS"** is a useful mnemonic device for remembering the dry eye categories. *L* stands for lipid abnormality, *A* for aqueous abnormality, *M* for mucin abnormality, *B* for tear base or epitheliopathy, and *S* for surfacing abnormality due to lid or blink problems.[10]

G. The **NEI** has classified dry eyes into major categories: **tear deficient** and **evaporative.** Sjögren's syndrome and lacrimal gland problems, including innervation disorders, are considered to be tear-deficient causes of dry eye. Contact lens–associated problems as well as lid-related and oil deficiencies are considered evaporative causes of dry eyes.[3]

III. **Causes** of marginal dry eyes should be ascertained so that the most effective treatments can be prescribed.[9] Several underlying conditions are associated with dry eyes and should be differentially diagnosed.

A. **Lacrimal gland dysfunction** can cause reduced tear flow and KCS.[11] Viruses, autoimmune disease; aging; and systemic medications such as diuretics, antihistamines, and antidepressants can all cause lacrimal gland dysfunction.

B. **Meibomian glands** secrete the lipid layer of the tear film. The meibum should be clear and resemble motor oil in appearance. When the gland is expressed, the meibum should puddle at the orifice. The orifices should not be pouting or distorted.[6] If the meibum is waxy, cloudy, or toothpastelike, there is **MGD.**[3] Foaming of tears is also indicative of MGD.[12] Native bacteria such as *Staphylococcus*, systemic conditions such as acne rosacea, and pollution and make-up can cause malfunctioning meibomian glands. Other signs of MGD are rapid tear break-up time (TBUT), papillary hypertrophy, injection, contact lens deposits, and fluorescein staining.

C. **Blepharitis** is associated with dry eyes. The tear evaporation rate is often 10 times faster than normal. There is a high correlation between blepharitis, MGD, and marginal dry eyes.[6] A typical sign is an accumulation of scruff on the lids. Lid massages and scrubs are prescribed to clean up the dead cells.

D.   The **environment** can exert a strong influence on tear film stability. Pollution, toxic fumes, and high levels of dust and fiber can disrupt the tear film. The majority of dry-eye soft lens patients indicate a sensitivity to cigarette smoke, smog, air conditioning, central heating, or some combination of these.[13]

E.   **Blinking** should be relaxed and frequent. Poor blinking has a detrimental effect on contact lenses. Proper blinking is important to replenish the tear film. Incorrect blinking has been related to dry eyes, corneal staining, and poor vision from soft lens dehydration. Proper blinking can be taught with blink exercises.[14]

Pearl: The tear film would not be stable if not for frequent blinking.[8]

1.   The **types** of blinks are forced, twitch, incomplete, and complete.[14]
   a.   A **forced blink** occurs when the lower lid rises to complete the lid closure. The patient can detect forced blinking by placing the index finger just lateral to the outer canthus. Contraction of the muscle can be felt with the finger if there is forced blinking. This type of blinking is not correct for contact lens wear.
   b.   A **twitch blink** involves a small movement of the upper lid. A twitch blink does not sufficiently cover the eye for contact lens wear.
   c.   An **incomplete blink** occurs when the upper lid covers less than two-thirds of the cornea. Incomplete blinking leads to exposure and fluorescein staining.
   d.   A **complete blink** is ideal for contact lens wear. The upper lid covers more than two-thirds of the cornea. There is sufficient coverage of the ocular tissues and contact lens.

2.   **Blink exercises** are prescribed to train proper blinking. Normal blinking should occur at the rate of three times per minute.[12] Normal blinks need to be relaxed, without any forced movement. Practicing correct blinking entails first relaxing, closing for a count of three, and then opening the eye momentarily (slightly wider than usual). The process is then repeated. Each practice period consists of 10 correct blinks. Ten practice periods per day are typically prescribed to correct poor blinking.[15]

3.   **Reading** reduces the frequency and completeness of blinking. Learning to blink properly during reading is important.[16] If problems with blinking are suspected, consider the patient's reading habits.

IV. It is important to become familiar with **risk factors.** Many dry-eye problems can be prevented if the clinician has a working knowledge of potential risk factors. Many of these risk factors are covered in the highly regarded **Mc-Monnis questionnaire.**[17] The questionnaire is based on a compilation of past literature regarding dry-eye risk factors.

Pearl: Clinical history is one of the "gold standards" for diagnosis of dry eyes.[18]

A. **Age and sex** are predispositioning factors for dry eyes. There is a reduction of tear flow for patients older than age 40 years. The incidence of MGD increases with age.[19] Women who are older than 40 are more likely to have postmenopausal reduction of tear flow and **Sjögren's syndrome.**[12,17]

B. **Different types of contact lenses** pose different risk factors. Contact lens wear in itself requires a higher-quality tear film. If there are dryness symptoms with no lenses, dryness will certainly worsen with lenses. Rigid lenses are better for dry eyes than soft lenses. Any type of lens stresses the tear film, however. Normally, the tear film is meant to cover the back of the lid and ocular surface. Contact lenses need enough tears to cover the back of the lid, the front of the lens, the back of the lens, the edge meniscus, and the ocular surface. If the lenses are soft, additional tears are necessary to wet the lens itself.[2,7]

C. A **past history** of dry-eye treatment, such as use of drops, usually indicates a preexisting condition. Knowledge of past treatment strategies and their effectiveness is very helpful.

D. **Symptoms** indicative of dry eyes include foreign body sensation, tearing, burning, and dryness. The symptoms are usually worse at the end of the day.[2] Patients suspected of having dry eye should be asked if any of the following nine key words describes how their eyes feel: **hot, dry, burning, itching, smarting, scratchy, gritty, water,** and **tear.**[20] Be aware that, unfortunately, the signs do not always correlate with the symptoms. Different signs appear with different types of dry eyes, making diagnosis confusing and difficult.[17]

Pearl: Ninety-eight percent of watery eyes are related to dryness, not an overabundance of tears.[21]

E. **Sensitivity to irritants** sometimes translates into a dryness problem. Influential factors are cigarette smoke, smog, air conditioning, central heating, swimming, and drinking alcohol. All of these factors have been shown to be related to dry eyes.[17]

F. **Medications** can produce dry eyes as a common side effect. Antihistamines, diuretics, tranquilizers, isotretinoin, and oral contraceptives cause dryness. Medications for high blood pressure, digestive problems, and glaucoma are also related to dry eyes.[12,17]

G. **Rheumatoid arthritis** is related to dry eyes. A history of arthritis with dryness in the eyes, nose, mouth, chest, or vagina constitutes **Sjögren's syndrome.**

Pearl: *Anyone with dry-eye symptoms who cannot eat dry crackers with-out drinking water probably has Sjögren's syndrome.*[22]

   H.   **Corneal exposure** clearly places the patient at risk for dry eyes and damage to the ocular surface.
       1.   **Graves' disease** and **other thyroid problems** are associated with corneal exposure. Exophthalmos and upper lid retraction cause incomplete corneal coverage by the lids. The tear film thins and the cornea can become damaged.
       2.   **Lagophthalmos** is incomplete lid closure when sleeping. The patient is usually unaware of the condition. Many times, family members report that the patient "sleeps with the eyes open."[17] Patients typically report itching, burning, or a foreign body sensation on awakening.[21]
       3.   **Epithelial basement membrane disorders** are often associated with dry eyes. Irritation or foreign body sensations in the morning on awakening are classic symptoms.
   I.   **Allergies** predispose a patient to dry-eye problems with contact lenses. Treatment of the allergy should be the first priority before any other measures are taken. Decongestants such as naphazoline (Naphcon) by Alcon (Fort Worth, Texas) are useful.[10]

V.   **Tear tests** are necessary for dry-eye diagnosis. The tests commonly used in clinical situations are covered here. Some experts recommend a battery of tests to diagnose dry eyes. It is advisable to examine the eye in the biomicroscope with white light first before performing any tests. Manipulation of the lids can unintentionally express the meibomian glands. Even blinking increases the thickness of the lipid layer.[8]
   A.   **Schirmer's test** involves applying a paper strip to the lower lid and measuring the amount of wetting occurring over a 5-minute period.[23,24] Readings of 5 mm or less are indicative of tear production problems. **Schirmer's I** test is done without anesthesia. **Schirmer's II** is performed with anesthesia and deliberate irritation of the nasal mucosa.[2] Numerous studies have shown Schirmer's test to be unreliable and of little clinical value.
   B.   **TBUT** is widely used by practitioners to diagnose dry eye, but the validity of results is under question. Fluorescein is placed into the eye and the time it takes for dark areas to form is measured. Full-beam observation of the cornea is preferable to scanning the cornea with a narrow slit.[25] Results of less than 10 seconds indicate a mucin deficiency and probable contact lens intolerance.[2,7,26] Reliability questions arise because the instillation of fluorescein can destabilize the tear film and affect results. **Noninvasive TBUT** (NITBUT) circumvents this problem.[27,28]
   C.   **NITBUT** entails projecting a grid or mire onto the tear layer and measuring the time it takes to disrupt. Typically, NITBUT is higher than TBUT because the application of fluorescein is circumvented. The NITBUT test is considered more reliable. A 10-second or less NITBUT test

result indicates a suspect dry eye with a grid.[2] Five seconds or less may indicate a dry eye with a keratometric mire.[2,7]

D. **Rose bengal** was thought to stain dead or degenerated cells and mucus. Rose bengal actually stains areas of inadequate mucus protection of the corneal epithelium, not necessarily dead cells.[29] A 1% drop is applied to the eye. A problem with rose bengal is the irritating nature of the drop. Applying the drop with a cotton-tip applicator reduces the amount of dye and provides less irritation. With a green biomicroscopic filter, corneal and conjunctival staining can be seen in dry-eye patients. The stain usually appears in the inferior nasal bulbar conjunctiva.[2,20]

Pearl: Dry-eye damage can be demonstrated to the patient by having the patient look in the mirror after rose bengal staining.[20]

E. The **phenol red test,** also called the **cotton thread test** and commercially available as **Zone-Quick,** is is similar to Schirmer's test. Instead of a cumbersome paper strip, a 70-mm thread impregnated with phenol red is inserted into the lower lid for 15 seconds. When the thread absorbs the tears, color changes from red to yellow due to tear pH, and the amount of string that turns yellow is measured. The test is much less irritating and more indicative of the basal tear function than Schirmer's test. The results are more reliable. A normal readings is 16.7 mm. Lower than 9 mm is diagnostic for dry eyes.[2]

F. **Lacrimal equilibration time (LET)** is a simple test for dry eyes. It involves the instillation of drop of Celluvisc (Allergan, Irvine, California) in each eye and timing how long it takes to regain predrop visual acuity. Asymptomatic patients take an average of 2.57 minutes to clear, and symptomatic patients take a longer 10.84 minutes to clear.[30] High LET results may be due to poor drainage of the lacrimal system or ineffective blinking.[30]

G. The **specular appearance of the lipid layer** can help in determining the quality and thickness of the tear film. A gray, thin layer may be too sensitive to evaporation.[31,32] A thick, colorful layer may leave lipid deposits.[7,33] Guillon's Tearscope (Keeler Instruments, Broomall, Pennsylvania) uses the same principle (see Chapter 3). There are different methods of classification.

    1. **Hamano** described three categories of patterns: marmoreal, flow, and amorphous.

        a. **Marmoreal patterns** are marblelike and gray in color. The lipid layer is 13–70 nm thick. Marmoreal patterns are the most common. If contamination is present, there can be excessive drying and deposits. Contamination appears as dark mucus strands and lumps in the lipid layer.

        b. A **flow pattern** (also known as a wave pattern) looks wavy and is 10–90 nm thick. The waviness is caused by the spread-

Table 16.1   Lipid Layer Colors

Lipid Layer Color	Thickness (nm)
White	30
Gray (white)	45
Gray	60
Gray (yellow)	75
Yellow	90
Yellow (brown)	105
Brown (yellow)	120
Brown	135
Brown (blue)	150
Blue (brown)	165
Blue	180

Note: The interference fringe colors seen in specular reflection can indicate the thickness of the lipid layer. Overly thick layers and insufficiently thin layers can lead to dryness and deposits.
Source: Adapted from DR Korb, JV Grenier. Increase in Tear Film Lipid Layer Thickness Following Treatment of Meibomian Gland Dysfunction. In DA Sullivan. Lacrimal Gland, Tear Film, and Dry Eye Syndromes. New York: Plenum, 1994;295.

ing of lipid across the surface. Patients with this pattern are good candidates for contact lenses.

   c. **Amorphous patterns** are blue-gray. They represent a stable, thick tear lipid layer. These patients show good tolerance for contact lenses but may suffer from lipid deposits.[7]

  2. **Guillon** further divided the marmoreal category into open meshwork and closed meshwork. Colored fringe pattern category was added.

   a. The **open meshwork,** or **open marmoreal,** pattern has a gray marblelike pattern over a thin, lighter-colored main layer. The meshwork appears open and sparse. An open meshwork indicates a very thin lipid layer. The patient is at risk for dryness problems with contact lenses.

   b. A **closed meshwork,** or **closed marmoreal,** pattern is similar to the open meshwork except that the meshwork is closed and tight. This is a thicker, more stable pattern. The patient is a good contact lens candidate.

   c. A **colored fringe pattern** appears in only 5% of tear films; it indicates a very thick tear film of more than 86 nm. Yellow, brown, blue, and purple appear in this pattern. Contact lens wear is possible, but the high lipid volume may cause deposits.[34]

  3. **Korb** has defined lipid layer thickness by interference fringe color. The thinnest layers are white, while the thickest layers are blue[31] (Table 16.1).

4. **Observation of sea slicks** on the ocean's surface may shed light on the actual composition of the lipid layer. The meibomian lipids do not have adequate spreading action. Like the foam and flotsam on the ocean surface, the meibomian lipids tend to clump together rather than dispersing evenly. Specular reflection may actually be showing a surface gel composed of mucin instead of a layer composed of lipid.[35]

H. The **tear meniscus**, or **tear prism height**, can be seen resting on the lower lid. The tear meniscus can be evaluated according to four characteristics: height, width, regularity, and curvature.[34] A height of 0.3 mm is considered normal. An abnormal tear prism has a lower height and appears uneven or scalloped.[2]

   1. **An aqueous deficiency or lipid abnormality** will affect the tear meniscus. A scanty meniscus appearance and areas of discontinuity are signs of tear abnormalities.
   2. **Taylor** classified tear meniscus with regard to zones of irregularity.
      a. The **intact** category has no zones of irregularity and appears in the normal eye.
      b. The **intermittently nonintact** category has zones of irregularity, but these are not always present. This is an abnormal meniscus.
      c. In the **permanently nonintact** category, zones of irregularity are present at all times. A meniscus of this type indicates a risk for many dry-eye problems.
   3. **Peripheral height measurements** are a simple and effective clinical technique described by Guillon. Central height (under the pupil) and peripheral heights (5 mm nasally and temporally) should be about equal. Differences between heights indicate irregularity.[34]
   4. A **pillarlike flare image** can be detected by the patient as a result of the meniscus. When looking at a bare light bulb against a black background, the tear meniscus forms a flare image. The patient can report the time it takes for the pillarlike image to disappear. Dry-eye patients report disappearance in a short 3–10 seconds.[36]
   5. **Black line formation** can be seen on the ocular surface immediately adjacent to the meniscus. Application of fluorescein enhances its appearance.[37] The anterior and posterior surfaces of the tear in this thin area cancel each other out, forming the black line. The black line area is the most unstable part of the entire tear film.[34] The black line can also be seen at the edge of rigid lenses while on the eye.[38]

I. **Fluorescein staining** is a very simple and easy test that reveals dry-eye problems. Dry-eye staining has been reported with one-third of soft lens wearers. Desiccation staining usually appears in the inferior portion of the cornea for lens wearers. Sometimes it takes the form of a "smile-shaped" stain in the inferior midperipheral cornea. Other times it is located in the central cornea. It is, however, rarely seen in the superior cornea. Desiccation staining can be light and punctate or progress to confluent patches. The most severe cases can progress even further to full-thickness erosions. Thin lenses are more likely to have desiccation staining than thicker lenses. High humidity and midwater thick lenses help alleviate dry-eye staining.[2,7]

    1. **Peripheral corneal desiccation,** or **3 o'clock and 9 o'clock staining,** can be related to dry eyes in rigid lenses. Numerous factors cause 3 o'clock and 9 o'clock staining. If a tear abnormality is one of the predominant causes, treatment with lubricating drops should be initiated (see Chapter 14).

    2. **Bacterial infections** have a pathway to invade the cornea when staining is present. Correlations between contact lens–related corneal infections and dry eyes have been reported.[21]

    3. **Bulbar conjunctival staining** is commonly seen with dry eyes, with or without contact lenses. The staining usually appears along the exposed horizontal bulbar conjunctiva.[8] Conjunctival staining indicative of dry eyes can occur without the presence of corneal staining.

    4. **Loss of corneal luster** is another sign of dry eyes. The cornea appears dull and is accompanied by staining and a hyperemic conjunctiva.

J. A **lactoferrin test** measures the amount of lactoferrin in the tears. Lactoferrin comes from the lacrimal gland. Decreased lactoferrin in the tears usually indicates poor production from the lacrimal gland. The Lactoplate test is used to measure lactoferrin. A filter paper circle is placed into the eye to absorb tears. The paper is then placed on an immunoreactive plate, and a ring forms. The larger the ring, the greater the amount of lactoferrin in the tears. Dry-eye patients have small amounts.[2,7]

K. **Hypofluorescence** occurs when the eye does not fluoresce on the instillation of fluorescein. If the eye is dry, the dye accumulates in flakes on the conjunctiva. Fluorescence does not occur unless a saline drop is added or the patient forces blinking. The severity of dryness can be categorized by the time required for fluorescence after a saline drop is instilled. Immediate fluorescence is normal, and gradual fluorescence is considered subnormal.[39,40]

L. **Tear osmolarity** measures the tonicity or salt content of tears. Although it is not a clinical test, it is highly sensitive for dry eyes.[18] Increased osmolarity means a decreased tear production.[6,7]

VI. **Management** of CLIDE usually involves wetting agents. If wetting agents are not effective, more complex options are necessary. Sometimes, the dry eye may be so intractable that lenses cannot be worn.

    A. **Wetting agents** are commonly the first treatment prescribed for dry eyes with or without contact lenses. The disadvantage of drops is their short time of effect. A common complaint is that the drops work only for a few minutes after instillation.[41,42] Some preservatives, such as benzalkonium chloride, can compromise the epithelial surface.

Pearl: *Soft lens dry-eye patients prefer nonpreserved wetting drops over drops with preservatives.[21,43]*

Components of drops should be considered when prescribing for dry eyes. Many drops have similar components and can be categorized accordingly. A trial-and-error method can be used to choose the best drop for the patient. One drop can be chosen from each category and applied according to a schedule.[44] Patients can then choose the best drops for their needs. Keep in mind, however, that saline has been shown to be just as effective as other lubricants.[45] Patients should avoid using the drops more than 10 times a day. Overuse of wetting drops can lead to development of medicamentosa, a toxic keratitis.[2]

Pearl: *Prevention is the key when using drops. Use the drops frequently, **before** the eye dries out.[21]*

1. **Methylcellulose** is a colorless, water-soluble colloid that can produce solutions of varying viscosity. It is nonirritating and nontoxic to ocular tissues. Methylcellulose prolongs the ocular retention time and enhances wetting. TBUT shows significant increases.[4] It is in Tears Naturale (preserved; Alcon), Tears Naturale Free (nonpreserved; Alcon), and Cellufresh (nonpreserved; Allergan).[44] Celluvisc also contains methylcellulose, but it is very viscous and should be used for severe or pathologic dry eyes.[21] Nonpreserved cellulose-containing tear supplements are **Bion** from Alcon and **GenTeal** from CIBA Vision. Bion is an ion-containing tear supplement. GenTeal is preserved with low amounts of hydrogen peroxide that convert to water and oxygen in the tear film.[46]

Pearl: *Occlude the puncta with an index finger for 30 seconds to prolong contact time and effect.[44]*

2. **Polyvinyl alcohol (PVA)** is a nonirritating, colorless wetting agent. PVA is not as viscous as methylcellulose, and it also increases TBUT. There are some incompatibilities with other commonly used solution components. Borate, found in some irrigating solutions, can cause a reaction when used with a PVA-containing drop.[4] PVA is in Liquifilm (preserved) and Refresh (nonpreserved) (both by Allergan).[44]

3. **AquaSite** (CIBA Vision) contains polycarbophil. The solution has a longer retention time than PVA or carboxymethylcellulose.

4. **Vitamin A–containing drops** such as **VIVA-DROPS** (Vision Pharmaceuticals, Mitchell, South Dakota) contain retinol with polysorbate 80. Retinol regenerates goblet cells and enhances mucus production. Subjective and objective improvement has been demonstrated with VIVA-DROPS.[4]

5. **Hypotonic** drops such as HypoTears (CIBA Vision) are the most popular tear substitute according to one study.[5] Hypotonic tears have been shown to bring effective subjective relief of symptoms.[6] Hypotonic saline has been found to decrease dryness and enhance wearing times for soft lens wearers. The osmotic gradient causes more water to flow into the lens in a hypotonic environment.

B. **Ointments** are usually composed of petrolatum, mineral oil, and sometimes lanolin. Patients allergic to wool may react to lanolin. Ointments are meant to melt at eye temperature and disperse into the tears. Ointments have much longer retention times than drops.[4] Unfortunately, vision is temporarily blurred after instillation. The ointments are best used before sleeping, which makes them especially useful for **lagophthalmos.** If used during the day, a very small amount of ointment may be sufficient. **Lacrisert** (Merck and Company, West Point, Pennsylvania) is a rod of water-soluble hydroxypropyl cellulose that is placed in the lower cul-de-sac. The preservative-free polymer is released into the tears for 12–24 hours, during which time vision may be blurred and the eye may have a foreign-body sensation.

C. **Changes in lens material and design** are sometimes effective for symptoms of dryness.

1. **Medium-water-content and thick soft lenses** are preferred over thin lenses.[12,47] Use of lenses with a water content of 55% and a thickness of 0.10–0.12 mm seems to retain water better than use of lenses with lower water content.[12] Thinner lenses are more prone to dehydration.

2. **Disposable lenses** are helpful. Patients with older lenses are more likely to complain of dryness.[48] Unstable tear films usually cause soft lenses to deposit more.[2,7] Comfort can be improved by frequent replacement. One-day disposable lenses may be the best soft lens option yet for dry eyes.

3. **Rigid gas-permeable (RGP) lenses** are very effective for dry eyes. RGP lenses do not need to be hydrated by the tear film. Lens awareness, however, may be a problem for some patients.

4. **Prism sphere soft lenses** with 3 diopters of prism can reduce the lens dehydration caused by evaporation.[49,50] The ballast acts like a wick and slows tear movement into the puncta. Some patients report relief with prism sphere lenses. The design should be used in conjunction with artificial tears and night ointment to resolve symptoms of contact lens intolerance.

5. **Bandage lenses** and **collagen corneal shields** have been used with sporadic success but are especially useful when filaments or mucus strands are present. The increased risk associated with continuous lens wear must be balanced with the benefits to be gained through this approach.

D. **Lid massages** are the most effective treatment for **MGD.**[19,31,51] Lid massages should be combined with warm compresses and gland expression. A small washcloth wrung after being soaked in warm water is applied to the closed lids. The lids are massaged for approximately 30 seconds. Meibum in blocked glands usually has a high melting point. Application of heat and massage serves to loosen the waxy meibum in the blocked glands. The washcloth can also be used to clean the lids of any of the scruff and flakes commonly seen with an associated blepharitis. Lid massage should be repeated one or two more times (for a total of two or three times). The glands are then expressed with firm digital pressure on the lower and upper lids. Lid massages should be performed at least twice a day. Unfortunately, there is no cure for MGD. Lid massages are a palliative measure and will probably be required as long as the patient wears lenses.

E. **Punctal occlusion** is used for tear preservation. It can be explained to patient that the tear film system is like a sink, with the inflow from the tear glands and the outflow through the puncta. Plugging the drain better allows the tears to remain on the surface of the eye.[52] **Collagen plugs** that dissolve are useful as temporary plugs to determine the effectiveness of punctal occlusion in preserving tears.[2]

1. The **procedure** is to place the plugs in both the upper and lower puncta of the most symptomatic eye. Both puncta should be occluded because the outflow from the nonoccluded punctum can compensate for the occluded punctum. The plugs are 3 mm long and available in several diameters. Anesthesia drops should be used to reduce blink reflex and make the lids more flaccid.[52,53] Holding the plug with a jeweler's forceps in one hand and pulling the lid laterally to straighten the canaliculus with the other hand, the clinician advances the plug until it disappears. The plugs should be pushed below the lid margin.

2. **After instillation,** the patient should be warned that the plugs may be itchy. The plugs may be noticeable on extreme angles of gaze. An antibiotic drop can be instilled in each eye after the procedure. Lubrication therapy should be continued.[52] The plugs dissolve in a few days, resulting first in immediate relief, then a decline in comfort.

3. **Permanent silicone plugs** can be used if the temporary plugs are successful. Herrick plugs require no dilation and come with their own insertion kit. Other procedures include thermal cautery, electrodesiccation, laser punctal occlusion, and surgical repositioning of the punctum anteriorly. Relief should be felt in 24 hours.[53,54]

4. Possible **disadvantages** are epiphora and irritation from a dislodged plug. Thirty-seven percent of patients experience corneal and conjunctival abrasions. There is also a question of effectiveness. In one study in which plugs were placed in only one eye, patients perceived no advantage of one eye over the other. Plugs were also shown to be ineffective in terms of TBUT, tear prism height, fluorescein staining, and tear lactoferrin.[55,56]

F. **Saline soaks** can prolong wearing time. The soft lens is rehydrated at midday. It is soaked in saline for 15 minutes, then reapplied.[50] A variation is keeping an extra set of lenses. At mid-day, the other pair of lenses is applied to the eye.

G. **Environmental** factors can be altered to optimize conditions for the dry-eye patient.[57] Low humidity, low atmospheric pressure, air pollution, and moving air promote more lens dehydration.[58,59] Irritating factors such as wind and dust can create dryness.[12]

1. **Humidifying** the environment has been shown to relieve symptoms. The lipid layers inhibiting evaporation on soft lenses are very sensitive to humidity. Use of humidifiers for the home and office is recommended. Air purifiers are also useful to remove particles that irritate the eye.

Pearl: More than 75% of soft lens wearers reported alleviation of all dry-eye symptoms with high humidity.[8]

2. **Avoiding drafts** and **excessive air conditioning** is helpful. Exposing the eyes to direct ventilation hastens drying.[2]

3. **Spectacles** increase humidity at the ocular surface. Larger wrap-around spectacles give the best results. Wearing spectacles for indoors and outdoors is also very helpful.

Pearl: Sometimes dry eyes can be alleviated with something as simple as wearing sunglasses outdoors.[12]

4. **Shields and goggles** can be prescribed for severe dry eyes. The humidity shields attach to the spectacles. The main drawback is the unusual appearance. Airtight goggles such as those used for swimming are the most effective.

H. **Tarsorrhaphy** is a surgical closure of the lids reserved for cases of severe, unresponsive disease, especially in nerve paralysis. Initially, the lateral third of the palpebral fissure is sutured shut. When this measure is insufficient, a complete tarsorrhaphy is performed.

I. **Estrogen replacement therapy** may be beneficial in patients with KCS.

J. **Salivary glands transplant** can produce preocular secretion. Placing salivary gland tissue in the conjunctiva has been attempted.

    K. It is useful to **group the various dry-eye therapies into stages.** The first stage is tried first, and if the treatments are ineffective, the treatments in the next stage should be initiated.[10]

        1. First-stage dry-eye therapy consists of artificial tears and lid massages for MGD.

        2. Second-stage dry-eye therapy consists of moist-chamber spectacles (shields and goggles) and medications.

        3. Third-stage dry-eye therapy consists of punctal occlusion.[10]

VII. The **prognosis** for dry eye is guarded in many cases. The treatment may represent only a maintenance strategy. **Multiple evaluations** may be necessary to establish the diagnosis and to determine the minimum treatment that produces results. Once a treatment plan has been shown to be effective, the clinician should provide follow-up care at appropriate intervals to encourage compliance and continued effectiveness.

REFERENCES

1. LaFerla JD. Punctal occlusion induces excessive soft toric rotation. CL Spectrum 1995;10(2):19.
2. Tomlinson A. Contact Lens-Induced Dry Eye. In A Tomlinson (ed), Complications of Contact Lens Wear. St. Louis: Mosby, 1992;195–218.
3. Caffrey BE. The diagnosis of dry eye. Optom Today 1996;4(3):26–30.
4. Jaanus SD. Lubricants and Other Preparations for Ocular Surface Disease. In JD Bartlett, SD Jaanus (eds), Clinical Ocular Pharmacology. Boston: Butterworth–Heinemann, 1995;355–367.
5. Holly FJ. Diagnosis and treatment of dry eye syndrome. CL Spectrum 1989;4(7):37–44.
6. Farris RL. The dry eye: its mechanism and therapy, with evidence that the contact lens is the cause. CLAO J 1986;12:234–246.
7. Tomlinson A. Tear Film Changes with Contact Lens Wear. In A Tomlinson (ed), Complications of Contact Lens Wear. St. Louis: Mosby, 1992;159–194.
8. Korb DR. Tear Film–Contact Lens Interactions. In DA Sullivan (ed), Lacrimal Gland, Tear Film, and Dry Eye Syndromes. New York: Plenum, 1994;403–410.
9. Caffrey B. Understanding the most common causes of dry eye. CL Spectrum 1993;8(11):51.
10. Farris RL. Staged therapy for the dry eye. CLAO J 1991;17:207–215.
11. Caffrey B. Take a closer look at "dry eye." CL Spectrum 1993;8(10):73.
12. Finnemore VM. Is the dry eye contact lens wearer at risk? Not usually. Cornea 1990(suppl);9:51–53.
13. Lowther GE. Comparison of hydrogel contact lens patients with and without the symptoms of dryness. ICLC 1993;20:191–194.
14. Collins M, Heron H, Larsen R, et al. Blinking patterns in soft contact lens wearers can be altered with training. Am J Optom Physiol Optics 1987;64:100–103.
15. Stein HA, Slatt BJ, Stein RM (eds). Fitting Guide for Rigid and Soft Contact Lenses (3rd ed). St. Louis: Mosby, 1990;234.

16. Korb D, Korb JE. Fitting to achieve normal blinking and lid action. ICLC 1974;1:57–70.
17. McMonnies CW. Key questions in dry-eye history. J Am Optom Assoc 1986;57:512–517.
18. Lucca JA, Nunez JN, Farris RL. A comparison of diagnostic tests for keratoconjunctivitis sicca: lactoplate, Schirmer and tear osmolarity. CLAO J 1990;16:109–112.
19. Hom MM, Martinson JR, Knapp LL, et al. Prevalence of meibomian gland dysfunction. Optom Vis Sci 1990;67(9):710–712.
20. Shenon P. Why you need to know about punctal occlusion. CL Spectrum 1990;5(7):43–49.
21. Shenon PW. Handouts for patients with dry eyes. CL Spectrum 1990;5(6):31–34.
22. Caffrey B. Digging below the surface of dry eye syndrome. CL Spectrum 1994;9(10):59.
23. Cho P, Yap M. Schirmer test. I. A review. Optom Vis Sci 1993;70(2):152–156.
24. Cho P, Yap M. Schirmer test. II. A clinical study of its repeatability. Optom Vis Sci 1993;70(2):157–159.
25. Cho P, Brown B, Chan I, et al. Reliability of the tear break-up time technique of assessing tear stability and the locations of the tear break-up in Hong Kong Chinese. Optom Vis Sci 1992;69:879–885.
26. Andres S, Henriquez A, Garcia ML, et al. Factors of precorneal tear film break-up time (BUT) and tolerance of contact lenses. ICLC 1987;14:103–107.
27. Cho P, Douthwaite W. The relation between invasive and noninvasive tear break-up time. Optom Vis Sci 1995;72(1):17–22.
28. Mengher LS, Bron AJ, Tonge SR, et al. A noninvasive instrument for clinical assessment of the pre-corneal tear film stability. Curr Eye Res 1985;4:1–7.
29. Feenstra RGP, Tseng S. What is actually stained by rose bengal? Arch Ophthalmol 1992;110:984–989.
30. Lavaux JE, Keller WD. Lacrimal equilibration time (LET): a quick and simple dry eye test. Optom Vis Sci 1993;70(10):832–838.
31. Korb DR, Grenier JV. Increase in Tear Film Lipid Layer Thickness Following Treatment of Meibomian Gland Dysfunction. In DA Sullivan (ed), Lacrimal Gland, Tear Film, and Dry Eye Syndromes. New York: Plenum, 1994;293–298.
32. Forst G. The precorneal tear film and "dry eyes." ICLC 1992;19:136–140.
33. Schnider CM. Extended Wear Soft Lenses. In CA Schwartz (ed), Specialty Contact Lenses: A Fitter's Guide. Philadelphia: Saunders, 1996;94–100.
34. Guillon JP, Guillon M. The Role of Tears in Contact Lens Performance and its Measurement. In M Ruben, M Guillon (eds), Contact Lens Practice. London: Chapman & Hall, 1994;453–483.
35. Baier RE, Thomas EB. The ocean: the eye of the earth. CL Spectrum 1996;11(1):37–44.
36. Fatt I. A measurable subjective patient response to the dry eye. CLAO J 1994;20:249–252.
37. Bennett ES, Gordon JM. The borderline dry-eye patient and contact lens wear. CL Forum 1989;19(7):52–74.
38. Benjamin WJ. Examination of the tear fluid meniscus surrounding the rigid lens on the eye. ICLC 1988;15:390–391.
39. Farris RL. Staged therapy for the dry eye. CLAO J 1991;17:207–215.
40. Soper JW. Method of diagnosing deficiency of aqueous tears. CL Spectrum 1993;8(1):31–35.
41. Campbell RC, Caroline PJ. Factors in alleviating dryness. CL Spectrum 1991;6(8):64.

42. Golding TR, Efron N, Brennan NA. Soft lens lubricants and prelens tear film stability. Optom Vis Sci 1990;67:461–465.

43. Caffrey BE, Josephson JE. Is there a better "comfort drop"? J Am Optom Assoc 1990;61(3):178–182.

44. Caffrey B. Finding the best drops for your dry-eye patients. CL Spectrum 1994;9(7):55.

45. Efron N, Golding TR, Brennan N. The effect of soft lens lubricants on symptoms and lens dehydration. CLAO J 1991;17:114–119.

46. Semes LP. Understanding dry-eye management. Optom Today 1996;4(3):32–36.

47. Orsborn GN, Zantos SG. Corneal desiccation staining with thin high water content contact lenses. CLAO J 1988;14:81–85.

48. Brennan NA, Efron N. Symptomatology of HEMA contact lens wear. Optom Vis Sci 1989;66:834–838.

49. Campbell R. Caroline PJ. Prism-sphere lens design reduces corneal staining. CL Spectrum 1994;9(4):56.

50. Lowther GE. The marginal dry eye and contact lens wear. ICLC 1988;15:333.

51. Shuley V, Collins M. Lid massage and symptoms of dryness in soft contact lens wearers. ICLC 1992;19:121–124.

52. Bockin DG. How to perform punctal occlusion. CL Spectrum 1993;8(11):30–32.

53. Caffrey B. How to approach punctal occlusion. CL Spectrum 1994;9(8):49.

54. Scott CA, Catania LJ, Larkin KM, et al. Care of the patient with ocular surface disease. St. Louis: American Optometric Association, 1995;1–49.

55. Lowther GE, Semes L. Effect of absorbable intracanicular collagen implants in hydrogel contact lens patients with the symptoms of dryness. ICLC 1995;22:238–243.

56. Slusser TG. A review of hydrogel contact lens-related dry eye and lacrimal occlusion. ICLC 1995;22:250–254.

57. Caffrey B. Creating the best environment for dry-eyed patients. CL Spectrum 1994;9(9):55.

58. Timberlake GT, Doane MG, Bertera JH. Short-term, low-contrast visual acuity reduction associated with in vivo contact lens drying. Optom Vis Sci 1992;69(10):755–760.

59. Andres S, Garcia ML, Espina M, et al. Tear pH, air pollution and contact lenses. Optom Vis Sci 1988;65:627–631.

Chapter 17

Keratoconus

Milton M. Hom

I. **Keratoconus** was usually treated in the past with scleral lenses. In 1823, **Sir John Herschel** described the neutralization of an **irregular cornea** using an animal jelly and a spherical capsule of glass. Today, keratoconus patients benefit from rigid gas-permeable (RGP) lenses. Even patients who were once thought to be candidates for corneal surgery can be refitted successfully with rigid lenses.[1]

    A. **Keratoconus** has no precise **definition.**[2] Authors disagree as to what is pathognomonic. Some consider the presence of Vogt's striae or Fleischer's ring along with irregular corneal astigmatism to be sufficient to diagnose keratoconus.[3] Others believe that Vogt's striae are not diagnostic because of their presence in other conditions, such as pellucid degeneration.[2]

    B. According to the **Collaborative Longitudinal Evaluation of Keratoconus (CLEK) study,** the severity of keratoconus is characterized by the presence of **Vogt's striae** in deep stroma, **Fleischer's ring,** and **corneal scarring.**[4]

    C. The **etiology** of keratoconus is not entirely known.

        1. **Proposed causes** are collagen alterations of the biochemical nature and proteoglycan physiologic activity.[5]

        2. **Systemic diseases** are associated with keratoconus. These diseases include Crouzon's syndrome, Ehlers-Danlos syndrome, osteogenesis imperfecta, oculodentodigital syndrome, Rieger's syndrome, Marfan's syndrome, atopy, Leber's congenital amaurosis, Down syndrome, focal dermal hypoplasia, and connective tissue disorders.

        3. **Other associated factors** are decreased ocular rigidity, collagen type III presence, high amounts of lysinonorleucine, and possibly hereditary factors.[6,7]

        4. **Eye rubbing** and **hard contact lens wear** have been shown to be associated with keratoconus. A link between keratoconus and wearing polymethyl methacrylate lenses is controversial.[5,7] Blunt ocular trauma has been described as a risk factor.[5]

    D. The **incidence** of keratoconus is between 50 and 230 per 100,000 of the general population.[8]

    E. **Unilateral keratoconus** may or may not exist. There is a reported incidence of 3%. Videokeratoscopy showed that what was once thought to be unilateral keratoconus was actually bilateral.[9] The keratoconus in the other eye was subclinical, perhaps representing an incomplete expression of the keratoconus gene.[8] Corneal topography can reveal early signs of inferior steepening.[9,10] Amsler used the term **keratoconus fruste** to describe an incomplete form that may slowly progress.[11,12]

    F. **Cone advancement** usually occurs in rapid stages followed by slower, quieter stages. The rapid stages usually last no more than 5 years at a time.[13]

        1. **Classic onset** is during puberty or in the late 20s.[4,14] The average age of a keratoconus patient is 27 years, according to the CLEK study.[15]

        2. The **spiral progression** or the steepening path in keratoconus begins in the inferotemporal quadrant and then spreads nasally to the inferonasal cornea. At or above the midline, the steepening rotates from temporal cornea up to superotemporal, superior cornea and finally to the superonasal area[16] (Figure 17.1).

II. A number of techniques are used in the **detection and diagnosis of keratoconus.**

    A. The **symptoms** are decreased vision, monocular diplopia or ghost images, multiple images, distortion, asthenopia, polyopia, photophobia, and halos.[17] Sometimes written words appear confusing, missing, or altered.[7] Two-thirds of mild to moderate keratoconus patients experience pain.[4,18]

        Pearl: *Even when visual acuity is good, it is normal for keratoconics to describe visual distortion. Studies show that keratoconics have dysfunctional vision despite adequate Snellen acuity with contact lenses.[19]*

    B. The **biomicroscopic signs** of keratoconus are well documented.

        1. **Apical thinning** can be viewed with an optic section.[20] Corneal thickness measurements by ultrasonic pachymetry show a significant loss.[21]

        2. **Fleischer's ring,** or **line,** is a yellow-brown to olive-green ring encircling the base of the cone. Iron deposition forms the superficial epithelial ring. The ring itself is rarely complete. Use of a cobalt filter can enhance detection of Fleischer's ring.[2,7,22]

        3. **Ruptures in Bowman's membrane** are clear spaces or interruptions appearing as anterior clear, networked lines.[10,17]

        4. **Vertical striae** or **Vogt's striae** are present at the level of Descemet's membrane. There are fine striations in the deep stroma, probably caused by the lamellar stretching.[12,17,22] Vogt's striae are closely packed, usually vertical, and relieved by digital pressure.[2,10] The striae can be oriented at any angle.

        5. The **visibility of corneal nerves** is more pronounced with keratoconus. Nerves are seen as grayish lines with corpuscle-like nodes at the point of branching. The fibers are not more numerous, but just more easily seen due to thinning.

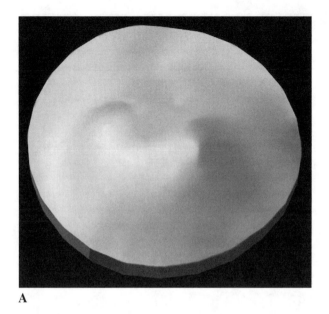

A

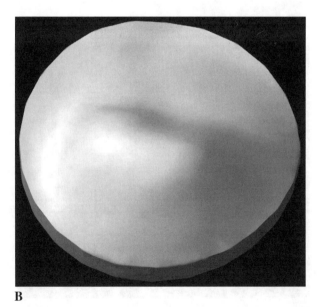

B

FIGURE 17.1 *Spiral progression. A. The path an oval cone takes is shown with computer-rendered models. The cone usually starts in the inferotemporal quadrant. It is relatively small at this stage. B. The cone enlarges and spreads in the nasal direction, still keeping below the midline. The inferior half of the cornea becomes involved. There are still normal areas in the superior half of the cornea.*

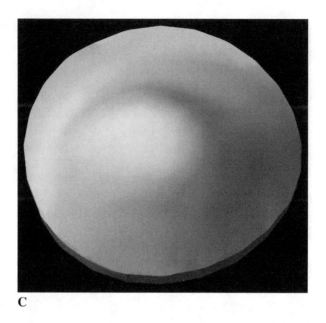

C

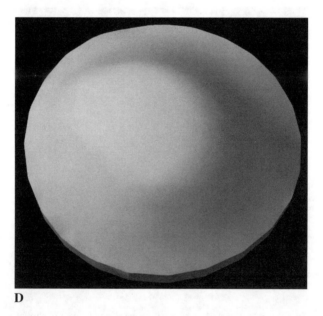

D

FIGURE 17.1   *(continued) C. The cone starts to encroach over the temporal midline as it becomes steeper and larger. The normal areas are shrinking, remaining in the superonasal quadrant of the cornea. D. The cone is very large, encompassing virtually the entire cornea. Normal areas are no longer apparent.*

6. **Ruptures in Descemet's membrane** are found in 5% of keratoconus patients. A crescent-shaped tear in the endothelium and Descemet's is seen at the apex of the cone. Anterior chamber aqueous passes through, causing edema and opacification called **hydrops.** Rolled edges of the tear are seen in Descemet's membrane. The loss of transparency is permanent, and the patient may require a corneal transplant.

7. An **endothelial cup reflex** is seen at the cone apex. The reflex resembles a "dewdrop."[23] The increased curvature of the posterior corneal surface may reflect like a mirror.

8. **Corneal abrasions** are seen in keratoconus.[24] Keratoconic patients are more likely to have contact lens–related abrasions than are nonkeratoconic patients.

9. **Munson's sign** indicates advanced keratoconus.[7] When the patient looks down, the shape of the lower lid markedly shows the curved profile of the advanced cone.

10. **Fine pigment on the endothelium** has been seen with keratoconus.[14]

11. **Anterior corneal mosaic** has been described in keratoconics. Brightly fluorescent lines in a honeycomb pattern with intervening polygonal areas appear because of the corneal flattening caused by a contact lens.[19] It may be described as resembling Schweitzer's polygonal staining.[11]

12. **Subepithelial fibrillary lines** located just inside Fleischer's ring occur in one-third of keratoconics. These fine, white lines are in concentric bundles.[2,10]

13. **Staining** and **scarring** are common findings with keratoconus.[22] These characteristics may be related to the greater corneal fragility reported with keratoconus.[5] The incidence of scarring is high in moderate to advanced cases. Two-thirds of the keratoconus patients with K readings of more than 52 Dk have scarring.[25]

    a. The **causes of scarring** are unclear. It is not clear if corneal staining and scarring are part of the natural history of keratoconus or secondary to mechanical rubbing from a contact lens. Sometimes, severe superficial scarring appears without any history of contact lens wear. Natural scarring can be advanced by contact lenses, however.[11]

    b. It has been proposed that there are two characteristic forms of the disease: one form that originates in the **ectoderm** and another form that originates in the **mesoderm.** Patients with keratoconus originating from the ectodermal form may be more prone to scarring.[5]

    c. **Formation of a new basement membrane** with a lipid layer is another theory about the cause of scarring. The new layer stops the progression of scarring into the stroma, allowing some corneas to be unaffected by contact lenses.[26]

14. **Subepithelial scarring** commonly appears with a nodular configuration and occurs in the apex.[5] Starting as discrete dots in Bowman's membrane, they increase in size and density as the fibrillar connective tissue invades.[12] It is believed to be contact lens–induced and can occur within 90–120 days of beginning contact lens wear.[5] Scarring can also appear raised.[11] The staining that can precede scarring can sometimes be described as a whorl or hurricane pattern.[22,27,28] The whorl pattern may be due to restriction of tear flow underneath the lens.[15] A dimple veil staining pattern can also be seen.[28] When discussing fitting, much of the literature focuses on the reduction of apical staining. This is usually accomplished by lightening the amount of apical pressure induced by the contact lens.[22]

Pearl: Expect to see fluorescein staining of the cornea with keratoconics. Resist the temptation to immediately change lens design unless there is a change in fluorescein pattern.[29]

15. **Prefit,** or **natural, scarring** is located in the Bowman's membrane, anterior stroma, or pre-Descemet's membrane. The appearance is circular or reticular.[5]

Pearl: Expect to see more Vogt's striae, Fleischer's ring, and corneal scarring with higher K readings.[25]

C. **Keratometry** is a invaluable test for diagnosis and management of keratoconus. **Lack of parallelism,** or **doubling of the mires,** is an early sign. **Distorted mires** are another sign. The mires can be of different sizes and may be irregular or broken. **High keratomater readings,** especially outside the range of the keratometer, are significant. Adding a +1.25 D lens in front of the keratometer will extend the dioptric range 8–9 D.[7] The Extend-O-Lens device (Ocular Contact Lenses, Benicia, California) is also designed to accomplish this.[30]

D. **Rizzuti's light reflex** is a common finding[2,31] (Figure 17.2). A penlight is shined at the temporal side of the cornea anterior to the iris plane. The light, rather than spreading evenly on the nasal limbus, is focused by the cone.[10,31] The reflex can also be seen in high-myopic astigmats.[31]

E. **Refractive error** is usually highly myopic with keratoconus.[14] Astigmatism is either oblique or against the rule in early keratoconus.[32] Lack of correlation between refractive astigmatism and corneal toricity is common in early keratoconus. **Spectacle prescriptions** are known to change frequently in the early stages.[17] In the latter stages, spectacle visual acu-

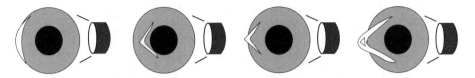

FIGURE 17.2 *Rizzuti's light reflex. The nasal aspect of the cornea is illuminated with a penlight. On a normal cornea, the reflex is spread evenly on the nasal aspect of the cornea in the shape of an arc. In mild keratoconus, the light converges sharply inside the limbus. In moderate keratoconus, the light focuses at or near the nasal limbus. In advanced keratoconus, the light focuses beyond the limbus.*

ity is poorer than with contact lenses. The presence of corneal scarring can adversely affect visual acuity.

Pearl: Prescribe spectacles for emergency or occasional use. Although the best corrected visual acuity is not perfect, the majority of patients can still obtain 20/40 vision.[33]

F. **Videokeratography** is increasingly important in detecting keratoconus.
  1. The **presence of keratoconus** may be evident before the appearance of biomicroscopic signs such as Fleischer's ring and Vogt's striae.[34] The best corrected spectacle acuity of some patients may be excellent, with little or no distortion in keratometric mires, but they may exhibit severe corneal distortion.[35] Steepening that develops below the visual axis revealed by videokeratography may indicate early keratoconus.[34,35] Discriminant analysis of topographic maps has been used successfully to diagnose keratoconus.[36]
  2. **Changing the fixation** of a keratoconus patient can drastically change the appearance of the corneal map and axial radius of curvature.[37] Centering the apex with a fixation adjustment results in a much more accurate map.
G. **Keratokyphosis** appears in keratoconus. The central ring of a keratograph appears to have a teardrop shape.[2] This helps in differentiating keratoconus from corneal warpage syndrome.
H. **Personality** characteristics such as anxiety, type A behavior, and neurologic and psychosomatic traits have been linked to keratoconus. Keratoconic patients have been shown to share traits in common with other chronic eye disease patients.[17]
I. **Other tests** produce findings characteristic of keratoconus. **Ophthalmoscopy** on a dilated pupil can reveal an advanced cone. A round, oval, or dumbbell-shaped shadow will appear in the red reflex.[7,35] **Retinoscopy** will show a "scissorslike" motion in early keratoconus.[7] It has been reported that compared with controls, keratoconics have a **lower intraocu-**

lar pressure of approximately 5–6 mm Hg. This finding may be disputable because the low ocular rigidity associated with keratoconus may generate false readings.[38]

III.   There are numerous **classification** schemes for keratoconus.

A.   The **shape** of the cone—nipple (or round), oval, or globus—can be used to classify keratoconus[39,40] (see Chapter 28). These shapes are evident when the mean K readings are more than 50 D.[32] Cone size may increase as the disease advances. The larger the cone, the more decentered the apex and the more difficult contact lens fitting becomes. The periphery of the cornea is often normal. There is a sudden change from cone area to normal periphery in the earlier stages.[14]

1.   **Caroline** relies on instrumentation such as the photokeratoscope or videokeratoscope for classification. Classification by shape is more clearly defined with corneal topographic maps.[40]

2.   In **nipple-shaped** topography, there is a central ectasia of less than 5 mm in diameter that is surrounded by almost 360 degrees of normal cornea. Nipple cones are often located centrally or decentered slightly inferiorly. The apex is in the lower nasal cornea, averaging 1.1 mm from the visual axis. Average K readings are greater than 65 D.[40] There is a rapid change between the central ectasia and flatter midperiphery.[16]

3.   **Oval-shaped** topography occurs below the corneal midline. Above the midline is an island of normal cornea. Oval cones are larger, and the apex lies in the midperipheral inferotemporal area of the cornea. The apex averages 2.3 mm from the visual axis. Compared with nipple cones, oval cones have more breaks in Bowman's membrane, more superior pannus formation, and more ruptures in Descemet's membrane. Average K readings are greater than 68 D.[40]

4.   A **globus-shaped** topography involves almost 75% of the corneal surface, and there are no islands of normal cornea. Globus cones are the largest cones; they are located inferiorly and are larger than 6 mm in size.[1]

B.   **Bennett** classifies keratoconus into four stages.[17]

1.   **Stage 1** is an early stage with normal keratometry readings and little or no mire distortion. Astigmatism can increase slightly and is correctable with spectacles. Spectacles are the first form of treatment for the disease.[17]

2.   **Stage 2** shows keratometric distortion, steepening of 1–4 D, and more refractive astigmatism.

3.   **Stage 3** has mire distortion, steepening of 5–10 D, and an irregular astigmatism increase of 2–8 D. Shadows are seen with retinoscopy and ophthalmoscopy. Best visual acuity is decreased with spectacles. Many biomicroscopic signs are evident, such as corneal thin-

ning, striae, and a pronounced cone shape. Placido's disk findings appear abnormal.

    4. **Stage 4** shows steepening of 55–60 D or more, apical opacities, Munson's sign, and overall worsening of the above signs.[7]

C. **Keratometry readings** have been used for classification. Depending on the author, mild keratoconus is below 45–48 D. Moderate keratoconus ranges from 45 to 54 D, and advanced keratoconus is above 52–54 D. Severe keratoconus is above 62 D.[1,40]

D. **Amsler** used a simple classification system.[12] Stage I showed oblique astigmatism with irregular mires. Stage II was an intensification of stage I. Stage III displayed a pronounced cone shape with thinning and no opacities. Stage IV was defined as having apical opacities.

IV. **Fitting philosophies** for keratoconus are many and varied.

A. **Three-point-touch,** or **divided support,** is a very common fitting philosophy. There is apical bearing with two other points of midperipheral touch, usually distributed 180 degrees from one another.[41] The central bearing area is 2–3 mm wide. The advantage of placing pressure on the apex to control disease progression is controversial.[7] That vision and comfort are better with flatter lenses has been reported but not proven conclusively.[42]

B. **Korb** advocates minimal **apical clearance fitting,** or opposing fit.[11,14] Apical clearance is most successful with early keratoconus. Permanent apical scarring was found with large and flat-fitting lenses. Scarring did not occur with apical clearance. The **lens parameters** are an 8.0-mm diameter and 5.8-mm optic zone (OZ). A smaller than usual OZ size and a flatter than usual secondary radius provide a desired edge lift of 0.28 mm. The initial base curves were equal to the steeper K reading, and a minimal apical clearance fluorescein pattern was sought with bearing on the paracentral areas.[11] Apical clearance is sometimes virtually impossible to fit and other approaches are necessary.[5]

Pearl: Choose an initial base curve midway between the average and steep K readings to obtain minimal apical touch or apical clearance.[43]

C. **Edrington** strives to achieve a minimal apical touch on the apex.[28] The initial lens is equal to or steeper than the average K readings. Most of the time, this initial lens touches the apex. Progressively steeper lenses are applied until apical clearance is seen. The final lens chosen is between the steepest apical touch lens and the first apical clearance lens. If the initial lens shows apical clearance, progressively flatter lenses are applied until bearing is seen. The final lens should be between the flattest apical clearance lens and the first apical touch lens. A diameter of 8.6 mm and an intrapalpebral fit are suggested. Secondary curve radii of 8–9 mm are recommended regardless of base curve.

Pearl: Set the OZ diameter equal to the base curve radius in millimeters.[29]

D. The **McGuire lens system** attempts a **"feather-touch,"** or mild bearing, on the apex.[39,44] There are three fitting sets in the McGuire system: **nipple** (8.1-mm diameter, 5.5-mm OZ), **oval** (8.6-mm diameter, 6-mm OZ), and **globus** (9.1-mm diameter, 6.5-mm OZ). The McGuire system has **four peripheral curves,** each 0.3 mm wide, with the most peripheral curve 0.4 mm wide. The curves are 3 (0.5 mm), 9 (1.5 mm), 17 (3 mm), and 27 (5 mm) diopters flatter than the base curve. The initial base curve is the **mean K reading.**[44]

E. **Aspheric lenses** work best with smaller nipple cones.[7,39] Average corneas have an eccentricity value (e value) of 0.65. Aspheric lenses are fit with a steeper base curve than three-point-touch because of higher e values. Central alignment or slight touch is seen with edge clearance. Paracentral bearing is eliminated with aspherics. Examples are KAS by GBF CL (Virginia Beach, Virginia) or Ellip-See-Con by Conforma (Norfolk, Virginia) (see Chapter 28).

F. A **large, flat design,** or **paracone fit,** is usually reserved for larger cones.[7,14,39] Diameters of 9–10 mm are fitted with lid attachment. Larger cones are usually displaced inferiorly, and centering the lens is problematic. Large and flat lenses rely on lid attachment to keep the lens in place on the eye. Smaller lenses will decenter and sometimes become displaced on blink. A lens that is too flat, however, can rock and be uncomfortable. An apical touch of 3.0–4.0 mm is used. The greatest disadvantage of the large flat lens is the possibility of exacerbating apical scarring. The advantage of a large lens is that it may be the only rigid corneal design to stay on the eye, especially with globus-type cones. Many practitioners prefer flat-fitting lenses because of better vision, increased wearing time, and superior comfort. The flat fit is also easier to maintain as the keratoconus progresses.[28]

G. **Offset** or **bicentric grinding** adds a flatter peripheral system to the superior portion of the lens. Three or four peripheral curves are added to the superior lens, whereas the inferior lens has only a secondary curve. The flatter superior periphery reduces inferior edge lift and allows better central alignment on some patients.[45]

H. A **duozone** lens has a central and annular zone on the back surface. The steep central zone centers the lens on the apex of the cone. The surrounding annular zone contains the power to correct the patient's refractive error. If the lens decenters because of the apex, the patient will still be able to see through the annular zone. Videokeratography is essential to determine the central and annular zone size and radius. The duozone lens works best for severely decentered cones.[46]

I. The **Soper lens system** uses bicurve lenses based on sagittal depth.[39] A steeper lens is selected by maintaining the same base curve but increasing the diameter.

1. **Three fitting sets** are available: mild (7.4-mm diameter, 6.0-mm OZ), moderate (8.5-mm diameter, 7.0-mm OZ), and advanced (9.5-mm diameter, 8.0-mm OZ). The smaller lenses are used for smaller, centrally located cones. The larger diameters are used for oval cones. The peripheral curve of this system is constant (7.5 mm) and does not change with base curve. This results in a steep peripheral system that is prone to sealing off.[25,39]

2. **Peripheral alignment** and **apical clearance** typify the Soper lens design.[19] Apical touch causes epithelial erosions and lens intolerance.[25]

Pearl: Expect to be humbled fitting keratoconic. Keratoconics often return with reduced wearing time related to corneal staining. Avoid the temptation to immediately change lens design unless the fluorescein pattern dictates a change.[29]

J. **SoftPerm** (Wesley-Jessen, Des Plaines, Illinois) lenses are a hybrid of soft and RGP materials. An RGP center is interwoven molecularly with a hydrogel skirt. The comfort is superior, although it is not as good as that of a soft toric.[47] Better centration is usually achieved with this lens. Many times the SoftPerm fits too tightly, resulting in inadequate lens movement. Also, the steepest base curve available is 7.1 mm, which may not be adequate for larger cones.[39,48] There are problems of lack of lens movement, corneal edema (when the material Dk is too low), and neovascularization.[39] Despite potential problems, the lens has been used on a long-term basis (8 years).[49]

K. A **"piggyback"** is a rigid lens fitted over a soft lens so that there are two lenses on the eye. The advantages of piggybacks are that there is no rigid lens decentration, excellent vision results from the centered lens, and excellent comfort is possible from the bandage effect of the soft lens.[50] Piggybacks can be used after penetrating keratoplasty, refractive corneal surgery, and corneal trauma.

1. **Adequate soft lens movement** is the key. Lens binding results in problems. The fit of the rigid lens should be checked for the presence of bubbles. Central bubbles indicate a steep lens; edge bubbles indicate a flat lens.

2. **Disinfection** should be kept simple. Instead of using two types of disinfection, soft lens solutions can be used for both types of lenses.

3. The **disadvantages** are the inconvenience of two lenses, edema, and neovascularization. A countersunk soft lens from Flexlens (Englewood, Colorado) forms a groove to hold the rigid lens in place. Unfortunately, the lens is prone to tearing at the groove junction.

L. **Soft lenses** for keratoconus are not commonly used but are sometimes indicated. Soft lenses are used because of rigid lens failure due to discomfort.

1. **Flexlens** soft lenses are 45% water and extremely thick (0.3–0.5 mm). These work well when there is difficulty in centering lenses. The soft lenses ride on the sclera and are less affected by a displaced corneal apex. Lens movement is vital for success.

2. **Freflex** from Optech (Englewood, Colorado) is another soft lens (55% water) for keratoconus. The 8.4-mm base curve and 14-mm diameter are available with a varied OZ. The larger the OZ, the steeper the lens. Three lenses are available: Cone A (5.9-mm OZ), Cone B (6.9-mm OZ), and Cone C (7.9-mm OZ). Cone A, the flattest, is tried first before using the steeper B and C.[39]

3. Morrison suggested that **soft toric lenses** should be preferred over rigid lenses.[51] Rigid lenses induce more trauma to the cornea in terms of scarring. Eye rubbing is also more likely with rigid lenses. Because of the need for better vision, spectacles over contact lenses or rigid lenses are required as an additional modality. Some patients even switch between soft and rigid lenses according to need.

4. **Advent lenses** have been successfully used on high-astigmat keratoconus patients.[52] The lens offers better comfort and large diameters.

V. A number of **complications** can occur.

A. **Hydrops** occurs when the aqueous penetrates the cornea because of a break in Descemet's membrane. The patient complains of blurred vision and a "white spot" on the eye. Hypertonic ointments are indicated.

B. **Atopy** is common in keratoconus. Twenty-four to forty-two percent of keratoconic patients have hay fever, allergies, eczema, or asthma.[17] This should be kept in mind when considering contact lens solutions.

C. **Cleaning** is a problem because keratoconics tend to develop abnormal amounts of deposits.[53,54] The keratoconic lens design with the high curvature and anterior flange also makes cleaning difficult. The central, highly curved area is easily cleaned but deposits can remain on the anterior flange.[13] Keratoconic patients should use enzyme cleaners. Sometimes a cotton swab for cleaning is useful.

D. **Lens adhesion** should be suspected if the lens is riding low with no movement.[55]

E. **Seal-off** of tears results in binding at the edge and poor movement.[13] A smaller OZ and a design with a flatter peripheral curve radius and greater edge clearance will minimize the risk of seal-off.[56] This is sometimes related to staining around the base of the cone.[28]

F. **Overminusing** is common, and when it occurs the patient has poor vision with the lenses. Profuse tearing during fitting often is the cause of accepting more minus than necessary. A topical anesthetic can be helpful.

G. **Lens flexure** is sometimes the cause of poor vision. Nonspherical over-keratometry reveals any flexure. Making the lens thicker with a moderate-Dk material is a solution.

H. Residual astigmatism is best corrected by prescribing the use of spectacles over the lenses. Bitoric lenses are not very effective because of difficulty in design.

I. Inferior decentration is common because of a sagging apex.[13] Large, flat lenses fitted with lid attachment may be the only alternative, although it is an imperfect one.

REFERENCES

1. Fowler WC, Belin MW, Chambers WA. Contact lenses in the visual correction of keratoconus. CLAO J 1988;14(4):203–206.

2. Shovlin JP, DePaolis MD, Kame RT. Contact lens–induced corneal warpage syndrome vs. keratoconus. CL Forum 1986;11(8):32–36.

3. Davis LJ, Barr JT, Vanotteren D. Transient rigid lens–induced striae in keratoconus. Optom Vis Sci 1993;70(3):216–219.

4. Zadnik K, Barr JT, Gordon MO, et al. Biomicroscopic signs and disease severity in keratoconus. Cornea 1996;15(2):139–146.

5. Shovlin JP. Keratoconus in patients wearing rigid contact lenses. Part I: a causal relationship. ICLC 1990;17:302–303.

6. Zadnik K. Keratoconus. In ES Bennett, BA Weissman (eds), Clinical Contact Lens Practice. Philadelphia: Lippincott, 1991(45);1–10.

7. Bennett ES. Keratoconus. In ES Bennett, RM Grohe (eds), Rigid Gas-Permeable Contact Lenses. New York: Professional Press, 1986;297–344.

8. Rabinowitz YS, Garbus JJ, McDonnell PJ. Computer-assisted corneal topography in family members of patients with keratoconus. Arch Ophthalmol 1990;108:365–371.

9. Siegel IM, Patalano S. Corneal topography evaluates "unilateral keratoconus." CL Spectrum 1995;10(4):33.

10. Krachmer JH, Feder RS, Belin MW. Keratoconus and related noninflammatory corneal thinning disorders. Surv Ophthalmol 1984;28(4):293–322.

11. Korb DR, Finnemore VM, Herman JP. Apical changes and scarring in keratoconus as related to contact lens fitting techniques. J Am Optom Assoc 1982;53:199–205.

12. Reinke AR. Keratoconus—a review of research and current fitting techniques, part 1. ICLC 1975;2:66–78.

13. Burger D, Barr JT. Effects of Contact Lenses in Keratoconus. In J Silbert (ed), Anterior Segment Contact Lens Complications. New York: Churchill Livingstone, 1994;379–399.

14. Ruben M. The Correction of Irregular Astigmatism with Contact Lenses. In M Ruben, M Guillon (eds), Contact Lens Practice. London: Chapman & Hall, 1994;8–863.

15. Edrington TE. Management of keratoconus with RGP contact lenses. Anaheim, California: 1996 California Optometric Association Congress, March 13–17, 1996.

16. Caroline PJ, Norman CW. Corneal Topography in the Diagnosis and Management of Keratoconus. In D Schanzlin, J Robin (eds), Corneal Topography: Measuring and Modifying the Cornea. New York: Springer, 1992;75–93.

17. Zadnik K, Edrington T. Keratoconus. In J Silbert (ed), Anterior Segment Complications of Contact Lens Wear. New York: Churchill Livingstone, 1994;367–377.

18. Barr JT, Gordon MO, Zadnik K, et al. Quality of life in keratoconus patients. Invest Ophthalmol Vis Sci 1995;36(4):S75.

19. Mannis MJ, Zadnik K. Contact lens fitting in keratoconus. CLAO J 1989;15(4):282–289.

20. Campbell R, Caroline P. Identifying characteristics of keratoconus (part 1 of 2). CL Spectrum 1995;10(4):56.

21. Insular MS, Cooper HD. New correlation in keratoconus using pachymetric and keratometric analysis. CLAO J 1986;12(2):101–105.

22. Weissman BA. Early superficial scarring in keratoconus. CL Spectrum 1993;8(3):43–45.

23. Campbell R, Caroline P. Identifying characteristics of keratoconus (part 2 of 2). CL Spectrum 1995;10(5):56.

24. Weissman B, Chun MW, Barnhart LA. Corneal abrasion associated with contact lens correction of keratoconus—a retrospective study. Optom Vis Sci 1994;71(11):677–681.

25. Raber IM. Fitting cellulose acetate butyrate lenses in keratoconus. Int Ophthalmol Clin 1986;26:91–99.

26. Nauheim JS, Perry HD. A clinicopathological study of contact-lens–related keratoconus. Am J Ophthalmol 1985;100:543–546.

27. Shovlin JP, Morrison RJ, DePaolis MD, et al. Does the Boston Lens II correct keratoconus? CL Forum 1983;8(7):21–32.

28. Edrington TB. Contact Lens Management of Keratoconus. In CA Schwartz (ed), Specialty Contact Lenses: A Fitter's Guide. Philadelphia: Saunders, 1996;142–151.

29. Bennett ES. Challenging RGP patients—6 steps to success. CL Spectrum 1995;10(5):15.

30. Scheid T, Eng J, Cohen S. Keratoconic keratometric measurements with the Extend-O-Lens. CL Spectrum 1993;8(4):28–31.

31. Rizzuti AB. Diagnostic illumination test for keratoconus. Am J Ophthalmol 1970;70:141–143.

32. Norman CW, Caroline PJ. Step-by-step approach to managing keratoconus patients with RGPs. CL Forum 1986;11(11):25–31.

33. Zadnik K, Barr JT, Edrington TB, et al. Scarring and visual acuity in keratoconus. Optom Vis Sci 1993;70(12s):22.

34. Weaver JL, Anderson AJ, Barr JT. Does this optometrist have keratoconus? CL Spectrum 1992;7(6):17–21.

35. Maguire LJ, Bourne WM. Corneal topography of early keratoconus. Am J Ophthalmol 1989;108:107–112.

36. Maeda N, Klyce SD, Smolek MK, et al. Automated keratoconus screening with corneal topographic analysis. Invest Ophthalmol Vis Sci 1994;35:2749–2757.

37. Mandell RB, Barsky BA, Klein SA. Taking a new angle on keratoconus. CL Spectrum 1994;9(4):44.

38. Edmonds CR. Accuracy of IOP measurement in keratoconus. ICLC 1993;20(1–2):29–31.

39. Burger DS. Contact lens alternatives for keratoconus: an overview. CL Spectrum 1993;8(3):49–55.

40. Perry HD, Buxton JN, Fine BS. Round and oval cones in keratoconus. Ophthalmology 1980;87(9):905–909.

41. Arias VC, Liberatore JC, Voss EH, et al. A new technique of fitting contact lenses on keratoconus. Contacto 1959;3:393–415.
42. Zadnik K, Mutti DO. Contact lens fitting relation and visual acuity in keratoconus. Am J Optom Physiol Opt 1987;64:698–702.
43. Edrington TB, Barr JT, Zadnik K, et al. Selection of initial trial-fitting RGP contact lens base curve radius in keratoconus. Optom Vis Sci 1993;70(12s):39.
44. Caroline PJ, McGuire JR, Doughman DJ. Preliminary report on a new contact lens design for keratoconus. Contact Intraocul Lens Med J 1978;4:69–73.
45. Miller L, Blaze PA, Baxter R. Rigid lens modifications for keratoconus and keratoplasty. CL Spectrum 1995;10(9):38–43.
46. Mandell RB, Barsky BA, Moore CF. A new lens for keratoconus. CL Spectrum 1995;10(12):17–22.
47. Tucker IS. Insights on using the Softperm lens. CL Spectrum 1993;8(10):53–56.
48. Maguen E, Martinez M, Rosner IR, et al. The use of Saturn II lenses in keratoconus. CLAO J 1991;17(1):41–43.
49. Boucher JA. Long-term use of Saturn II and Softperm contact lenses for keratoplasty and keratoconus: a case report. ICLC 1992;19(1–2):35–38.
50. Campbell R, Caroline P. Piggyback lens reverses lens disorientation. CL Spectrum 1995;10(3):47.
51. Morrison RJ. Caring for keratoconus patients. CL Spectrum 1988;3(2):55–58.
52. Keech P. Correcting the high astigmia of keratoconus and postkeratoplasty. CL Spectrum 1990;5(2):69–72.
53. Connelly S, Morgan B, Norman C, et al. Your most perplexing RGP lens complications—solved! CL Spectrum 1995;10(2):23–30.
54. Fowler SA, Korb DR, Finnemore VM. Coatings on the surface of siloxane gas-permeable lenses worn by keratoconic patients: a scanning electron microscope study. CLAO J 1987;13(4):207–210.
55. McLaughlin R. Modifying lens design in early keratoconus. CL Spectrum 1994;9(6):17.
56. Gruber E. Material vs. design: expand your fitting philosophy. CL Spectrum 1994;9(9):32–34.

Chapter 18

Monovision and Bifocals

Milton M. Hom

I. **Monovision** is defined as the designation of one eye for distance vision and the other eye for near vision. Single-vision contact lenses are used for each eye. The patient selectively suppresses one eye while using the other eye.

Pearl: Emmetropes make excellent monovision patients.[1]

A. **Success rates** of more than 50–75% have been reported for monovision.[2,3] Patients have shown a strong preference for monovision over bifocal soft lenses. It has been reported that both distance vision and near vision are better than those attained with simultaneous bifocals (center-near) and diffractive bifocals.[4,5] Monovision is also less expensive and easy to fit.

B. **Which patients will be successful** can be predicted by level of distance ghosting, distance stereoacuity, and age. Patients for whom monovision fails tend to be older and to have higher levels of ghosting at distance and greater loss of distance stereoacuity.[6]

C. **Personality traits** have been correlated with monovision success. Well-structured, detail-oriented individuals are not as successful as those who are adaptable, holistic, and optimistic.[7]

D. **Difficulties with night driving** are a major drawback of monovision; 33% of monovision patients report glare while night driving.[8] **Compromised stereoacuity** is evident with monovision.[5] **Contrast sensitivity** is also reduced, although simultaneous bifocals show about the same reduction.[9] **Liability** can be a problem if the practitioner fails to discuss and warn about the drawbacks of monovision in advance.[10,11] Effects of **suppression** during long-term binocular vision are also potential problems.

Pearl: Because of limitations such as decreased stereoacuity, refitting a successful monovision patient with bifocal contacts may be necessary. For these patients, the nondominant eye should be refitted first, at least 2 weeks before the dominant eye.[12]

E. **Fitting monovision** is virtually identical to fitting single-vision lenses. Both eyes are given the best lenses to maximize visual acuity.[4,5]

1. The **near eye** is usually the nondominant eye. The dominant eye is fitted with a distance lens. Studies have shown that choosing the dominant eye for distance does not necessarily produce better vision. Monovision visual acuity is not improved when eye dominancy is used as a guideline for selection.[13]

2. The **left eye** is sometimes chosen for distance. The rationale, disputed by some experts, is that while driving, the left eye is used for the side-view mirror.[11,12]

3. The **swinging-plus test** can be used to select the distance and near eyes. The patient holds a +1.50 D lens over one eye while walking around the room, then repeats the procedure with the lens on the other eye. The eye most comfortable with the lens is designated as the near eye.[14]

4. Performing the **near point of convergence** test can help in determining the best eye for distance vision. The eye that loses fixation first can be chosen as the distance eye.

F. **Management of monovision** may require several follow-up visits.

1. **Adaptation** time is usually 2 weeks, but patients may take up to 6 weeks. Normal adaptation includes **hazy vision, eye strain,** and **mild eye switching** in the first weeks of wear. Adapting patients should be limited to nondemanding visual activities.[10]

Pearl: Switching eye function (making the distance eye the near eye and the near eye the distance one) can relieve even the vaguest symptoms.[9]

2. **Common fitting problems** associated with single-vision lenses (residual cylinder, dry eyes, wrong powers, poor fit) should be ruled out first whenever there are problems.

*Pearl: If a patient is already wearing **soft toric lenses,** consider monovision as the best option.[1] Bifocal lenses that correct astigmatism are not commonly available.*

3. **Spectacle overcorrection** is another option for monovision patients. Spectacles are specifically prescribed over contact lenses for driving or reading blur. The overcorrection can be done for distance, reading, or bifocally.

4. **Adding minus to the near eye** can relieve intermediate blur. Near vision will probably be compromised, however. If unsuccessful, modified monovision II is an alternative strategy.

    5. **Low add power** is sometimes insufficient to enable suppression. Increasing the add will be helpful, but it may bring the working reading distance too close.

    6. **High-water-content** lenses are preferred over thin low-water-content lenses for low-plus monovision patients.[15] More striae and folds were found for the thin low-water-content lenses after 5 hours of daily wear.

  G. **Other options** include modified monovision and combinations therewith.

    1. **Modified monovision I** uses a different bifocal in each eye. The dominant eye is designated for distance, and the nondominant eye is for near. A better performing distance bifocal is used for the distance, dominant eye, and a better performing near lens is used in the near, nondominant eye. An example of this is a PA1 (Bausch & Lomb [B&L], Rochester, New York) for distance and Bisoft (CIBA Vision, Duluth, Georgia) for near.[12]

    2. **Modified monovision II** uses a single-vision lens on one eye and a bifocal on the other.[1,12] The distance eye is fitted with a single-vision lens, and the near eye is fitted with a simultaneous bifocal. This useful option is best for monovision patients who complain of **intermediate blur.** Myopes tend to do better with modified monovision because they prefer better binocularity. This is especially true in the higher add powers.[16]

    3. **Combinations of modified monovision** can be fitted. Following are examples of some combinations to improve distance vision in the dominant right eye[17]:

Right	*Left*
Distance single vision	*Center-near*
Center-distance	*Center-near*
Center-distance	*Near single vision*

    4. **Modified trivision** is correction for distance, near, and intermediate vision with contact lenses. A bifocal lens on one eye is fitted for two of the required distances and a single-vision lens is used for a third distance. Two bifocals can also be used for each of the three distances, creating an overlap or "binocularity" for one of the distances.[18]

II. **Bifocal contact lenses** are more complicated to fit but can offer many advantages over monovision.

  A. **Selection** involves careful screening that maximizes patient success for multifocals. The criteria for choosing rigid and soft multifocals are similar to those for choosing single-vision lenses. Usually, keeping the patient in the current type (soft or rigid) is advisable.[19]

1. **Low refractive errors** are not ideal for bifocal lens wearers. Patients with less than 1 D of hyperopia are poor candidates because they see "perfectly" without spectacles. Myopes with less than 1.25 D are accustomed to seeing without any correction for near.[12]
2. **Dry eyes** that affect contact lenses should be considered when dealing with the presbyope. Smaller pupil size, slower pupillary responsiveness, and flaccid lids also affect bifocal contact lenses and should be carefully screened when fitting the presbyope.[20]

B. **Adaptation** can take many weeks. Within 3–4 weeks, the patient and practitioner should be able to decide whether to continue with bifocal lenses. Wearing the lenses for 8–10 weeks is a good sign because few patients discontinue after that time. Motivation is an important key to success. Because of the longer, more difficult adaptation period, it is important that the patient be highly motivated. The patient should be informed that lens changes may be numerous. A follow-up visit should be scheduled about 1 week after dispensing each refit.[12]

*Pearl: Remember that even small, **0.25 changes** are significant to these patients.*[21]

C. **Bifocal fitting considerations** are sometimes different than those of fitting single-vision lenses.
1. **Which fitting sets to have?** This is an excellent question. Good fitting sets are essential for successful fitting, but it is not necessary to have every bifocal that is available. Many laboratories will loan the practitioner a needed trial lens.

Pearl: Having at least five trial sets on hand is recommended: aspheric soft, aspheric rigid, diffractive soft, segmented (alternating) rigid, and concentric soft.[1]

2. **Auxiliary glasses** are sometimes needed for extremely small print. Some authors tell the patient that the contact lenses will be adequate **at least 80% of the time.** At other times, however, spectacles are needed over the contact lenses.[1]

Pearl: Telling the patient "We'll either successfully fit you with contact lenses or prove that there is no appropriate lens available for you" is good, positive advice.[22] *Sometimes, a patient cannot be fit successfully with a presbyopic (bifocal or monovision) contact lens.*

3. **Use loose trial lenses** and over-refract each eye separately. The prescription should then be refined with both eyes open for bifocal contact lenses. Because many designs depend on pupil size, the

effect of **high and low illumination conditions** should be demonstrated to the patient.

III. **Rigid bifocals** usually afford better vision than soft bifocals.

    A.   **Selection** for rigid bifocal lenses entails many factors.[23] Prior experience with rigid lenses is a big advantage. Patients wearing rigid lenses prior to fitting with a rigid multifocal are the most successful.

Pearl: The best contact lens choice for a presbyopic rigid gas-permeable (RGP) lens is an RGP bifocal.

        1.   The **location of the corneal apex** is an important selection factor with RGP bifocals. For superior decentration of the apex relative to the pupil, **Lifestyle GP** (Permeable Technologies, Morganville, New Jersey) or translating designs are better than aspherics. Centered aspherics work best with centered apices.

        2.   **Pupil size** should be considered. Small pupils work best with aspherics. Very large pupils, greater than 6 mm in diameter, can have flare and poor visual acuity with both concentrics and aspherics.[19]

        3.   For those who **work on computers,** a simultaneous design is appropriate.[23] Generally, if the patient spends more than 30% of the day on the computer, a concentric or aspheric is recommended.

        4.   For patients who work at an **intermediate distance,** at "arm's length," a simultaneous design is appropriate. These patients include beauticians, electricians, plumbers, and mechanics.

        5.   **Lower-lid tangency** to the limbus strongly affects a translating design.[23] If the lower lid is below the limbus, a simultaneous design is better than an alternating lens. Translation depends partially on lower lid contact to enable movement on downgaze.

    B.   **Simultaneous designs** cast both the near and the distance images on the retina at the same time. The patient must selectively attend to either the distance or the near image. If the patient is looking at near, the out-of-focus distance image must be suppressed, and when looking far, the near image must be suppressed. Visual compromise is normal and adaptation is needed.

        1.   **Usability in all fields of gaze** is the most noted advantage of simultaneous designs. Patients appreciate the ease with which near objects can be viewed from any position.[24]

        2.   The **junction** between distance and near can be gradual (aspheric) or definite (concentric). The near portion can be central (center-near concentric or front aspheric) or peripheral (center-distance concentric or back aspheric).

        3.   **Problems** with simultaneous designs stem from **decentration** and **pupil size.** Vision is compromised when these lenses decenter. **Superior, inferior,** or **lateral decentration** causes poor vision in a

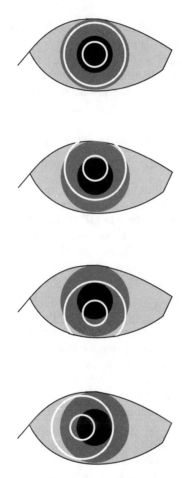

FIGURE 18.1 *Lens positioning. On the top is a properly centering lens. Below are superiorly, inferiorly, and laterally positioning lenses. Lens positioning for a concentric bifocal is absolutely critical. Superior, inferior, or lateral decentration will result in a decentered zone and subsequent poor vision.*

simultaneous-vision lens. The central zone should be centered within the pupil for best vision (Figure 18.1). Also, under different light conditions, vision can change due to pupillary size.

C. **Concentric lenses** have definitive distance and near zones. The center zone can be distance or near **(reverse centrad)**. The power can be two curves on the front or back surface. The polymethyl methacrylate (PMMA) **deCarle bifocal** has a center-distance zone and two curves ground on the back surface. The **ACC-Bivision** by Salvatori Ophthalmics (Sarasota, Florida) is a center-distance concentric.

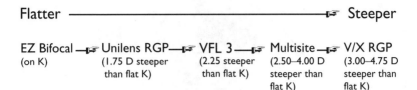

FIGURE 18.2 *Initial base curves of rigid aspherics. Aspheric lenses are usually fitted steeper than K. The initial base curve choices for various aspheric bifocals are shown in relative order from flat (on K) on the left to steep on the right. (Adapted from DW Hansen. For more natural vision try aspheric rigid gas-permeable multifocals. CL Spectrum 1995;10[6]:15.)*

D. **Aspheric lenses** can be either **center near** or **center distance.** E values (eccentricity values) are often used to specify different aspheric curvatures. Most aspheric lenses for presbyopia have e values of more than 1.0. A moderate to high degree of flattening is required to induce enough add power in the periphery.[25]

1. **Back aspherics** are center distance. The power progressively changes from center to periphery. Better distance vision is a noted advantage over front aspherics. Lower add powers and poor centration with decentered corneal apexes are limitations. For decentration problems, consider front aspherics with spherical base curves. Back aspheric lenses are **Unilens** (Unilens Corp USA, Largo, Florida); **Multisite** (Salvatori); the **VFL series** (Conforma Contact Lenses, Norfolk, Virginia); and **Tri-aspheric, ELS, V/X, V/X-2,** and **C-Rite** (GBF Contact Lenses, Virginia Beach, Virginia).[26]

2. **Front aspherics** are center-near lenses. Near vision is better with front aspherics than with back aspherics.

3. Most aspherics are fit **steeper than flat K** (Figure 18.2). Base curves can be adjusted to achieve the best possible correction. Steepen the base curve if the lens is too flat or moves temporally. Flatten the base curve if the lens is too steep or moves nasally.[27]

4. Patients sight through the **peripheral areas** of the aspheric lens when they look down. If they do not, they have insufficient near vision. If the lens moves too much with the eye on downgaze, a steeper or larger diameter can be used.[27]

E. **Alternating bifocals** usually offer the best vision among bifocal designs. The top part of the lens is meant for distance and the lower segment is for near. For adds +2.00 or higher, segmented bifocals are best.[1]
Tangent Streak (Fused Kontacts, Kansas City, Missouri) and **Fluo-**

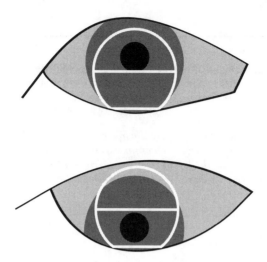

FIGURE 18.3   *Lens translation. The near portion of an alternating lens translates, or moves up into position, when the patient looks down. Above is the bifocal lens in primary gaze. Below is the lens translating on downgaze. The lower lid helps translation by catching the lens while the eye moves down.*

roperm **ST** (Paragon Vision Sciences, Mesa, Arizona) are both translating designs. These lenses offer superior vision and have high success rates.

1. The lens **translates** (moves) when the patient looks down. The patient looks through the lower, or near part, of the lens (Figure 18.3). Only one segment of the lens is meant to focus light on the retina at a time, so the patient views either distance or near light bundles, not both. In theory, the images are much clearer than in simultaneous vision, but this is not completely true when it comes to near vision. One lens usually does not translate perfectly, so there is a mild simultaneous effect at near.[24]

2. **Prism ballast** helps to position the bifocal. The lens is made thicker at the base. Gravity has little effect in keeping the prism ballast in the downward (6 o'clock) position; this occurs because of the **"watermelon seed" principle,**[28] in which the upper lid is largely responsible for squeezing the thick part of the lens downward. The squeezing effect helps to stabilize the lens.

3. The **upper lid** has the most effect on translation. Photographing the movement of a contact lens bifocal shows that lower-lid action accounts for only 1 mm of the total translation.[29,30]

4. **Diagnostic lens fitting** is the best, most common method of fitting. Most practitioners use diagnostic lenses supplied by the man-

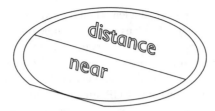

FIGURE 18.4 *The Tangent Streak Bifocal (Fused Kontacts, Kansas City, Missouri) is a monocentric, truncated, prism-ballasted translating bifocal. The near zone is located below the distance zone.*

ufacturer. There is no substitute for observing the dynamics of a trial alternating bifocals on the eye because patient-to-patient variability is considerable.[31,32]

F. **Tangent Streak Bifocal** by Fused Kontacts has a very high success rate (Figure 18.4) of 70–91%.[24,33–35] The lens is one-piece, monocentric, prism-ballasted, and truncated. Patients already wearing RGP lenses do very well with this lens.

1. **Fitting the Tangent Streak Bifocal** with a diagnostic fitting set is recommended.

a. The **base curves recommended** by the manufacturer[32] are as follows:

Corneal toricity	Base curve
0	*1 D flatter than K*
0.5 D	*0.50 flatter than K*
>1 D	*Not steeper than ¼ toricity*

b. A **lower lid positioned near the limbus** and an **alignment** fluorescein pattern are necessary for success with translating designs.[36] The ideal fit is an **inferiorly positioning** lens with a **lower lid at or just above the lower limbus.**[24] **Head position** must be erect or slightly downward for distance viewing. A natural downward gaze accompanied by blinking will position the lens for reading.[22] The base curve should be flatter than the superior cornea or translation will be inadequate. **Thirty percent of the pupil** can be covered by the segment line during distance viewing without interfering with vision.[1] The segment height should be set at 1.3 mm below the geometric center of the pupil.[37] **Lens movement** should be upward with moderately hard blinking, and the lens should drop quickly into position when looking straight ahead. When looking down, the lens should move up, covering part of the upper sclera. The lens position can be observed by gently lifting the upper lid while the patient is looking down.

2. **Discomfort** is a major factor in discontinuation. Translating designs are often thick and heavy.[38] A patient may have discomfort with a translating RGP bifocal because of the thickness and prism required. Patients with extra-sensitive lids and poor adapters are not ideal candidates for a Tangent Streak Bifocal. A thinner encapsulated segment such as the Fluoroperm ST Bifocal may be a better choice. A simultaneous-vision lens (especially aspheric) or monovision would provide better comfort.

3. **Three o'clock and 9 o'clock staining,** or peripheral corneal desiccation (PCD), is another disadvantage of the thick and heavy translating designs. Korb and Exford theorized that PCD was caused by a lid gap.[39] This occurs when the edge of the lens holds the lid away from the cornea. Lenses can be modified to enhance wetting and decrease staining. Solutions include thinning the edges, changing the diameter, or facilitating proper blinking (see Chapter 16).

4. **Encyclorotation** can cause poor near vision and is influenced by lid movement. The upper lid moves up and down like a windshield wiper.[40] The lower lid moves in a horizontal, transverse motion. As the upper lid moves downward, the lower lid moves toward the medial canthus. This lid action results in nasal rotation of a bifocal lens on blink. Rotation increases on downgaze.[32]

   a. **Changing the prism axis** helps achieve better lens orientation by adjusting the amount of rotation. This works well when the **rotation is stable** but not with an unstable lens. Increasing the prism does produce benefits with an unstable lens.[34] Some practitioners automatically assume there will be encyclorotation. Depending on the amount of rotation, a suggested adjusted axis would be 100–105 degrees for the right lens and 75–80 degrees for the left lens[41] (Figure 18.5). Both adjusted axes are 10–15 degrees base in. Changing the base apex changes the location of the prism apex (the thinnest part of the lens).[32] When placed at the proper axis, the base apex can be used to orient the lens in the desired location. The manufacturer suggests changing the base apex by no more than 20 degrees.[42,43]

   *Pearl: Order the prism axis in the **same direction** as the excessive rotation.*[44]

   b. **Reduction of the diameter** can decrease rotation on downgaze if lid capture is the cause.[32] Because of the upper lid forces, lessening the lid contact can help stabilize the lens.

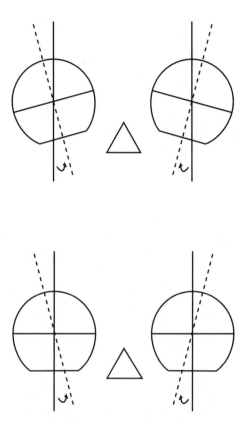

FIGURE 18.5 *Changing prism axis. Rotation of 15 degrees in each eye is shown above. The dotted line indicates a prism axis of 90 degrees. The solid lines are 90-degree reference lines. The prism axes have rotated 15 degrees nasal. To correct for this, assume that the next lens ordered will also rest at 15 degrees rotation. For 15 degrees nasal rotation, a prism axis of 105 degrees for the right eye and 75 degrees for the left eye should be ordered. Adjusted prism axes are shown below. The dotted lines are the adjusted prism axes. The truncation shows that the lenses are no longer rotating with the adjusted axes.*

       c. **Increasing the prism** can help stabilize rotation.[45] More prism especially will steady a fluctuating rotation.

       d. **Changing truncation orientation** will stabilize the lens whenever the lower lid is causing the rotation. Modifying the truncation can better fit an oblique **lid angle** or **lid slope** (Figure 18.6).

  5. **Inadequate translation** causes poor near vision. It occurs for a number of reasons.[45] The lens may be too large and unable to move upward; when this occurs, **excessive superior lens impingement** can be seen on downgaze with a fluorescein pattern.[42] This problem

FIGURE 18.6   *Changing truncation. If the lower lid is at an oblique angle and causes the lens to rotate, the truncation can be changed to help stabilize the lens. On the left, a lens is rotated because of the obliquely aligned lower lid. The dotted line indicates the prism axis of the lens at 90 degrees. On the right, truncation was changed to match the lower lid, allowing the lens to stabilize in the proper position.*

can be addressed by reducing the diameter. When the lower lid is not catching the lower lens edge, widening the truncation may help. Little or no movement on blink also results in poor translation. Flattening the lens is necessary if the fit is too tight; a steep lens resists the lower lid push. "Plussing" the edge or adding a minus carrier to the lens is an effective strategy. An optimal interaction between upper lid and lens edge is the key to adequate translation.

6. **Lateral decentration** of lenses, especially on downgaze, results in poor near vision. Macalister and Woods showed with video that increasing the size of the lens and steepening it are the most useful strategies. Of the two, increasing size is better than steepening the lens. Making the lens both larger and steeper is the most effective, however.

7. **Rotation** and **decentration** together commonly cause poor near vision. Macalister and Woods showed that increasing lens diameter reduces rotation and provides coverage for a lateral decentration.[32] If a stable rotation is the only problem, changing the prism axis is better than increasing lens diameter.

8. **Poor distance vision** occurs when the pupil is not within the distance zone on primary gaze. Close observations can determine the cause.

   a. If the **segment height is too high,** it can be lowered by truncation. Whenever possible, aim high when ordering segment heights.[46] Segment heights are easier to lower (with modification) than raise.

   b. A **lens riding too high** must be lowered. Remember that the ideal fit is an inferiorly positioning lens. When there is no upper lid contact, flattening the periphery, base curve, or both can help.

   Pearl: Consider the Lifestyle GP if the upper lid holds the lens too high.

    c. A slow recovery after a blink is called **lens lifting** or **slow return**. The lens drops slowly into position, causing visual distress as the segment crosses the pupil. Increasing the prism adds mass and makes the lens drops faster.[34] A smaller lens also has a faster return.[32]

    d. **Superior flare** can be caused by a dilated pupil looking through the lens edge. Increasing the lens size solves the problem.

9. **Variable vision** can be caused by excessive movement of a flat lens. Make certain there is an alignment fit. If the fit is already aligned, check for unsteady rotation and consider increasing prism.[42]

10. Studying **reorders** and **lens modifications** will improve Tangent Streak Bifocal problem-solving. A study by Remba carefully reported the treatment strategies needed for refitting.[34]

    a. The most common reorder was for **increased prism** to remedy lens lifting and unsteady rotation (Figure 18.7).

    b. **Lens modifications** were most frequently done on the truncation (Figure 18.8). The truncation was reshaped to enable consistent translation. Truncation was recut to lower segment heights. The other most common modification was thinning or tapering the edges for comfort. Modification plays a key role in fitting the Tangent Streak Bifocal.

G. **The Fluoroperm ST Bifocal** is a translating monocentric lens[44] (Figure 18.9). The encapsulated segment resembles that of a straight-top spectacle bifocal. The segment is 6 mm wide and 3 mm high. Features such as prism ballast and truncation are also available.

1. **Alignment** and **inferior positioning** are the keys to fitting this lens. The segment should be 0.4–0.7 mm below the inferior pupillary margin. The segment is fit considerably lower than that of the Tangent Streak Bifocal. **Lens movement** should be a uniform 1 mm with blink and 2 mm of translation on downgaze.[42] **Flatter than K or on K** is the recommended initial base curve for spherical corneas.[47] If the lens is fitted too flat, it has a tendency to move more than other translating designs. The lens is designed to be lighter than other designs.

    Pearl: *Lens too high, lens too low, unstable rotation, excessive movement, insufficient movement, excessive translation, insufficient translation—what do these performance problems have in common? Answer: a nonalignment fit.*[42] *For all of these problems, checking the fit is the first step.*

2. **Initial size and segment height** can be empirically determined based on simple calculations[9] (Figure 18.10).

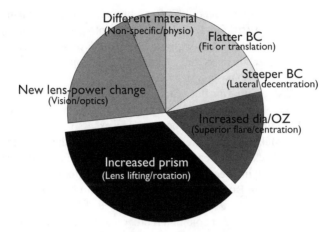

FIGURE 18.7   *Frequency of reorders for the Tangent Streak Bifocal by causes. There are many reasons to reorder the Tangent Streak Bifocal (Fused Kontacts, Kansas City, Missouri) during fitting and follow-up. Pictured are the changes made when reordering was needed. In parentheses are the reasons why each change was needed. One may note that increased prism due to lens lifting or rotation is the change most frequently ordered. (Adapted from MJ Remba. The Tangent Streak rigid gas-permeable bifocal contact lens. J Am Optom Assoc 1988;59:212–216.)*

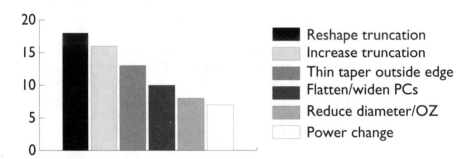

FIGURE 18.8   *Frequency of lens modifications. Many lens modifications are needed when fitting a rigid translating design. The most frequent modifications are reshaping or increasing truncation. (Adapted from MJ Remba. The Tangent Streak rigid gas-permeable bifocal contact lens. J Am Optom Assoc 1988;59:212–216.)*

3. A **slit lamp reticule** in the eyepiece is helpful to accurately measure the segment height. The slit aperture should be small so that the measurement is made on a **dark-adapted pupil.** A segment height set for a constricted pupil can result in too much height and subsequent flare at night.

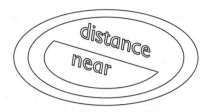

FIGURE 18.9   *Fluoroperm bifocal. The near segment is encapsulated, allowing for a thinner and lighter lens. The near portion is located below the distance zone. The Fluoroperm ST Bifocal (Paragon Vision Sciences, Mesa, Arizona) is available with truncation, prism ballast, different prism axes, front-surface toricity, or combinations of these characteristics.*

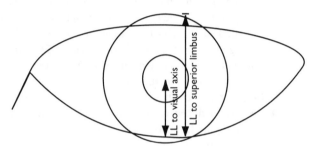

FIGURE 18.10   *Initial size and height. After taking measurements of the eye, the segment height and vertical and horizontal diameters can be calculated using the formulas shown. The horizontal and vertical diameters are different if truncation is ordered. Vertical lens size = lower lid (LL) to superior limbus – 2 mm; segment height = lower lid (LL) to visual axis – 1.3 mm; horizontal lens size = add 0.4 mm to vertical.*

> **Pearl:** *Segment height can be estimated by remembering that the encapsulated segment itself is 3 mm high.*

4. The **Fluoroperm ST Bifocal** is an alternative to the Tangent Streak Bifocal. There are many features in this encapsulated design.[48]

    a. **A large variety of parameters** is available. Segment heights are available from 3.3 mm to more than 5 mm. Truncation, prism amount, and axis can be customized.

    b. The **excellent physiologic response** to the Fluoroperm 60 material is not unlike that with a single-vision RGP lens.

    c. A **reduced center thickness** of approximately 30% results in 20% less lens mass. Other translating designs are thick and heavy. The Fluoroperm ST Bifocal is thinner and lighter and subsequently has less 3 o'clock and 9 o'clock staining. The thinner design is also more comfortable.[42]

    d. **Rotation and lateral movement** are less of a problem than with other translating designs. Even with tight lids, very little rotation has been reported.[49]

    e. A **high-index material** of thermoset styrene acrylate copolymer makes up the segment. The segment has an inherent fluorescence, making it easier to see when fitting.[47,48]

  5. The **disadvantages** of the Fluoroperm ST Bifocal are **lack of intermediate zones** and poor performance when using the lens for **computer work**.[48] This lens is similar to a segmented spectacle bifocal. Raising the segment height sometimes helps.

  6. **Adaptive symptoms** need to be explained to the patient prior to dispensing.[20] **Head posture** must be upright for distance viewing. The patient must learn to look downward for near. **Flare at night** is a problem if the segment height is too high or if the distance area is too small. The segment height can be lowered with truncation or by adding mass with prism.[48] **Mild corneal flattening** and **reduction of astigmatism** may occur. Waiting for several weeks to prescribe glasses may be prudent.

  7. **Fitting problems** can be solved because this lens can be customized.[48]

    a. **Superior decentration** caused by upper-lid capture can be resolved with truncation superiorly.

    b. **Residual astigmatism** can be corrected for with toricity ground on the front surface. A front-surface toricity up to 2 D is possible.

    c. A **round, nontruncated** lens is better for a lower lid below the limbus. Normally a risk factor for poor translation, a round lens may supply the contact needed for translation.

    d. **Rotation** of more than 5–10 degrees temporal or 30 degrees nasal on downgaze would probably result in near problems. If there is an alignment fit, changing the axis of the prism base is recommended.

H. The **VE-ACC-Translating bifocal** is a translating concentric bifocal made by Salvatori (Figure 18.11). The lens is truncated and prism-ballasted. The distance zone is 4 mm and is located in the upper mid-center of the lens. Fitting on flat K is the initial base curve of choice. In one study, discontinuance was mainly due to poor reproducibility of distance and near vision.[50]

I. The **Menicon Decentered Target Bifocal** (Menicon, USA, Clovis, California) is a center-distance prism-ballasted and truncated translating lens made in the highly permeable SF-P material. The distance segment is fitted centered on the pupil.[49] The peripheral curves are junctionless and aspheric (Figure 18.12).

J. The **Menicon Crescent Seg Bifocal** (Menicon, USA) is a translating lens made in the highly permeable SF-P material. Rotation is better tol-

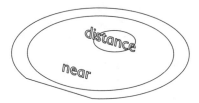

FIGURE 18.11   *VE-ACC-Translating bifocal (Salvatori Ophthalmics, Sarasota, Florida). The concentric distance zone is decentered and surrounded by the large near area. The lens relies on translation for near vision.*

FIGURE 18.12   *Menicon Decentered Target Bifocal (Menicon, USA, Clovis, California). The distance portion is a decentered zone surrounded by the near area. The lens is truncated and prism-ballasted.*

erated with this prism-ballasted, truncated lens. The major advantage of a crescent segment is that near vision is less likely to be compromised with lens rotation (Figure 18.13).

K.   The **Solitaire bifocal** is a segmented lens made by Tru-Form Optics (Euless, Texas). The lens is prism-ballasted, truncated, and meant to translate for near. In one study, 83% of the patients were satisfied with the Solitaire. Fifty-three percent of the patients did experience significant glare disability, however. Some dropped out because of the lack of intermediate vision.[51]

L.   The **Tangent Streak Trifocal** (Fused Kontacts) follows the same design guidelines as the Tangent Streak Bifocal. The difference is an intermediate zone 1 mm wide located between the distance and near areas. Of 16 patients dissatisfied with the Tangent Streak Bifocal, 12 were refitted successfully with the Tangent Streak Trifocal[52] (Figure 18.14).

M.   The **Lifestyle GP** lens is unique because it is a lid-attachment aspheric lens that uses translation to see through the distance, intermediate, and near zones. Patients whose lenses ride high with a lot of lid tension do well with this lens.[53] With-the-rule astigmats and prior RGP lens wearers are ideal candidates.[36] Computer users are also successful with this lens. Those with larger pupil sizes of 5 mm diameter or more may be marginal candidates, however.[38] The lens is considered to have a +1.75

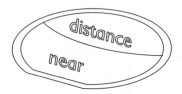

FIGURE 18.13   *Menicon Crescent Seg Bifocal (Menicon, USA, Clovis, California). The distance area is located above the segment. The near segment is crescent-shaped, making the near vision less susceptible to rotation.*

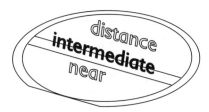

FIGURE 18.14   *The Tangent Streak Trifocal (Fused Kontacts, Kansas City, Missouri) is based on the Tangent Streak Bifocal (also by Fused Kontacts) with an additional 1 mm wide intermediate zone.*

add.[53] There are two diameters, 9.0 and 9.5 mm. The 9.0-mm diameter is the initial lens of choice.[54]

1. The **"equivalent base curve"** or secondary aspheric curve is the 1.2 mm wide fitting curve.[54] The goal is a midperipheral alignment fit. An equivalent base curve equal to or 0.1 mm flatter than flat K is the starting point.[27] The lens is designed to ride high under the upper lid and translate on downgaze (Figure 18.15).

2. **Inferior decentration** can be remedied by changing to a larger-diameter lens with a flatter base curve.

3. A **superiorly decentered** lens may result in blurred distance vision. A decentered lens can make the patient view through the near area.[54] The diameter can be decreased to 9.0 mm (if initially 9.5 mm) and slightly steepened.

4. **Poor translation** into reading position may be due to a steep lens. The reading vision will appear blurred.[54] The lens should be flattened.

N. **Diffractive** (holographic) bifocals use "full-aperture optics" and depend less on pupil size than on simultaneous designs.[20] Light that enters the pupil is divided into two equal packets (distance and near). **Decentration** has less of an effect on vision with diffractive bifocals than with refractive concentric designs.[55] A three-dimensional effect with shadowlike images seen around printed letters is commonly reported. Glare and ghosting

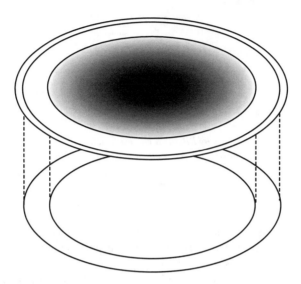

FIGURE 18.15 *The Lifestyle GP (Permeable Technologies, Morganville, New Jersey) has a central prescription zone for distance and near. The darker area represents distance power progressing outward to near power. The surrounding fitting zone or equivalent base curve on the back surface is shown below.*

around images also occur, inhibiting clear night-driving vision.[22] The **Diffrax** lens by PBH is a rigid diffractive bifocal (Figure 18.16).

IV. **Soft lens bifocals** have many designs similar to RGP bifocals.

    A. **Simultaneous vision** in soft lenses is similar to vision with RGP bifocals in that both the distance and near vision—both the distance and near bundles of light—are on the retina at the same time. The patient must learn to selectively suppress the unfocused image while looking at the properly focused image.

        1. **Superior distance stereoacuity** for simultaneous designs is the major performance advantage over monovision.[5] Being able to see near work in all fields of gaze is another advantage.

        2. **Reduction of visual acuity** related to **decentration** and **changes in illumination** is the major drawback. Simultaneous bifocals give a reduction of scotopic (dim illumination) vision.[56] There are two types of simultaneous bifocals: concentric and aspheric.

    B. **Concentric simultaneous bifocals** have a distance and near zone within the pupil. Concentric bifocals are available as **center-distance** or **center-near.**

        1. The **zone-check technique** is used to determine the location of the concentric zones while the lenses are on the eye. A +4-D trial lens

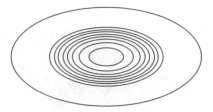

FIGURE 18.16   *The Diffrax lens by PBH is a rigid diffractive bifocal. The rings in the lens are echelettes that diffract the light rays into equal distance and near bundles.*

is hand-held over the eye while being viewed with a direct ophthalmoscope. The +4-D lens magnifies the reflex so that the zones can be seen within the pupil.

2. **Bi-soft** by CIBA Vision (Duluth, Georgia) is a **center-distance** concentric lens. Because it is a concentric, there are more higher add powers available than with aspherics.[9] In one study, however, a comparison with a pair of concentric distance lenses was not made because the pilot acceptance rate was too low (5%).[21]

3. **Alges** and **Simulvue**, both by Unilens, and **Spectrum** by CIBA Vision are **center-near** concentrics.

   a. **Pupil size** plays an important role with center-near designs. At near, the miosis associated with the near reflex helps to clear the near images. The unfocused distance rays are blocked, leaving the focused near rays of light.

   b. **Alges** is available in several near diameters. Almost any desired base curve can be custom-ordered.[57] **Simulvue** has an aspheric transition between the center-near and distance zones to reduce secondary visual images. The lens is meant for higher-add patients (+1.50 to +2.50).[58]

   c. **Spectrum** differs because it is 55% water and is approved for extended wear.[57]

      (1) An 8.6-mm base curve is the first-choice lens. The 2.3 mm segment is placed on the dominant eye and 3.0 mm on the nondominant eye. As with other simultaneous designs, lens centration is imperative.

      (2) Success rates have been raised by using two equal center zones rather than different zones. An increase to a 67% success rate from 50% has been reported when failures are refitted with the same center zones.[59] Moderate- to high-hyperopic presbyopes benefit from the highest Dk of any soft bifocal.

(3) Disadvantages of the Spectrum are material-related fragility and deposits. Ghosting at near is another disadvantage reported for center-near concentrics.[5] The most common reason for failure with the Spectrum is unacceptable near vision.[59]

(4) Lower adds are shown to work best with simultaneous vision. In one study, when add power is increased, simultaneous bifocals show significantly poorer low-contrast and low-illumination visual acuity.[60]

C. **Aspheric soft bifocals** are generally comparable.[16] One study compared monovision with an aspheric bifocal and found that 80% preferred the aspheric.[61] **Front aspheric lenses** such as **Unilens** and **Esstech PS Aspheric** (Blanchard Contact Lens, Manchester, New Hampshire) have central-near optics.[62,63]

1. The **Unilens** initial lens has a 9.0-mm base curve and 14.5-mm diameter. Spectacle sphere power plus one-half the add is the initial diagnostic power. Low to moderate adds to +1.75 D are the best candidates for the Unilens.[57]

2. **The Esstech PS Aspheric** has a front surface based on an S curve. The central zone is larger than that of a Unilens and has up to a +2.00 add.[64]

D. **Back aspheric** soft bifocals, such as **Occasions** (B&L), **PA1** (B&L), **Hydrocurve II** (Wesley-Jessen, Des Plaines, Illinois), **V/X** (GBF), **Allvue** (Salvatori), and **Fulfocus** (Premier Contact Lens Company, Memphis, Tennessee), have distance power in the center.[16] **Higher add powers** are a common goal among bifocal aspheric manufacturers. The inherent limitation of aspheric designs is low add powers. **Greater eccentricity** results in higher add powers for Hydrocurve II and V/X lenses.

1. **Central aspheric zones** allow higher eccentricity in the **Allvue**. A higher add results from a 7-mm central zone.

2. The **Fulfocus** has a spherical distance zone surrounded by an aspheric band and another larger spherical band.[9]

3. **B&L Occasions** has +1.50 add, which is greater than the +1.25 add in the **B&L PA1**. Occasions is a bifocal meant to be worn on an occasional basis. The B&L Occasions are available in multipacks.[16] The lens has been compared to the PA1 with favorable results[65] (Figure 18.17).

4. The **GBF V/X** has an eccentricity value of 1.6 and is hyperboloidal in the central section. The distance power is usually –0.25 to –0.50 higher because of the high eccentricity.[26]

5. **Special considerations** should be kept in mind with aspheric soft bifocals. **Pushing the plus** is highly recommended because add power is usually limited in asperics. The more plus prescribed, the

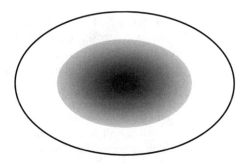

FIGURE 18.17   *The Bausch & Lomb (Rochester, New York) Occasions multifocal has distance power in the center and changes to near power in the periphery. The dark areas represent distance power.*

better it would be for near. Some manufacturers recommend pushing the plus at distance to an acceptable visual acuity of 20/25. Sometimes **more minus** at distance is necessary, however. The visual axis can be located nasal to the geometric center of the pupil and aspheric contact lens. This anatomic variation forces the patient to sight through additional plus, and more minus is needed to compensate.

  a. **Hyperopes** tend to have better success with aspherics than do myopes. Additional plus of a progressive add power is tolerated well because these patients may have a small amount of latent hyperopia.

  b. **Low-add** monovision patients needing better near-stereopsis may be good candidates for aspheric bifocals.[16]

  c. **Centration** and **pupillary sizes** are concerns for aspherics, as with other simultaneous lenses. The effects of decentration on an aspheric were calculated and graphed by Charman et al.[66,67] Use of centered lenses with smaller pupils obstructs the light rays that pass through the peripheral regions. Decentered lenses and larger pupils do not block the peripheral distortions, and vision is affected.

E. The **Lifestyle 4-Vue** (Permeable Technologies) is a soft aspheric multifocal with an additional **night zone** around the outer edge (Figure 18.18). The extra night zone helps the patient see better in dim illumination. The separate intermediate zone permits "arm's-length" (intermediate) vision in all fields of gaze. Starting with a +0.50 D over distance and pushing the plus is recommended.[68] The **Specialty Progressive** (Specialty Ultravision, Campbell, California) is a disposable lens of the same design.

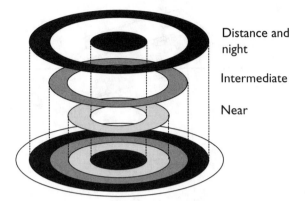

Distance and night

Intermediate

Near

FIGURE 18.18 *The Lifestyle 4-Vue (Permeable Technologies, Morganville, New Jersey) has an additional night zone surrounding the lens. A scotopic pupil can take advantage of this extra zone to afford the best vision under dim illumination. The lens is an aspheric bifocal with distance power in the center and periphery.*

F. The **Echelon Bifocal** from Ocular Sciences/American Hydron (South San Francisco, California) is a soft **diffractive** design (Figure 18.19). The diffractive phase plate is across the entire optic zone. A series of concentric grooves (echelettes) on the back surface forms the diffractive phase plate. Light is diffracted, and both distance (zero order) and near (first order) images are produced. Patients give quick responses regarding the acceptability of the vision—the lens either works or does not.[11,14]

1. Problems relating to **pupil size** and **centration** are less severe because of the design. If pupil size is too large (5–6 mm diameter) or the lens decenters, a diffractive lens is a superior choice over aspheric or concentric designs.[11]

2. With aspheric designs, movement produces more subjective fluctuations in vision than with diffractive designs. Although the contrast sensitivity of a diffractive design is less than with an aspheric, for decentration or excessive movement, a diffractive design is the better option.[69]

3. **Near vision** is similar to that with other simultaneous designs. Soft diffractive bifocals performed similarly to near-center concentric bifocals in a range of near tests.[5]

4. **Discontinuations** were mostly due to near-vision difficulties such as blur and ghosting. In one study, only 2% failed because of poor distance vision.[70] Because the light bundle is split evenly between distance and near, **dim illumination** has a negative effect. Diffractive lenses such as the Echelon have relatively poor low-contrast acuity.[71]

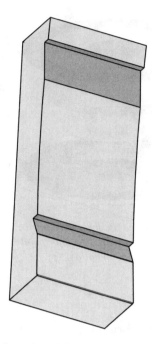

FIGURE 18.19   *The echelettes in a magnified view. A small portion of the back surface is pictured. The groovelike echelettes are located on the back surface and fill with tears. The change in indices and the shape of the echelettes diffract the light.*

    G. **Alternating soft bifocals** work similarly to RGP bifocals. Older soft translating designs include the **Durasoft 2** (Wesley-Jessen), **Synsoft** (Salvatori), **Crescent Softsite** (B&L), and **Bi-Tech** (B&L).

       Pearl: *Refitting failed bifocal lenses with monovision can be quite effective.*[21]

  V. **The optical mixture** describes the type of vision a contact lens bifocal lens patient experiences. Because of the many variability factors, a patient does not have pure bifocal vision at all times. Whether intentional or not, some form of modified monovision is taking place at some times. Realistically, most bifocal patients have an optical mixture of monovision, simultaneous, and alternating vision. The optical results are located somewhere on the "face of the pyramid" shown in Figure 18.20.[72]

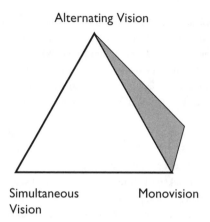

FIGURE 18.20 *Optical mixture. Vision with bifocal contact lenses is usually somewhere between monovision, simultaneous, or alternating vision. The type of vision is usually located somewhere on the face of the pyramid. (Adapted from WJ Benjamin, IM Borish. Presbyopia and the Influence of Aging on Prescription of Contact Lenses. In M Guillon, CM Ruben [eds], Contact Lens Practice. London: Chapman & Hall, 1994;828.)*

VI. **Best overall bifocal vision** is usually acheived with rigid gas permeable **translating** or **alternating designs**. Unfortunately, bifocal contact lenses are perceived by many practitioners as difficult to fit. Much of the contact lens literature is devoted to stepwise approaches to fitting. A video diagnostic fit may be the best way to learn how to fit alternating designs (CD-ROM: Translating bifocals: walk-through). Use of **additional prism**, as small as one-quarter diopter, can make a large difference in enhancing rigid alternating lens performance. Other key points demonstrated are the importance of an **alignment fit** and distinguishing between a **light blink** and a **full blink**.

REFERENCES

1. Weiner B. Dispelling the myths of multifocals. CL Spectrum 1993;8(10):22–29.
2. Gauthier CA, Holden BA, Grant T, et al. Interest of presbyopes in contact lens correction and their success with monovision. Optom Vis Sci 1992;69:858–862.
3. Shapiro MB, Bredson DC. Premarket evaluation of Unilens RGP aspheric multifocal contact lens. CL Spectrum 1992;7(5):21–24.
4. Harris MG, Sheedy JE, Gan CM. Vision and task performance with monovision and diffractive bifocal contact lenses. Optom Vis Sci 1992;69(8):609–614.
5. Back A, Grant T, Hine N. Comparative visual performance of three presbyopic contact lens corrections. Optom Vis Sci 1992;69:474–480.
6. Back A. Factors influencing success and failure in monovision. ICLC 1995;22:165–172.

7. Erickson DB. Self-efficacy may determine monovision success. CL Spectrum 1995;10(9):51.
8. Schor CM, Carson M, Peterson G, et al. Effects of interocular blur suppression ability on monovision tasks performance. J Am Optom Assoc 1989;60:188–192.
9. Bennett ES, Henry VA. Bifocal Contact Lenses. In ES Bennett, VA Henry (eds), Clinical Manual of Contact Lenses. Philadelphia: Lippincott, 1994;362–398.
10. Harris MG, Classé JG. Clinicolegal considerations of monovision. J Am Optom Assoc 1988;59:491–495.
11. Blanks G. Literature review of hydrogel presbyopic correction. ICLC 1991;18:142–147.
12. Josephson JE, Caffrey BE. Bifocal Hydrogel Lenses. In ES Bennett, BA Weissman (eds), Clinical Contact Lens Practice. Philadelphia: Lippincott, 1991(43);1–20.
13. Robboy MW, Cox IA, Erickson P. Effects of sighting and sensory dominance on monovision high- and low-contrast visual acuity. ICLC 1990;17:299–301.
14. Stein HA. The management of presbyopia with contact lenses: a review. CLAO J 1990;16:33–38.
15. Hine N, Holden BA. Performance of low- versus high-water-content plus lenses for presbyopes. ICLC 1992;19(11–12):257–263.
16. Pence NA. Strategies for success with presbyopes. CL Spectrum 1994;9(5):30–39.
17. Gasson A, Morris J. Presbyopes and Bifocals. In A Gasson, J Morris (eds), The Contact Lens Manual. Oxford: Butterworth–Heinemann, 1992;209–223.
18. Pence NA. Modified trivision: a modified monovision technique specifically for trifocal candidates. ICLC 1987;14:484–488.
19. Hansen DW. Evaluations for a successful multifocal fit. CL Spectrum 1995;10(4):13.
20. Norman CW. Managing presbyopes with soft contact lenses. EyeQuest 1994;4(3):76–89.
21. Back A, Holden BA, Hine N. Correction of presbyopia with contact lenses: comparative success rates with three systems. Optom Vis Sci 1989;66(8):518–525.
22. Norman CW, Lotzkat U. Stressing success with your presbyopic contact lens patients. CL Spectrum 1995;10(5):29–36.
23. Hansen DW. RGP multifocals: they really work! CL Spectrum 1995;10(2):15.
24. Josephson JE, Caffrey BE. Rigid Bifocal Lens Correction. In ES Bennett, BA Weissman (eds), Clinical Contact Lens Practice. Philadelphia: Lippincott, 1991(42);1–12.
25. Ames K. Aspheric Rigid Gas-Permeable Lenses. In CA Schwartz (ed), Specialty Contact Lenses: A Fitter's Guide. Philadelphia: Saunders, 1996;49–57.
26. Goldberg J. The V/X aspheric progressive add soft contact lens. CL Spectrum 1992;7(7):26–27.
27. Hansen DW. For more natural vision try aspheric RGP multifocals. CL Spectrum 1995;10(6):15.
28. Hanks AJ. The watermelon seed principle. CL Forum 1983;8(9):31–35.
29. Borish IM, Soni PS. Bifocal contact lenses. J Am Optom Assoc 1982;53:219–229.
30. Borish IM, Perrigin DM. Observations of bifocal contact lenses. Int Eyecare 1985;1:241–248.
31. Bennett ES. Basic Fitting. In ES Bennett, BA Weissman (eds), Clinical Contact Lens Practice. Philadelphia: Lippincott, 1991(23);1–22.
32. Macalister G, Woods C. Translating rigid bifocals: choosing fitting parameters to optimize visual performance. ICLC 1992;19:199–203.
33. Kirman ST, Kirman GS. The Tangent Streak Bifocal contact lens. CL Forum 1988;13(6):38–40.

34. Remba MJ. The Tangent Streak rigid gas-permeable bifocal contact lens. J Am Optom Assoc 1988;59:212–216.

35. Josephson JE, Wong M, Caffrey BE. Clinical experience with the Tangent Streak RGP bifocal contact lens. J Am Optom Assoc 1989;60:166–170.

36. Bennett E. RGP multifocal contact lens fitting pearls. CL Spectrum 1994;9(4):17.

37. Fluorex/Tangent Streak panel discussion. CL Spectrum 1990;5(5):61–68.

38. Hansen DW. How to fit the Lifestyle Hi-Rider. CL Spectrum 1993;8(10):36–38.

39. Korb DR, Exford JM. A study of three and nine o'clock staining after unilateral lens removal. J Am Optom Assoc 1970;41:7–10.

40. Doane MG, Gleason WJ. Tear Layer Mechanics. In ES Bennett, BA Weissman (eds), Clinical Contact Lens Practice. Philadelphia: Lippincott, 1993(2);1–17.

41. Mandell RB. Toric Lenses. In RB Mandell (ed), Contact Lens Practice (4th ed). Springfield, IL: Thomas, 1988;284–309.

42. Bridgewater BA. Troubleshooting the FluoroPerm ST Bifocal contact lens. CL Spectrum 1992;7(9):37–43.

43. McLaughlin R. How to stabilize a rotated bifocal lens. CL Spectrum 1993;8(12):15.

44. Bridgewater BA. The Fluoroperm ST bifocal. CL Spectrum 1992;7(5):24–31.

45. Mandell RB. Presbyopia. In RB Mandell (ed), Contact Lens Practice (4th ed). Springfield, IL: Thomas, 1988;785–823.

46. Remba MJ. Presbyopia. In ES Bennett (ed), Contact Lens Problem Solving. St. Louis: Mosby, 1995;109–139.

47. Ghormley NR. The Fluoroperm 60 bifocal. ICLC 1992;19:150–152.

48. Kame R, Bridgewater B, Hansen D, et al. An introduction to the Fluoroperm bifocal lens. Prescriber's Panel 11 [audiotape]. Mesa, Arizona: Paragon Vision Sciences, 1995.

49. Hansen DW. Translating designs for sharp visual acuity. CL Spectrum 1995;10(8):13.

50. Van Meter WS, Gussler JR, Litteral G. Clinical evaluation of three bifocal contact lenses. CLAO J 1990;16:203–207.

51. Birely JR, Lim ES, Litteral G, et al. A quantitative and qualitative assessment of the Solitaire bifocal contact lens. CLAO J 1995;21:20–23.

52. Gussler JR, Litteral G, VanMeter WS. Clinical evaluation of the Tangent Streak Trifocal. CLAO J 1991;17:160–163.

53. McLaughlin R. RGP bifocals: selecting the optimal design. CL Spectrum 1994;9(7):19.

54. Hansen DW. Presbyopia: Rigid Gas-Permeable Bifocal Lenses. In CA Schwartz (ed), Specialty Contact Lenses: A Fitter's Guide. Philadelphia: Saunders, 1996;58–78.

55. Woods RL, Saunders JE, Port MJA. Optical performance of decentered bifocal contact lenses. Optom Vis Sci 1993;70:171–184.

56. Cagnolati W. Acceptance of different multifocal contact lenses depending on the binocular findings. Optom Vis Sci 1993;70:315–322.

57. Ghormley NR. Bifocal soft contact lenses—clinical management. ICLC 1990;17:166–167.

58. Ghormley NR. A soft bifocal contact lens system—Unilens Corporation. ICLC 1992;19:102–103.

59. LaPierre M, St-Armaud F. Success rate evaluation of a simultaneous center add soft contact lens. ICLC 1992;19:157–161.

60. Cox I, Apollonia A, Erickson P. The effect of add power on simultaneous vision, monocentric, bifocal, soft lens visual performance. ICLC 1993;20:18–21.

61. Josephson JE, Caffrey BE. Monovision vs. bifocal contact lenses: a crossover study. J Am Optom Assoc 1987;58:652–654.
62. Shapiro MB, Bredeson DC. A prospective evaluation of Unilens soft multifocal contact lenses in 100 patients. CLAO J 1994;20:189–191.
63. Eiden SB. Aspheric hydrogel contact lens correction for presbyopia. CL Spectrum 1991;6(5):19–23.
64. Levy B. Clinical evaluation of the PS45 lens in presbyopia. CL Spectrum 1990;5(6):59–61.
65. Ghormley NR. The Occasions multifocal contact lens. ICLC 1993;20:134.
66. Charman WN. Optical characteristics of Bausch and Lomb Soflens (PA1) bifocals. ICLC 1984;11:564–575.
67. Charman WN, Walsh G. Retinal images with centered, aspheric varifocal contact lenses. ICLC 1988;15:87–94.
68. Shovlin JP. Cornea and contact lens Q&A. Rev Optom 1995;132(5):93.
69. Brenner MB. An objective and subjective comparative analysis of diffractive and front surface aspheric contact lens designs used to correct presbyopia. CLAO J 1994;20:19–22.
70. Back A, Grant T, Hine N, et al. Twelve-month success rates with a hydrogel diffractive bifocal contact lens. Optom Vis Sci 1992;69:941–947.
71. Papas E, Young G, Hearn K. Monovision vs soft diffractive bifocal contact lenses: a crossover study. ICLC 1990;17:181–186.
72. Benjamin WJ, Borish IM. Presbyopia and the Influence of Aging on Prescription of Contact Lenses. In M Guillon, CM Ruben (eds), Contact Lens Practice. London: Chapman & Hall, 1994;828.

Chapter 19

Aphakia and Postsurgical Corneas

Christine L. K. Astin

I. For **aphakia,** fitting of contact lenses is a preferred method of vision correction.
    A. Contact lenses have several **advantages** over spectacles for aphakes.
        1. Spectacles produce a **large increase in magnification,** so the image from one eye is difficult to fuse with that of the fellow eye. A significant difference in spectacle power between right and left lenses also causes **binocular fusion problems** due to relative prismatic effect and image aberration.
        2. Spectacles restrict the field of corrected vision. There is an apparent **"ring scotoma"** due to deviation of light rays at the lens periphery.
        3. Spectacles are **heavy** and give a differing power at the eye plane if the lens position relative to the eye alters.
    B. After cataract surgery, an intraocular lens is implanted. There are basically **two intraocular lens types for aphakes: posterior-chamber** and **anterior-chamber.** Posterior-chamber lenses are supported in the capsular bag remaining after extracapsular extraction. Anterior-chamber lenses are used after intracapsular extraction. Pediatric patients can be fit 1–2 days postoperatively because the small incision heals quickly. Patients who have had phacoemulsification with extracapsular extraction can be fitted with lenses 4–6 weeks postoperatively. The types of incisions currently performed are scleral tunnel or pocket, limbal, and clear corneal.
    C. **Rigid gas-permeable (RGP) lenses** allow clearer visual acuity in patients with aphakia because more corneal astigmatism is corrected than with soft lenses. RGP lenses are less likely to be affected by deposits. In manufacture, extra care is taken to avoid lens thickness; one method uses the **lenticular form** on the anterior surface, well blended to avoid a step.
        1. **Aphakia power trial lens sets** are strongly recommended for fitting. The lens thickness and behavior should be similar to those of the final lens prescribed. Use of trial lenses decreases the chance of mistakes in the final power calculation.[1]

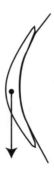

FIGURE 19.1   *Center of gravity of contact lens.*

2. An **"on K" alignment fit** tends to ride low because of the increased thickness of the lens and the fact that the lens center of gravity is anterior to the cornea[2] (Figure 19.1). A **steeper curve lens** is required for stability, but good tear flow beneath the lens must be maintained. A **negative-edge carrier** grasped by the upper lid can improve lens position in some cases.

3. **Against-the-rule astigmatism** is sometimes present in aphakes. This contour encourages the lens to drift laterally off center, resulting in inadequate pupil coverage. A **larger lens diameter** or **a toric peripheral curve** can improve lens centration.

4. An **aspheric-back-surface design** lens allows smoother lens movement and masks more astigmatism. This lens type is fit near the flatter keratometry reading and the fluorescein appearance shows little central pooling and minimal edge clearance.

   D. **Soft (hydrophilic) lenses** wrap around the globe and more easily achieve a central position. The first lens **total diameter** is 1.5–2.0 mm larger than the visible iris diameter, and the curvature is 0.70 mm (3–4 D) flatter than the flattest keratometry reading. After a 15-minute settling period, the lens fit is judged regarding position. The lens should be centrally fitting with good corneal coverage. Movement should be 0.50–1.0 mm on blink and eye movement. If an astigmatic residual correction is required, this can be incorporated into the **multifocal spectacle correction** worn over the contact lens. Some aspheric lens designs reduce lens bulk, improving comfort and fit, but thin lenses may be more difficult for older patients to handle.

   E. **Extended-wear lenses** fitted for aphakes should be high-water-content soft lenses of adequate oxygen permeability. Care must be taken that the fit does not tighten excessively as the lens loses water. In some cases, RGP lenses of high oxygen transmissibility can be worn for extended wear. The practitioner should watch out for signs of RGP lens binding on the patient's epithelium overnight.

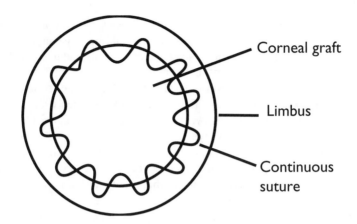

FIGURE 19.2   *Continuous suture method in penetrating keratoplasty.*

    F.   **Frequent aftercare visits** of aphakic patients are needed to watch for signs of corneal hypoxia and edema, blurred vision, limbal vessel hyperemia, vessel growth, epithelial erosions, and endothelial folds.

    G.   **Incomplete blinks** are likely to lead to areas of drying and increased lens deposits. These interfere with vision, decrease comfort, and increase the risk of infections.

  II. Contact lens fitting after **full-thickness penetrating keratoplasty (PK)** is sometimes necessary for adequate vision (see Chapter 29).

    A.   After trephination from the cadaver eye, the donor button of corneal tissue is transplanted into the circular aperture of the host cornea. With careful control of the anterior chamber fluids, the surgeon eases the button into place to align the edge with the host margin. Sutures are inserted at a suitable depth to keep the transplant (graft) in place. There are at least eight radial interrupted sutures or a single continuous suture (Figure 19.2). A combination of four to eight cardinal sutures with a running suture of nylon can also be used. Frequent aftercare and appropriate medical treatment with steroids and prophylactic antibiotics are provided.

    B.   **Indications** for PK include keratoconus, corneal dystrophy, corneal decompensation (e.g., bullous keratopathy), and significant corneal scarring after trauma or inflammation.

    C.   Although a lamellar keratoplasty patient may be referred for lens fit **3–6 months postoperatively,** in the case of full-thickness penetrating keratoplasty, the period is often **12 months postoperatively,** after the removal of sutures. Corneal sensitivity is still significantly below normal levels 12 months postoperatively, so if the patient begins lens wear before adequate sensitivity returns, he or she may be unaware of debris beneath the lens, which can cause **epithelial erosions.** The patient may continue lens wear, not realizing the damage that is being caused by the debris. At 1 year postoperatively, however, wound healing from full-thickness penetrating keratoplasty should be satisfactory, and there is less concern that minor epithelial erosions will lead to corneal transplant rejection or to penetrating infection.[3]

D. Compared with the normal cornea, the PK eye has **differences in topography** and **physiology.**[4] Extra care should be taken with lens fit and aftercare because the PK eye responds differently to contact lens wear than does the nonoperated eye[5] (see Chapter 29). Contact lenses are useful for optimizing vision after PK, but the visual improvement may tempt the patient to overwear the lens and to risk the development of corneal edema and epithelial erosions, which could lead to serious problems and stimulate vessel ingrowth.[6]

E. The **soft lens** of choice is a medium- to high-water-content lens. Good oxygen transmissibility is important. The lens material is preferably deposit resistant to reduce the chance of **epithelial erosions** caused by deposits. The lens of first choice would have diameter 2.0 mm larger than the visible iris diameter and have a radius of curvature 0.50 mm (2.50 D) greater than the flattest keratometry reading. Lens fit is judged after approximately 15 minutes settling time, aiming for good centration, corneal coverage on eye movements, 0.5-mm movement on blinks, and absence of limbal indentation or disturbance to limbal vessels.

F. **High residual astigmatism** may necessitate the use of a toric lens. Care should be taken to achieve a stable-position lens fit. Excess lens thickness and a tight fit should be avoided. Tight-fit lenses are likely to inhibit oxygen supply to the cornea and to restrict limbal blood flow. These effects result in corneal hypoxia, which encourages neovascularization.

G. An **irregular corneal contour** can sometimes be successfully fitted using a soft lens or a combination lens such as a soft lens with a central RGP portion.[7–9] The flexible periphery of the lens wraps around the eye to provide good lens centration and comfort; the RGP lens center corrects the corneal astigmatism. Use of combination lenses can be risky in patients who have had PK, however. A silicone rubber lens can also give the best fit, and such lenses have good oxygen permeability.[10]

H. **Extended wear in PK patients** should be avoided because of the increased risks of chronic corneal edema, infection, and stimulation of neovascularization.[4] In cases in which lens handling and daily wear are not achievable, a high-water-content soft lens can be fitted. The first-choice lens would have parameters of about 8.80/14.50. If, after 20–30 minutes of settling, the lens has tightened such that lens movement is inadequate, a looser lens fit should be chosen. If lens mobility is excessive, a tighter fit is tried.

I. **Aftercare visits** are at 1 day after initial lens fitting, 1 week, and 4 weeks to assess corneal tolerance of extended wear. The practitioner notes vision and lens condition and fit and conducts a slit-lamp biomicroscope examination with particular attention to **corneal clarity** and **epithelial integrity.** If, with time, the lens fit becomes too tight, leading to conjunctival hyperemia or inadequate lens movement, the lens should be replaced by one of a looser fit.

J. **Extra power correction** and **prescribing spectacles** can be done at the 4-week aftercare visit. Follow-up visits for ocular assessment and disinfection of the lens would be arranged for every 4–8 weeks. If early signs of neovascularization are noted, the lens should be refitted loosely. If vessel growth persists, a reduction in lens wear time is necessary. The extended-wear patient should be advised of the importance of obtaining an eye examination without delay if redness, pain, or decreased vision occurs.

K. **RGP lenses** must be fit using trial lenses (see Chapter 29). The graft-host interface can cause problems during lens wear, since this is where irregular astigmatism may be induced secondary to irregularities of suture tension, healing, and scar formation.

1. **Central keratometry** is important, not only to assess corneal curvature and the type of irregular astigmatism, if present, but also as part of the follow-up routine to monitor corneal changes. In addition, detailed examination with slit-lamp biomicroscopy and the use of videokeratography give valuable information about the corneal topography. Thorough analysis of the PK patient and cornea before lens fitting can minimize the time taken for a proper fitting.

2. The **corneal contour** may have a **flat plateau,** so a standard-design rigid lens would vault too high and trap excess tears and bubbles beneath the lens. A good starting point is using the steep K for base-curve selection. A special-design PK lens with flat central curvature but steeper peripheral curves than those of standard designs may be needed. If the donor button was significantly oversized, the graft can have a **relatively steep curvature.** This enhances the curvature change at the graft margin and necessitates fitting a special lens design whose edge would not indent the peripheral cornea. Against-the-rule toricity also makes the fitting more difficult.

3. A **high degree of corneal astigmatism** can remain, even if the corneal transplant appears clear. A tilted or projecting profile or an irregular host-to-donor margin produces an irregular corneal topography on which it is difficult to fit a suitable lens.[11] Together with the influence of the lids, this can give rise to variable vision, reduced lens tolerance, and increased risk of lens decentration and loss.

4. **Large total diameters**—for example, 10.0–11.0 mm—are recommended to give good coverage over the transplant and to avoid the lens edge rubbing the transplant margin during lens movement. Smooth lens surfaces with good wettability, well-blended transitions, and rounded edges are also required. These allow a gliding lens movement and encourage good flow of tears beneath the lens, lubri-

cating the cornea and minimizing epithelial erosions caused by the lens or by debris. A good oxygen supply to the transplant is essential.

5. **Several aftercare visits** and **lens changes** may be needed. The patient should be warned that RGP lens fitting after PK is complex and may require several extra trial lenses and clinic visits. Also, since the corneal condition has changed, lens wear time may be rather limited.

6. The **first-choice lens** should have a back central curve radius on or near the steepest keratometry reading, and the fluorescein picture should demonstrate light central touch with good tear flow beneath the lens. The lens will show good centration over the graft. If movement is excessive, fit a lens with a larger diameter or a slightly steeper curve. After lens settling for about 10 minutes, over-refraction and visual acuity are determined. In most cases, the astigmatism is corrected by the spherical central curve of the RGP lens. If irregular topography disturbs lens fit, an aspheric design lens whose curve flattens smoothly from center to edge may fit better. Constad recommends a first lens slightly flatter than the mean keratometry; for example, for Ks of 45.00 D/48.00 D, try a 46.00-D curve 9.0-mm diameter trial lens.[12] Often a larger lens with a flatter curve has more stable centration.

7. **Videokeratography** has been used by Lopatynsky et al. to facilitate RGP lens fitting on 19 eyes after PK.[13] Nine of the eyes required modifications in the fit 3 months later. Keratography is useful in fitting and aftercare but can be misleading if the patient's fixation is variable.

8. **Another special PK lens design** has a central base curve with four peripheral curves designed to simulate the aspheric shape of a normal peripheral cornea. A trial on 25 subjects by Koffler et al. showed 93% success by 1 year, and 82% achieved at least 20/40 vision.[14] Weiner and Nirankari obtained 81% wearing success using a type of **biaspheric RGP lens** with minimal lens-related complications.[15]

9. Care should be taken to avoid **increasing irregular astigmatism** by RGP lens wear. A few studies have shown beneficial manipulation of corneal topography using lenses, however.[16,17]

10. **Proper lens care** is especially important for these patients because any trauma or prolonged corneal edema can initiate an inflammatory response and possibly increase the risk of corneal rejection. Even if the patients have worn lenses before PK, they can benefit from further education regarding correct lens handling, hygiene, and the need for suitable follow-up visits.

11. A number of **lens-related complications** may occur.

    a. **Epithelial indentation** may result from a tight lens edge.

b. **Corneal edema and hypoxia** may result from, for example, a tight fit, poor oxygen transfer, or overwear.[18]

c. There may be **vessel ingrowth** to and along the graft margin. If the vessels grow into the graft, there is a significant risk of inflammation and edema, which could lead to rejection.

d. **Wound gape** at the graft margin may result from trauma, particularly if lens fit is attempted too soon postoperatively.

e. Lenses may cause **persistent epithelial erosions.**

f. **Infection** is a possibility, particularly if lens wear persists in the presence of lens-related complications. Soft lens wearers are especially at risk for infection. Spectacles may be a preferable alternative for PK patients.

REFERENCES

1. Port MJA. Contact Lenses in Abnormal Ocular Conditions—Aphakia. In AJ Phillips, J Stone (eds), Contact Lenses. London: Butterworth, 1989;757–763.

2. Astin CLK. Fitting aphakic patients with contact lenses. CL J 1992;20(1):16–19.

3. Astin CLK. Contact lens fitting after anterior segment disease. CL J 1992;20(4):8–10.

4. Cohen EJ, Adams CP. Postkeratoplasty Fitting for Visual Rehabilitation. In OH Dabezies (ed), Contact Lenses: The CLAO Basic Guide to Science and Clinical Practice. Orlando, FL: Grune & Stratton, 1984;1–7.

5. Woodward EG. Contact lens fitting after keratoplasty. J Br CL Assoc 1981;4(2):42–49.

6. Smiddy WE, Hamburg TR, Kracher GP, et al. Visual correction following penetrating keratoplasty. Ophthalmic Surg 1992;23(2):90–93.

7. Campbell R, Caroline P. A soft lens option for post-op graft/host bulge. CL Spectrum 1994;9(10):64–65.

8. Astin CLK. The use of Saturn II lenses following penetrating keratoplasty. J Br CL Assoc 1985;8:2–5.

9. Zadnik K, Mannis MJ. Use of the Saturn II lens in keratoconus and corneal transplant patients. ICLC 1987;14(8):312–315.

10. Astin CLK. Fitting corneal grafts—some unusual cases. J Br CL Assoc 1990;13(1):88–90.

11. Beekhius H, van Rij G, Eggnik FAGJ, et al. Contact lenses following keratoplasty. CLAO J 1991;17(1):27–29.

12. Constad WH. Fitting post-op keratoplasty patients with RGP CLs. CL Forum 1988;13(12):40–43.

13. Lopatynsky M, Cohen EJ, Leavitt KG, et al. Corneal topography for rigid gas-permeable lens fitting after penetrating keratoplasty. CLAO J 1993;19(1):41–44.

14. Koffler BH, Clements LD, Litteral GL, et al. A new contact lens design for postkeratoplasty patients. CLAO J 1994;20(3):170–175.

15. Weiner BM, Nirankari VS. A new biaspheric contact lens for severe astigmatism following penetrating keratoplasty. CLAO J 1992;18(1):29–33.

16. Wilson SE, Friedman RS, Klyce SD. Contact lens manipulation of corneal topography after penetrating keratoplasty: a preliminary study. CLAO J 1992;18(3):177–182.

17. Campbell R, Caroline P. Managing irregular astigmatism after penetrating keratoplasty. CL Spectrum 1993;8(3):64–66.

18. Bourne WM, Shearer DR. Effects of long-term rigid contact lens wear on the endothelium of corneal transplants for keratoconus 10 years after penetrating keratoplasty. CLAO J 1995;21(4):265–267.

Chapter 20

Refractive Surgery and Contact Lenses

Christine L. K. Astin

I. **Radial keratotomy (RK)** is the surgical procedure for reducing myopia by incision into the cornea, avoiding a central zone of more than 3 mm in diameter (Figure 20.1). The procedure and the effect of the number of incisions (three to eight) have been described in several papers.[1,2]

   A. **Patients may request RK** to improve unaided vision for professional, cosmetic, or psychological reasons or for convenience, even if their visual acuity (VA) can be corrected to 20/20 by spectacles or contact lenses. **Pre-RK counseling** is most important.

   B. The **outcome of RK** is variable.

   1. Kraff et al. reported that 75% of the surgeons in their study used the **Casebeer nomogram** to improve predictability of RK outcome.[3]

   2. The **incision depth** is usually 90% of the previously measured central corneal thickness; deeper incisions increase the risk of perforating Descemet's membrane.

   3. The **rigidity** of the cornea is decreased by RK such that intraocular forces acting on the cornea cause midperipheral regions to "bulge" forward.

   4. The **radius of curvature** of the apical cap becomes longer than that measured preoperatively. This flatter central curvature has **less refractive power** and results in a hypermetropic shift, reducing the original myopia. The extent of the shift and its relation to the curvature changes have been investigated by numerous researchers.[4–7]

   5. The **corneal power change** is usually greatest within the first few days postoperatively. During the following months (in some cases 12 months), **corneal rigidity** can increase and induce a change in the corneal shape.

   6. **Central keratometry** readings at intervals show the radius of curvature gradually decreasing from the postoperative value. There is

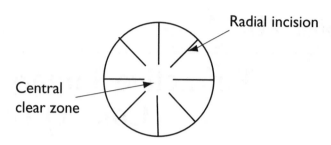

FIGURE 20.1   *Radial keratotomy corneal incision pattern.*

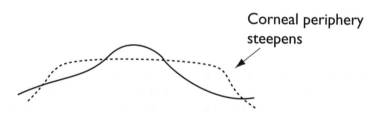

FIGURE 20.2   *Corneal shape changes after radial keratotomy.*

not, however, a one-to-one correlation between radius of curvature decrease and decrease in myopia. Following is an example of keratometry readings.

Keratometry	Preoperative	Postoperative	1 Year Later
Horizontal	45.45 D	42.72 D	42.86 D
	(7.42 mm)	(7.90 mm)	(7.88 mm)
Vertical	46.23 D	43.55 D	43.68 D
	(7.29 mm)	(7.75 mm)	(7.73 mm)

7. The **cornea shape** changes from a prolate to an oblate elliptic form—that is, from the flat center it becomes steeply curved toward the periphery (Figure 20.2).

C. The **selection criteria** listed below were defined in the Prospective Evaluation of Radial Keratotomy (PERK) study.[8]

1. The patient should have tried **spectacle or contact lens** correction and understand that optic correction may be necessary after surgery. There are potential complications of RK surgery, and a presbyopic correction may be needed earlier than without surgery because of the hyperopic shift.

2. The patient is 21 years old or older. The progression of physiologic myopia is less likely after this age.

3. The patient has no residual, recurrent, or active ocular disease or abnormality.

4. The patient's **myopia** is physiologic, without ophthalmic signs of progressive myopia.

5. The patient does not have a **systemic disease,** such as lupus or rheumatoid arthritis, that can produce dry eyes, which are likely to influence corneal healing.

6. **Previous contact lens wearers** must demonstrate stable keratometry readings with regularly shaped mires 1–4 weeks after ceasing lens wear. Consistent readings during two subsequent visits can confirm a stable cornea. This helps to screen out those with corneal warpage or keratoconus.

D. After RK, there may be **problems with vision.**[9]

1. **Anisometropia** of up to 9.0 D between the two eyes may lead to diplopia and disturbed binocular fusion. The visual disturbance results from the unequal retinal image sizes and the relative prismatic effect of corrective spectacles.

2. **Diurnal fluctuation of vision** is caused by diurnal changes in refraction and corneal curvature.[10] Generally, anterior corneal curvature increases during the day, so a stronger myopic correction is required for evenings. The **PERK study** found that approximately 35% of subjects had this problem.[11] It has been speculated that corneal hydration and lid squeezing are factors. There are patients who still experience diurnal variation 4 years after RK.[12] Shovlin suggested that an alternative RK method reduces fluctuation.[13]

3. **Astigmatism** may increase and cause unsatisfactory vision even when the degree of myopia is reduced by RK. Diurnal variation and irregular astigmatism may result in vision problems even with spectacle correction.

4. **Increased sensitivity to glare,** together with problems with contrast sensitivity, may occur. These problems seem to correlate with the size of the **optic zone (OZ)**, the width of the incision scars, and the pupil size. Glare gradually diminishes as the scar density decreases in the first 6 months, but it may persist for some patients.

5. **Residual ametropia** due to the regression of the RK effect on corneal power as the incisions heal may be larger than the patient hoped. Up to 15% of patients have residual myopia. **Steroid treatment** slows the healing process and may elevate the intraocular pressure, both of which may enhance the myopia reduction. It is rarely advisable to remain on prolonged steroid treatment because of the side effects, such as rise in intraocular pressure and cataract formation.

E. **Retreatment with RK** is sometimes performed.

1. **Residual myopes** complain that their unaided vision is unsatisfactory, and some demand a repeat RK procedure. The surgeon should

decide whether **RK "enhancement"** is advisable. Sometimes, the enhancement entails reopening the incisions at the OZ and making them longer and deeper.[14] Again, the RK surgeon should take care to avoid corneal microperforations and inclusion cysts or debris in the incisions.

2. **Regression** can relate to inadequate incision depth or aggressive stromal wound healing. Some patients become **hypermetropic** and have difficulty adapting, especially if presbyopic.

3. **Corrective surgery** has unpredictable results, so these patients may need lenses.

F. **Counseling** is essential before patients undergo RK. Patients should be warned of the possible need for lenses and potential difficulties with fitting them, particularly if they previously had a limited tolerance for lens wear.[9]

G. **Soft lens fitting** can vary with hydration of the lens and with different peripheral corneal contours. Individuals can vary even if their central keratometry is similar.

1. **Diurnal fluctuation** in an RK patient may produce problems pertaining to corneal shape, power changes, and limbal disturbance when the soft lens drapes over the abnormal corneal contour.

2. **Wait several months** until the contour has stabilized before attempting to fit the patient, and always avoid a tight fit.

3. The **cornea should not be fitted** if there is wound gaping, significant staining or neovascularization, or inclusion plugs or cysts in the incisions.[15] There may be an increased risk of ulcerative keratitis in these cases.

4. **Lens choice** by the practitioner should not be based on preoperative keratometry. The RK surgical method differs slightly for each case, and corneas vary in their rigidity and wound-healing response; any of these factors can influence the curvature that results after RK.

5. **Lens fit** must be judged based on the stabilized topography and the lens behavior on the eye during trial fitting.

6. **Videokeratoscopy** is helpful; it indicates the width of the central corneal flat plateau over which the soft lens must drape.

7. The recommended **lens design** is a thin, high-water-content lens, which will have good oxygen transmissibility and flexibility. Compared with a low-water-content or thick lens, it will be less likely to cause hypoxia, undue pressure, or neovascularization on the cornea and limbus.

8. Vickery recommends that **flat-fit** lenses align more closely to the RK corneal contour to avoid limbal compression.[16]

9. **Examples of soft lens–fit patients**
   a. **Patient H,** 2 years after RK, had a VA of 20/60.

Refraction	$-1.00 -1.00 \times 170$, VA 20/20
Keratometry	43.83 D (7.70 mm) at 5 and 44.41 D
	(7.60 mm) at 110
Lens fit	8.70/–1.00 D/13.5 mm, VA 20/17

After 15 minutes of settling time, the patient had a good fit with central positioning, 0.5-mm lens movement on full blinks, and no conjunctival indentation. The patient preferred a soft lens to a rigid gas-permeable (RGP) lens because the lens position remained stable throughout a very active workday and was easily tolerated. Wearing time was controlled to minimize limbal hyperemia. At a follow-up visit 2 months later, a surprising result was that after 5 hours of uncomplicated daily lens wear, the keratometry was 43.32 D (7.97 mm) at 180 and 42.98 D (7.84 mm) at 90, and the unaided vision was 20/17. Lens wear had caused a central corneal flattening effect, reducing the myopia.

b. Patient E, 2 years after RK, had a VA of 20/200.

Refraction	$-0.50 -5.00 \times 20$, VA 20/30
Keratometry	36.69 D (9.20 mm) at 15 and 39.94 D
	(8.45 mm) at 105
Lens fit	9.0/–0.50/–4.00 × 15 mm/14.00 × 12.50,
	VA 20/25

The patient had good fit and coverage, stable positioning, and no indentation. At a 3-month follow-up visit, after 6 hours of daily lens wear, the keratometry was 36.20 D (9.32 mm) at 15 and 39.47 D (8.56 mm) at 105.

Refraction is +0.50 D–3.50 × 20; VA is 20/20, unaided 20/80.

10. Unintentional orthokeratology may result from lens wear even when the RK cornea shape has been presumed to be stabilized.[17]

  a. Myopia reduction has resulted from the peripheral corneal swelling and central flattening induced by **soft-bandage lenses.**[14] These lenses were used in the first weeks after RK to assist healing of epithelial defects or microperforation.

  b. It is during the **postoperative** period of up to 3 months that the cornea is most malleable and prone to warpage. Lens fitting should not be carried out during this period unless it is medically necessary for short-term use to aid wound healing.

H. Complications of contact lens wear can occur on an RK cornea.

  1. Lens wear can stimulate **corneal vessel** growth.

      a. The **prevalence** of **corneal** stromal neovascularization increases after soft lens fitting.[18,19]

      b. **RK** may alter corneal oxygen requirements or the mode of oxygen flow through the stroma.

  2. **Polymegethism** leading to a decreased cell density has been revealed by several studies.[20] Polymegethism may reduce corneal ability to cope with hypoxia, one of the stimulants of vessel growth.

  3. The **lens fit** becoming tighter, even when a lens of high oxygen transmissibility is fitted, may cause lens pressure and epithelial indentation at the limbus (or negative fluid pressure between the lens and the eye), which could affect the corneal contour and metabolism. Localized corneal swelling and irregular astigmatism could result.

  4. **Flexing** of imperfectly healed stromal segments stimulates neovascularization.

  5. **Extended wear** is not recommended because it leads to corneal hypoxia, stromal swelling, and longer periods of lens flexing under the influence of lid pressure. A greater prevalence of rapid vessel growth has been shown after extended wear.[21]

I. **Fitting with RGP lenses** after RK results in fewer complications than fitting with soft lenses.

  1. Choose a **lens material** with moderate to high oxygen transmissibility. Use of a material with low transmissibility can lead to corneal swelling if the lens fit is tight or wear time is prolonged.

  2. Recovery from **corneal edema** may be slow in an RK patient who has suffered **endothelial cell loss;** the result may be disturbed vision, corneal irregular steepening, and neovascularization. An RK cornea is susceptible to lens-induced warping.

  3. The **topography of the RK cornea** is unusual; there is a flat central curve and steep "knee" of the periphery, which complicates lens fitting (Figure 20.3).

  4. **Lens fitting** from standard sets generally demonstrates excessive edge clearance and mobility on the RK eye, since these sets are designed for normal ametrope corneal contours that increasingly flatten toward the limbus.

      a. **Excess lens mobility** on an RK eye leads to lid discomfort, lens decentration, and either a low-riding position or a high position held by the upper lid.

      b. A **small, steeply fit lens** would precipitate the problem of excessive central tear pooling and trapping of debris and bubbles beneath the lens. A flatter-fit lens with a minimum edge clearance design is recommended, such as an elliptical design or a redesigned blended multicurve lens. Trying several lenses can take a lot of clinical chair time, but it is worthwhile to obtain an acceptable fit and counsel the patient.

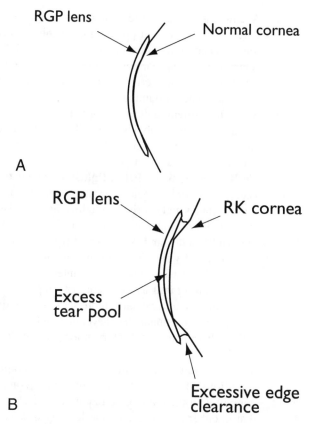

FIGURE 20.3   *Radial keratotomy (RK) corneal topography. A. Prelens fit. B. Post-radial kera-totomy, standard design lens shows excess central tear pool and excessive edge clearance. (RGP = rigid gas-permeable.)*

    c. Special RK lens designs have been introduced. These designs reduce the excess lens edge stand-off, improve comfort, and stabilize lens movement.

    d. Aspheric lenses can often mask astigmatism. Goldberg describes a RK-aspheric design whose ellipsoidal back surface has an eccentricity value of 0.6.[22] The fluorescein picture shows central tear pooling with a slight green rim of tears at the lens edge. Goldberg recommends fitting 1.75 D steeper than the flattest preoperative keratometry and choosing the overall lens diameter as 2.0 mm larger than the base curve radius. The design aims to give improved centration over the pupil and minimal displacement on blinking.

5. Certain complications may occur when fitting RK lenses.

a. A **chafing effect** at the limbus can occur in fitting after RK.[23,24] In the corneal profile, midperipheral steepness surrounds a central flat area, and some lenses vault high over the central cornea and bear down on the midperiphery. If this pressure persists, particularly if there is friction, epithelial rubbing by the lens causes staining.

b. **Soft-lens tightening** during wear may also induce friction and pressure on the limbal vessels. These effects can lead to chronic epithelial erosion and vessel blanching, which stimulate corneal vascularization.

c. An **RGP lens, when fitted tightly** to center the lens, may vault the central cornea excessively and trap a pool of tear fluid. Bubbles and debris are retained beneath the lens. There is also a risk of central corneal edema. The lens edge can press too firmly on the corneal midperiphery, causing epithelial indentation and wrinkling. Chronic erosions are especially a problem for incisions that cross or intersect.

d. **Lens handling and hygiene** are very important. Corneal infection and trauma can have more serious consequences in an RK eye than in a nonoperated eye. In both RK and contact lens fitting, there is physical intervention on a healthy ametropic eye. Both procedures require good assessment and measurements before the procedure, an accurate operation, and conscientious aftercare. Patients must also comprehend and comply with these aftercare requirements. They must accept that in either procedure and particularly in lens fit after RK, quality of vision may be disturbed even if the VA seems reasonable on the Snellen chart.

II. Fitting contact lenses after **photorefractive keratectomy (PRK)** is easier than fitting lenses after other corneal surgical procedures.

A. The **PRK procedure** uses an **excimer laser** that emits highly energetic photons (at a wavelength of 193 nm) to break molecular bonds at the target surface. This process, called **photoablation,** removes a thin layer of molecules over the 5.0-mm or larger diameter zone at each laser pulse. This essentially nonthermal process has been well investigated for ophthalmic use.[25,26]

1. **Myopia** is treated by adjusting the characteristics of the laser beam (e.g., by inserting a computer-controlled iris diaphragm in its path) to remove more central corneal tissue within the beam zone. This procedure results in a flatter central corneal curvature. A topical anesthetic is used, and the epithelium is scraped from the cornea or removed by the laser before the photoablation procedure.

2. **Computer programs** have been created to calculate ablation depth and corneal power changes.[27] These changes depend on the ablation method and zone—for example, for a –7.00-D power change, the

axial depth of ablation is 45 µm over a 4.0-mm diameter zone, but over a 6.0-mm zone it is 100 µm (about one-fifth of the corneal thickness). For 6.0 mm, a **multizone technique** with more gradual curvature changes would be advisable. The 6.0-mm zone has recently been approved by the U.S. Food and Drug Administration.

B. In terms of **outcome, tissue healing** in the first few weeks after PRK produces thickening of the ablated zone due to subepithelial deposition and growth of new layers of epithelial cells. Various grades of corneal haze have been recorded. PRK for myopia results in a **hypermetropic shift** followed by a partial regression of the refractive effect over a period that can range from a few weeks to a few months depending on medical treatment and healing response. This second phase relates to delayed stromal remodeling and produces a myopic shift.[28]

   1. A **stabilization** time of 6–12 months after PRK should be allowed for the refraction and corneal topography to settle before fitting lenses. Fitting sooner may affect corneal healing and refraction changes.

   2. **PRK research studies** on "sighted eyes" began in 1989. Worldwide, many thousands have undergone PRK, and generally the results have been encouraging.[29–32]

   3. **Caution** should be exercised because some studies report significant individual variation in wound-healing response, particularly for PRK treatments of **greater than 6.00 D** of myopia.[33,34] In addition to receiving appropriate pre-PRK screening, patients must be counseled regarding this variation.

   4. **Corneal curvature** becomes steeper 1–2 weeks postoperatively. An example of corneal curvature measurements after PRK is as follows:

Curvature	Preoperative	1 Week	8 Weeks	6 Months
Horizontal	40.65 D	35.15 D	38.40 D	37.92 D
Vertical	40.50 D	35.10 D	38.40 D	38.14 D
Refraction	−5.50	+6.00	−1.25	−1.25
Astigmatism	−0.50 × 20	−1.00 × 10	−0.50 × 50	−0.25 × 70

C. **Selection criteria** for PRK are based on current research.[35]

   1. Patients should be 21 years of age or older. Patients should be warned about presbyopia.

   2. An **ocular history** of significant ocular disease or surgery leads to exclusion, including a history of herpes simplex, lupus, and rheumatoid disease.

   3. Patients whose **occupations** depend on exacting visual ability (e.g., pilots, professional night drivers) are excluded from having the procedure.

4. The individual's **sex** is not significant in determining who is eligible for the procedure, but PRK is not advised during pregnancy.

5. **Refraction** must be stable and preferably less than –6.00 D of myopia. Patients with higher degrees of myopia have significantly greater risks of regression of treatment effect and of complications.

6. **Astigmatism** should be less than 1.00 D, depending on myopia. Astigmatic PRK treatments are still rather variable, **depending on the procedure.**

7. The best corrected **VA** should be 20/30 or better. A dominant eye should not have PRK if the fellow eye has limited visual potential.

8. A **contact lens history** demonstrating the patient's ability to wear lenses can be an indication of improved tolerance of post-treatment anisometropia, but patients with variable refraction due to corneal distortion should be excluded. An assessment of corneal topography is recommended when PRK is considered for a patient.

9. **Motivation** is important, and only patients with realistic visual aims and expectations should be included.

D. **PRK and RK share some features but have important differences.**

1. A **postoperative hyperopic shift** is produced by both procedures due to central curvature flattening, followed by a myopic drift or regression toward the original power. Some RK patients experience a small hyperopic drift even several years after operation.

2. **PRK equipment** is more expensive than RK equipment.

3. **PRK affects the central cornea,** so haze in some patients restricts the best corrected VA. RK affects the peripheral cornea.

4. Some surgeons using computer calculations have claimed that the **PRK outcome predictability** is lower than that of RK.

5. The **PRK procedure is rapid,** requiring a shorter operating time, topical medication, and less surgical preparation than RK.

6. PRK affects a **limited corneal area**—approximately 10% of the depth of the cornea—but RK affects the whole cornea area to 90% depth (entailing a risk of globe microperforation).

7. **Wound healing** is faster with PRK, and the risk of corneal rupture from trauma is smaller than for RK, even many years after surgery.

8. There is less **glare** and **diurnal fluctuation of vision** with PRK than with RK.

9. **Contact lens fitting** is easier on the PRK eye than on an RK eye.

E. There are **several reasons** for fitting contact lenses after PRK.[36]

1. **Residual ametropia** may result from hyperopia due to overcorrection, and myopia may result from miscalculation, or an aggressive wound-healing corneal response. Lenses are supplied either temporarily until a repeat PRK procedure has been performed or for longer-term use because further refractive surgery is refused or inadvisable.

2. **Anisometropia** may result from significant under- or overcorrection of PRK effects. Binocular visual coordination is severely disturbed.
3. **Irregular astigmatism** may arise for reasons related to laser characteristics or irregular healing patterns (e.g., **central island syndrome**).
4. A **decentered PRK zone** usually results from unstable fixation or patient misalignment during ablation. Visual flare and irregular astigmatism result.

Pearl: Demonstrate the expected visual result by placing a diagnostic RGP lens on the eye. This may work even if the corneal power is still changing.

5. A **feeling of dryness** is relieved by lubricating eye drops.
6. **Corneal hazing** is often more noticeable 6–8 weeks after PRK but should recede. Patients should be warned that contact lenses will not remove haze.
7. **Complications of epithelial healing** are rare, but epithelial irregularity or a persistent epithelial defect may arise, necessitating the use of a thin therapeutic soft lens.
8. **Lens fit time** for refractive correction should be **9–12 months** after PRK, allowing time for the corneal response to stabilize. After the first few aftercare visits, the follow-up should continue every 6 months for normal cases.
9. When fitting a **soft hydrophilic lens,** the practitioner should keep in mind a number of issues.
   a. A **lens diameter** of 14 mm is often chosen to provide good corneal coverage in all positions of gaze.
   b. A **thin lens** gives good comfort and satisfactory oxygen transmissibility to minimize corneal edema due to lens wear. Some patients prefer slightly thicker lenses, however, which can mask corneal astigmatism and are easier to handle. In such cases, a material with high water content is selected to maintain the good corneal oxygen supply.
   c. The **best choice of a trial lens** has a radius of curvature **1.50 D** flatter than the flattest keratometry reading.[37] The **lens fit** after 15 minutes on the eye should show good lens centration, lens movement of 0.5–1.0 mm on blink, an absence of conjunctival indentation or vessel blanching, and stable over-refraction and VA.
   d. The **original peripheral contour** is retained after PRK, so a standard-design soft lens is fitted to vault the PRK zone and bear on the corneal periphery and limbus. A wide zone with relatively deep ablation is more difficult to vault, so variable vision with the soft lens may result.

10. **Patients should be given instructions regarding lens wear.**
   a. Once the correct lens is issued, **wear time** should be gradually increased, even if lenses were worn before PRK.
   b. **Good lens hygiene and handling** methods should be practiced.
   c. Overwear can lead to **corneal edema** and should be avoided.
   d. **Extended-wear lenses** should be fitted only when medically necessary and should be correctly monitored.
   e. **Regular follow-up appointments** are important.

11. **RGP lens fitting** on the PRK patient is similar to fitting a normal patient.
   a. **RGP lens fitting** is simplified when the ablation zone has a relatively **small diameter** of about 5.0 mm and a gradual curvature change at the zone margin. With RGP lenses, there is no excess edge clearance or instability of lens movement problems encountered in post-RK eyes.[38,39] Fortunately, in PRK the corneal peripheral region does not change.
   b. **Central corneal thickness** returns to 90% of the original value by the 6-month postoperative stage, so there is reduced likelihood of excess tear pooling beneath the lens center.
   c. An **RGP lens** vaults the ablation zone and rests on the normal contour of the corneal periphery. When the zone diameter is wider or significantly decentered or irregular, obtaining satisfactory stability of lens centration and movement is more problematic.
   d. **Choose the appropriate trial fitting lens.** Fitting experience by the author was gained with patients who had PRK by excimer laser.[40]
      (1) The best-choice trial lens has a back OZ radius of curvature 0.50 D (0.10 mm) steeper than the mean keratometry reading. The overall lens diameter should be 9.2–10.0 mm, depending on the influence of the lids on the fit.[41] Often the original lens can be used with a slightly lower power and a smaller ablation zone between 5 and 6 mm.
      (2) Lens fit is assessed using fluorescein; there should be good lens centration on the cornea, adequate pupil coverage, and 1.0–2.0 mm of movement on blinking. There should be slight central tear pooling with good tear exchange beneath the lens. The midperiphery should appear to be aligned with the cornea and the green rim of tears at the lens edge should indicate a small degree of edge clearance (Figure 20.4).
   e. **Over-refraction** may require incorporating an extra –0.50 D of power in the lens ordered to cancel out the positive power effect of the central tear pool. Allow time for the patient to adapt to the

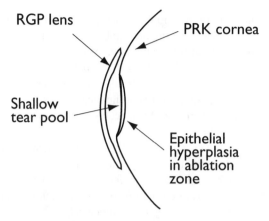

FIGURE 20.4   *Cross-section of a rigid gas-permeable (RGP) lens on a photorefractive keratectomy (PRK) cornea. There is slight central fluorescein pooling because the lens vaults the ablation zone.*

trial lens before refraction. As there should have been no lens wear since before the PRK procedure, the patient may experience increased lacrimation on RGP lens insertion. Excess lens movement would give variable VA and misleading over-refraction.

    f. **Lens design** is important in obtaining lens tolerance.

        (1) Aspheric back surface designs are preferred because they distribute the lens pressure more evenly on the cornea and glide smoothly over the PRK zone margins.[42]

        (2) Special computer-assisted designs for PRK fits are being investigated. Designs use a flat central curve to more closely follow the corneal contour and use a relatively steep peripheral curve to arch around the comparatively steeper midperipheral corneal region. Such corneal modeling cannot take into account the influence of lens movement, however. As on normal corneas, lid tension and lens thickness also affect lens fit.

    g. Choice of **lens material** should be considered.

        (1) Good oxygen transmissibility is important to avoid corneal hypoxia.

        (2) The lens should resist deposition, scratching, and breakage.

        (3) Good lens surface wettability is desired to encourage lens movement and adequate tear flow beneath the lens. As the patient is monitored at follow-up visits, wearing time and lens type may need to be altered.

  12. **Follow-up visits** should include monitoring for signs of adverse responses to lens wear.

    a. Biomicroscopic signs include conjunctival hyperemia, epithelial staining, and limbal disturbance.

    b. Corneal shape should be monitored.

    c. Corneal edema is likely with overwear. Some patients need to wear their lenses to obtain their best corrected VA and are tempted to overwear the lenses.

13. Persistent stromal haze occurs in some patients post-PRK and can take years to fade.

    a. Patients with worse VA than that obtained before PRK are very disappointed. They may be annoyed that they need to wear contact lenses to achieve adequate VA, particularly when escape from the nuisance of lens wear and care was one of the reasons they opted to undergo PRK.

    b. Careful comanagement with the ophthalmologist and counseling of such patients are important. A proportion of patients may become suitable for repeat PRK treatment at a later date.

III. In **phototherapeutic keratectomy (PTK), superficial keratectomy** is performed using the excimer laser. An **unfocused wide beam** with a circular profile is passed through an aperture. **Each laser pulse** ablates a layer of tissue only a few molecules thick, and large areas of tissue can be ablated.

A. The **original surface contour** is reproduced in the base of the ablated disc. The uneven surface must be "smoothed" by applying a liquid whose ablation properties are similar to those of the cornea. Collagen gel is an example.[43]

B. There are several **indications for PTK,** including the following:

    1. Anterior corneal conditions include dystrophies, degenerations, scars, and recurrent erosions.

    2. Irregular astigmatism in a stabilized eye may arise after trauma or surgery.

C. Exclusion criteria must be considered. Patients can be excluded for the **same conditions as for PRK,** and for significant dry eyes or severe blepharitis as well.

D. Regarding **outcome, PTK can be effective** for a variety of corneal conditions. Rapuano and Laibson treated 20 eyes and reported that 75% functionally improved and 5% deteriorated.[44]

    1. Corneal opacity treatment shows varying results.

    2. A number of **problems may occur with PTK.**

        a. Vision may not be improved, depending on the patient's original condition.

        b. Vision may become worse, and irregular astigmatism may increase.

        c. A **hyperopic shift** may occur.

       d. **Scar tissue** may resist ablation.

       e. **Infection** may be reactivated.

E. **Contact lenses** may be fit after PTK to **reduce discomfort, to optically correct induced anisometropia, or to provide ocular protection** as an epithelial defect heals.

F. A variety of **lens types** may be fitted.

    1. A **soft therapeutic lens** is fitted to promote comfort and epithelial healing.[45]

    2. After the epithelium becomes stable, an **RGP lens** is used to correct astigmatism and residual ametropia.

IV. **Automated lamellar keratectomy (ALK) and laser in situ keratomileusis (LASIK)** are other procedures sometimes used.

A. **The ALK procedure** was developed using keratomileusis technology. **Keratomileusis** involves lathing a frozen disc of corneal tissue to create a powered lens; myopic and hyperopic correction is possible, but **irregular astigmatism** can result.

    1. The ALK procedure, rather than using **corneal freezing,** uses a microkeratome to remove a cap of central corneal tissue. A thin layer is removed, and the cap is replaced.

    2. **ALK** show impressive results in cases of moderate to high degrees of myopia.

B. A **combination of ALK and PRK** technologies has been used in the **LASIK procedure.**

    1. The **"flap and zap"** method uses a microkeratome to resect a corneal cap, which is folded back on a "hinge" of tissue. PRK is performed on the bare stromal bed. The cap is returned to the original position without suturing.

    2. The **advantages of LASIK** include the following:

       a. The patient has **less pain** and discomfort. Recovery times are faster.

       b. A **higher degree of myopia** can be corrected than by PRK alone.

       c. **Bowman's layer** and epithelium are retained.

       d. **Keratocyte disturbance** and postoperative haze are minimal.

    3. In terms of **outcome, LASIK** can significantly reduce **high-degree myopia.** The amount of **astigmatism** usually does not change markedly,[46] and the **best corrected VA** is unchanged in most patients.

C. **Complications** include irregular and increased astigmatism, haze, debris, and epithelial invasion in the interface.

D. Several **contact lens requirements** should be kept in mind.

    1. A **soft therapeutic lens** assists wound healing and cap positioning.

    2. An **RGP lens** can correct irregular astigmatism.

    3. **Residual ametropia** can be corrected by daily-wear RGP or a soft lens after corneal healing is complete.

    4. **Trauma** related to lens handling should be avoided.

V. A variety of **other refractive procedures** have been used to surgically correct ametropia.[47]

A. **Keratectomy** in many patterns has been used to reduce corneal astigmatism. Predictability is unsatisfactory. Postkeratoplasty astigmatism can be carefully treated with this method.

B. **Hyperopia has been reduced** by thermokeratoplasty, excimer laser, and the holmium laser. Results are unreliable.

C. **Intrastromal implants** are still under investigation.

D. **Epikeratoplasty,** using a lathed tissue lens on top of a de-epithelialized cornea, can help in aphakia and keratoconus.

E. A **corneal stromal ring** made of rigid clear material is implanted into the stroma and adjusted to create a steepening or flattening effect on the cornea, depending on the patient's refractive error.

F. **Phakic intraocular lenses** are used in Europe to correct high refractive errors (plus or minus). This is another form of refractive surgery that is an alternative to corneal refractive surgery.

G. **Multiple procedures** may also be used in refractive surgery.

1. **PRK after RK** has improved residual myopia but can produce problems with haze in some cases.

2. **Irregular corneal topography** is likely to result after multiple refractive surgery, which may require RGP lens fitting to obtain the best VA.

3. **Diurnal variation** of refraction may be more likely after multiple refractive surgery.

REFERENCES

1. Nirankari VS, Katzen LE, Richards RD, et al. Prospective clinical study of radial keratotomy. Ophthalmology 1982;89(6):677–683.

2. Fyodorov SN, Durnev VV. Operation of dosaged dissection of corneal circular ligament in cases of myopia of mild degree. Ann Ophthalmol 1979;11:1885–1890.

3. Kraff MC, Sanders DR, Krachmer D, et al. Results of a survey of the American Society of Cataract and Refractive Surgery. J Cataract Refract Surg 1994;20(2):172–178.

4. Hoffer KJ, Darin JJ, Pettit TH, et al. UCLA clinical trial of radial keratotomy: preliminary report. Ophthalmology 1981;88:729–736.

5. Arrowsmith PN, Sanders DR, Marks RG. Visual, refractive, and keratometric results of radial keratotomy. Arch Ophthalmol 1983;101:873–888.

6. Bores LD, Myer W, Cowden J. Radial keratotomy—an analysis of the American experience. Am J Ophthalmol 1981;13:941–948.

7. Steele AD. An introductory review of refractive keratoplasty. Trans Ophthalmol Soc UK 1984;104:26–27.

8. Waring GO, Moffit SD, Gelender H, et al. Rationale for and design of National Eye Institute for Prospective Evaluation of Radial Keratotomy (PERK) study. Ophthalmology 1983;90:40–58.

9. Astin CLK. Considerations in fitting contact lenses to patients who have undergone radial keratotomy. Trans Br CL Assoc 1986;1:2–7.

10. Schanzlin DJ, Santos VR, Waring GO, et al. Diurnal change in refraction, corneal curvature, visual acuity, and intraocular pressure after radial keratotomy in the PERK study. Ophthalmology 1986;93:167–175.

11. Waring GO, Bourque L, Cartwright CS, et al. Summary of initial results of the prospective evaluation of radial keratotomy (PERK) study. Ophthalmol For 1985;3:177–185.

12. Santos VR, Waring GO, Lynn MJ, et al. Morning to evening change in refraction, corneal curvature and visual acuity 2 to 4 years after radial keratotomy in the PERK study. Ophthalmology 1988;95:1487–1493.

13. Shovlin JP. Lasso technique solves fluctuation with radial keratotomy. Rev Optom 1995;132:119.

14. DePaolis MD, Aquavella J. When is additional surgery necessary? Part 1. CL Spectrum 1995;10(2):55–56.

15. DePaolis MD, Shovlin JP, Ryan RA. The state of refractive surgery: a clinician's guide to post-op care. Rev Optom 1995;132:93–96.

16. Vickery J. Post RK and the soft lens. CL Forum 1986;11(10):34–35.

17. Astin CLK. Keratoreformation by contact lenses after radial keratotomy. Ophthalmic Physiol Opt 1991;11(2):156–162.

18. Shivitz IA, Russell BM, Arrowsmith PN, et al. Optical correction of postoperative radial keratotomy patients with contact lenses. CLAO J 1986;12:59–62.

19. DePaolis MD. The role of contact lenses in the management of the radial keratotomy patient. Optom Clin 1994;4(1):25–34.

20. Binder PS, Zavala EY, Baumgartner S, et al. Radial keratotomy and keratophakia in a non-human primate. Arch Ophthalmol 1984;102:1671–1675.

21. Janes JA, Reichie RN. Refractive surgery and contact lenses. CL Forum 1986;11(10):28–32.

22. Goldberg JB. The RK-aspheric RGP corneal lens for radial keratotomy. CL Spectrum 1993;8(3):23–24.

23. Grohe RM. A complete guide to detecting and managing limbal complications. CL Spectrum 1994;9(6):26–29.

24. Astin CLK. Contact Lenses in Abnormal Conditions—Post Radial Keratotomy. In AJ Phillips, J Stone (eds), Contact Lenses. London: Butterworth, 1989;772–782.

25. Trokel SL, Srinivasan R, Braren B. Excimer laser surgery of the cornea. Am J Ophthalmol 1983;96:710–715.

26. Marshall J, Trokel SL, Rothery S, et al. An ultrastructural study of corneal incisions induced by an excimer laser at 193 nm. Ophthalmology 1985;92:749–758.

27. Munnerlyn CR, Koons SJ, Marshall J. Photorefractive keratectomy: a technique for laser refractive surgery. J Cataract Refract Surg 1988;14:46–52.

28. Piebenga LW, Matta CS, Deitz MR, et al. Excimer photorefractive keratectomy for myopia. Ophthalmology 1993;100(9):1335–1345.

29. Seiler T, Wollensak J. Myopic photorefractive keratectomy with the excimer laser. One year follow-up. Ophthalmology 1991;98:1156–1163.

30. Gartry DS, Kerr-Muir MG, Marshall J. Photorefractive keratectomy with an argon fluoride excimer laser: a clinical study. J Refract Corneal Surg 1991;7:420–435.

31. McDonald MB, Lui JC, Byrd TJ, et al. Central photorefractive keratectomy for myopia. Ophthalmology 1991;98:1327–1337.

32. Ficker LA, Bates AK, Steele AD, et al. Excimer laser photorefractive keratectomy for myopia: 12-month follow-up. Eye 1993;7:617–624.

33. Gartry DS, Kerr-Muir MG, Marshall J. Excimer laser photorefractive keratectomy—18 month follow-up. Ophthalmology 1992;99:1209–1219.

34. Salz JJ, Maguen E, Nesburn AB, et al. A two-year experience with excimer laser photorefractive keratectomy for myopia. Ophthalmology 1993;100:873–882.

35. Gartry DS. Treating myopia with the excimer laser: the present position. BMJ 1995;310:979–985.

36. Astin CLK. Contact Lens Fitting Post-Refractive Surgery. In M Ruben, M Guillon (eds), Contact Lens Practice. London: Butterworth–Heinemann 1994;843–854.

37. Astin CLK. Considerations in contact lens fitting following photorefractive keratectomy. Practical Optom (Canada) 1995;6(3):94–96.

38. Shovlin JP. A comparison between patients wearing contact lenses following radial karatotomy and myopic photorefractive keratectomy with the excimer laser. ICLC 1992;19:141–142.

39. Astin CLK. Contact Lenses in Abnormal Conditions—Radial Keratotomy and Photorefractive Keratectomy. In AJ Phillips, L Speedwell (eds), Contact Lenses. Boston: Butterworth–Heinemann, 1996.

40. Stevens JD, Steele ADMcG, et al. Comparison of the Summit Excimed UV200 & VisX 20:20 excimer laser systems at one site. Arch Ophthalmol 1996 (in press).

41. Astin CLK. Contact lens fitting after photorefractive keratectomy—a comparison of two groups. Ophthalmol Physiol Optom 1995;15:371–374.

42. Schipper I, Businger U, Pfarrer R. Fitting contact lenses after excimer laser photorefractive keratectomy for myopia. CLAO J 1995;21(4):281–284.

43. Gartry DS, Kerr-Muir MG, Marshall J. Excimer laser superficial keratectomy: a laboratory and clinical study. Br J Ophthalmol 1991;75:258–269.

44. Rapuano CJ, Laibson PR. Excimer laser phototherapeutic keratectomy for anterior corneal pathology. CLAO J 1994;20(4):253–257.

45. McLaughlin R. Phototherapeutic laser keratectomy patients require special treatment. CL Spectrum 1995;10(3):47–48.

46. Buratto L, Ferrari M, Rama P. Excimer laser intrastromal keratomileusis. Am J Ophthalmol 1992;113:291–295.

47. Flowers CW, McDonnell. Mechanical methods in refractive corneal surgery. Curr Opin Ophthalmol 1994;5(4):81–89.

Chapter 21

Orthokeratology Concepts

Milton M. Hom

I. **Orthokeratology (OK)** is the manipulation of the fitting characteristics of a rigid lens to flatten the cornea, and decrease myopia, astigmatism, or both.[1] It is a safe and practical alternative to refractive surgery.[2,3]

    A. OK shifts an aspheric cornea to a spherical contour through the use of the mechanical pressures of a properly designed rigid lens. For a myopic eye, the apex is flattened, and the midperiphery is steepened.

    B. **Excellent quality of vision** has been reported with OK. When myopia is sufficiently reduced, uncorrected visual acuity is usually good. OK compares favorably to radial keratotomy, which not uncommonly produces poor acuity, glare, and unstable vision through spectacles.[2]

    C. That **changes may not be permanent** is one of the major criticisms of OK. When the lenses are no longer worn, the refractive changes dissipate over time.[4] Retainer lenses are necessary to preserve any reduction of myopia.[5]

II. The **effectiveness** of OK has been proven by studies. OK subjects have shown significant reduction in corneal power. **Previous rigid lens wearers** may not respond well to OK, however, because their corneas may already have adopted a more spherical form.[6]

    A. **Lack of predictability** is a disadvantage of OK. Reported findings vary greatly. Previous studies have reported average decreases of 0.75–2.0 D of myopia, although it has been suggested that a reduction of 5–6 D is possible. Corneal curvature averages between 0.03 D and 1.36 D of change. Snellen acuity increases average between 5.5 and 9 lines of acuity.[5] One study showed that there is no correlation between corneal eccentricity, subjective refraction, and autorefraction.[7]

    B. **Corneal rigidity** has been reported as an important influence on the amount of myopia reduction and how long it takes. A cornea with low rigidity can sustain more reduction for longer periods. A highly rigid cornea may not respond to any OK procedures. Ocular rigidity, however, has not been shown to be a significant factor in OK success.[8]

III. **Selection** includes patients with myopic or astigmatic refractive errors. Low myopes with an occasional need for correction are usually good candidates. Other good candidates are police officers and pilots with myopia. High myopes with realistic expectations are also good candidates.[9] Those with more than 3 D of astigmatism are not considered good candidates.[6,10] The ability to wear rigid lenses is an absolute requirement for OK.

A. **Myopia in children** can be controlled with rigid lenses. Children fitted with rigid gas-permeable (RGP) lenses experience an increase in myopia about one-third as much as myopic children who do not wear lenses.[6]

B. A **realistic endpoint** for the patient's visual acuity should be established at the outset. Given that a reduction of 2 D of myopia is reasonable, a 4-D myope cannot expect 20/15 vision without wearing lenses or glasses.

1. **Functional vision** can be presented as a realistic goal for the patient. Some experts refer to functional vision as 20/40 without wearing lenses or glasses.

   Pearl: Present vision goals to the patient as a range of values. For example, a 2-D myope has a 90% chance of reaching functional vision.[6]

2. **Keratometry readings** have been used to determine an endpoint. Corneas with definite flattening in the periphery have a **positive shape factor** and respond better to OK than spherical corneas.[2,6,10,11] The temporal (peripheral) K readings can be compared with the central K readings; flatter temporal readings indicate a positive shape factor. The temporal horizontal K can be taken while the patient fixates on the plus mire.[2] **One diopter plus twice the difference** between the temporal and central K readings has been reported to give the maximum change possible. The reliability of this guideline is questionable, however.[2,6]

C. Patients who have corneas with **moderate curvatures** are better candidates for OK than those with flat or steep corneas.[12] Patients who have very steep corneas of 46–49 Dk or flat corneas of 36–39 Dk do not respond as well.[10]

D. **Increased chair time** with many visits and lens changes is usually necessary. The patient must be available and agree to these requirements. Fees should be set appropriately higher.

   Pearl: Expect a dropout rate of 25%. Expenses, lens fit, insufficient reduction of myopia, and other problems contribute to patients' dropping out.[2,13]

IV. The **OK lens designs** commonly used today are normal RGP spherical lenses and reverse-geometry lenses. **Conventional spherical lenses** are fitted large and flat. The May-Grant method utilizes typical total diameters of 10 mm with 8.4–8.6 mm optic zone diameters (OZDs).

A. **Conventional OK** uses conventional lenses. The initial base curves used in studies have been approximately 0.12–2.50 D flatter than flat K, de-

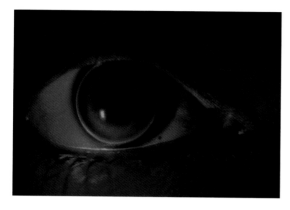

COLOR PLATE 21.1 *Orthokeratology lens fit. An orthokeratology fluorescein pattern is shown. There is apical bearing with sufficient tear exchange between the central and peripheral areas. (Courtesy of Harue J. Marsden, O.D., M.S., Southern California College of Optometry, Fullerton, California.)*

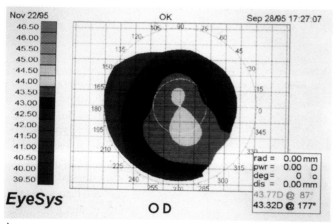

A

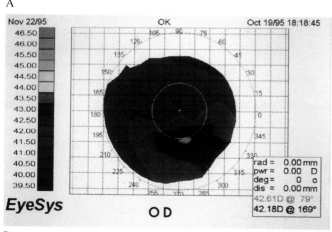

B

COLOR PLATE 21.2 *A. Cornea before orthokeratology. B. Cornea after orthokeratology. Notice the lack of steep areas. (Courtesy of Harue J. Marsden, O.D., M.S., Southern California College of Optometry, Fullerton, California.)*

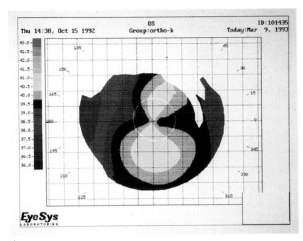

A

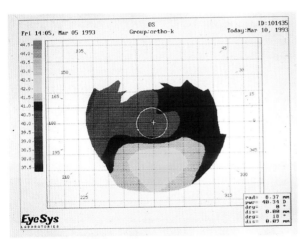

B

COLOR PLATE 21.3 *Decentered apex. A. With-the-rule cornea before orthokeratology. B. Cornea with a decentered steep area after orthokeratology. Some practitioners consider this an ideal result. (Courtesy of Harue J. Marsden, O.D., M.S., Southern California College of Optometry, Fullerton, California.)*

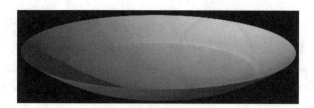

FIGURE 21.1   *A computer-rendered model of the orthokeratology lens. The lens has a reverse-geometry design with a secondary curve steeper than the base curve. The wider and steeper secondary curve results in more rapid flattening of the cornea with twice the efficiency. It is difficult to detect the steeper-than-normal secondary curve with the naked eye.*

pending on the fitting philosophy.[2] It has been suggested that 0.50 D flatter than alignment is a useful starting point.[14] A middle to high Dk with a thicker center is recommended.

    B. **Decentering of lenses** is a potential problem because of the flat-fitting relationship. Astigmatism can be induced because of the superior decentration.[2] Larger diameters, prism ballasting, and truncation may be needed.

V. **Reverse-geometry** lenses are manufactured with the secondary curve steeper than the base curve. Reverse geometry lenses are twice as efficient and take half the time of conventional lenses to correct myopia. Dr. Richard Wlodyga and Nick Stoyan of Contex (Sherman Oaks, California) devised reverse-geometry lenses, or the OK series (Figure 21.1). The steeper secondary curve enables concomitant steepening of the midperipheral cornea in a more rapid fashion. Use of these lenses is known as **accelerated OK**.[6] Other reverse-geometry lenses are the Plateau (Menicon, USA, Clovis, California) and RK/Bridge (Conforma Contact Lenses, Norfolk, Virginia).

    A. The **expected reduction** for reverse-geometry lenses is approximately 2 D of myopia and 50% of the refractive astigmatism and corneal toricity.[2]

    B. The **initial base curves** are 1.00–1.50 D flatter than flat K.[10] This amount is adjusted depending on the patient. Low amounts such as 1 D of myopia can be fit 1–2 D flatter than K. High amounts such as 6 D of myopia can be fit with 2–3 D flatter than K.[6]

    C. The **OZD** should be small (6.0–6.5 mm), with a total diameter of 9.5 mm.[14] The smaller the OZD, the greater the flattening and the better the effect. This is because smaller OZDs have smaller sag heights and a flatter fit. Although sometimes necessary, an increased OZD is not desirable because it results in a large sag height and a subsequently steeper lens.

    D. The **fluorescein pattern** should have an apical bearing of 2–3 mm and a midperipheral clearance band that is 2 mm wide under the steep secondary curve. The clearance band is surrounded first by peripheral bearing area and then by peripheral pooling under the edge. There must be a clear channel of tear exchange between the edge pool and clearance

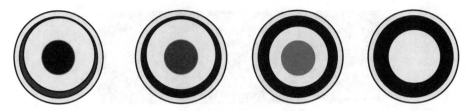

FIGURE 21.2   *The fluorescein patterns of the orthokeratology lens. From left to right, the lens steepens. On the left is the ideal fit before flattening with apical bearing. There is sufficient tear exchange between the outer ring of fluorescein and the midperipheral clearance area. To the right is a steeper lens with lighter apical bearing. The cornea has flattened. Although the midperipheral clearance area is starting to diminish, there is still sufficient tear exchange. The next image to the right shows a lens with seal-off of tear exchange. The peripheral bearing area has increased in width. The lens needs to be changed to a flatter fit. The lens on the far right is very steep and not commonly seen.*

band under the secondary curve to avoid seal-off. Movement should be 1–2 mm.[6] The **central fluorescein pattern** should appear flat. The apical bearing area lightens as the cornea flattens. When the peripheral bearing area widens to the point of blocking any tear exchange between the central area and far periphery, the lens is too steep and needs to be changed. Some sources indicate that the lens should be changed when there is no longer apical bearing and the **midperipheral clearance band** diminishes. This is rarely seen during an actual course of reverse-geometry fitting (HJ Marsden, personal communication, 1996) (Color Plate 21.1, Figure 21.2).

E.   **Power in reverse-geometry lenses** is determined with an over-refraction. Determining power in reverse-geometry lenses is similar to determining power when prescribing normal rigid lenses. The power of the tear lens depends on K readings, and the base curve should correlate to yield the proper lens power. For example, a –2.00-D myope with a base curve 1.50 D flatter than K should yield a lens power of –0.50 D.[6]

F.   **Centering** during OK is imperative to gain the best result. The flattest lens that centers well provides the maximum myopic reduction. Trial lens fitting must be done to evaluate centration.

   Pearl: A centered slightly tight lens is preferred over a noncentered slightly flat lens (N Stoyan, personal communication, 1996).

G.   **Corneal topography** shows the changes induced by OK. The ideal cornea after OK appears flat, with no steep areas. A decentered steep area sometimes results, however. Although there is functional vision, this type of topography is probably induced by a lens riding too high (Color

Plates 21.2, 21.3). The lens needs to be made larger (10.0 mm diameter) or have prism added.

H. **Lid attachment** is necessary when performing OK. Much of the pressure placed on the cornea during contact lens wear is due to the lens being pressed onto the eye by the upper lid. If the lids are loose or if there is no lid attachment, the effect will be diminished. Sometimes 10.5-mm diameters are needed.

I. **Tighter fit** and **flare** may be problems associated with reverse geometry. Smaller OZDs are the cause of these side effects. A larger OZ should be used first. If a larger OZ does not work, changing to conventional lenses may be the best option for a tight fit or flare.

VI. **Aftercare** of patients is similar to that provided for those with spherical rigid lenses. The entire program should take 3–12 months, with four to five progressively flatter lenses for each eye.[10]

A. The **wearing schedule** is a minimum of 8–10 hours to a maximum of 14–16 hours a day for the first week. The longer the wearing time, the greater the OK effect. The patient should begin with 4–5 hours the first day and increase 1–2 hours per day. A patient already wearing RGP lenses can continue the current wearing schedule.

B. **At the dispensing visit** the lenses should be examined closely for tightening within 5 hours of wear. Sometimes the lenses need changing hours after being dispensed. An improvement in vision without lenses can also be demonstrated to the patient. The patient should return in 1–2 days.

Pearl: For high myopes, demonstrating vision improvement may be difficult with a 20/400 E. Showing the change in the patient's farpoint more effectively demonstrates vision improvement.[6]

C. **Follow-up appointments** should be scheduled at the end of the day, when the most tightening is apparent. Look at the patient's eyes under white light before instilling fluorescein. Addition of fluorescein may disguise a nonmoving lens by lubricating the eye. **OK-2,** which has a less steep 2-D secondary curve, should be used if frequent follow-up is not possible. The risk of lens tightening is reduced compared with a 3- to 5-D steep secondary curve lens. The changes will not be as rapid with an OK-2.

Pearl: An OK-2 is 0.5 mm steeper than an OK-3. Thus, if an OK-3 is 1.5 mm flatter than K, the equivalent OK-2 lens would be 1.0 mm flatter than K (N Stoyan, personal communication, 1996).

D. **Multiple pairs** may be ordered in advance, each lens ordered being 0.50–1.00 mm flatter than the prior lens. Experts recommend ordering two to four pairs of lenses initially. Each pair is commonly worn for 1–3 weeks.[10]

> ***Pearl:*** *In determining the number of lenses needed during the course of OK, a useful guideline is to order one pair of lenses per diopter of OK.*[6]

E. **Rapid changes** slow down after the first 2 weeks of OK. As the changes slow, the visits can be less frequent. When the cornea stops changing, the maximum change has probably occurred, and going flatter will not induce more change. This is a proper time to prescribe retainer lenses. A low plus refraction of +0.50 D is an ideal endpoint, if it is possible. Most improvement occurs in 2–3 months.[2,4,6]

> ***Pearl:*** *Often, the faster the changes, the faster the regression.*[6]

F. **Night therapy** offers several benefits: little adaptation, more rapid changes, and elimination of environmental irritants. Using lubricating drops and wearing lenses for 1 more hour after awakening helps to restore tear film quality. Lenses should otherwise not be worn during the day. The fewer hours the lenses are worn, the less the risk of corneal compromise.
   1. The **follow-up schedule** includes a 1-day morning visit after the first night of wear. The second lens should be ready to dispense immediately in the event that the lens tightens. If there are no changes after 2 weeks, night therapy should be discontinued.
   2. **Lens adherence** is a potential problem. A newer **OK-A** (Contex) lens is designed to fit looser and reduce adherence. The secondary zone is aspheric.

VII. **Retainer lenses** are worn to maintain the OK effect. For conventional lenses, the retainer is 0.50 D flatter than central K. For reverse-geometry lenses, the last lens worn can be used if it fits properly.
   A. The **fluorescein pattern** of a reverse-geometry retainer lens should indicate minimal central touch.[2]
   B. The **wearing time** of the retainer lenses should be the amount of normal daily wear time minus 3–4 hours. After each reduction, patients can check their vision acuity at home. The time it takes to first show a reduction in acuity should be noted. Retainers should then be worn the minimal amount of time required to maintain the patient's visual goals. Some patients prefer to wear lenses a few hours in the morning and in the evening.
   C. **Overnight retainers** can be worn using high-Dk materials. This additional wearing time can enhance the effect of OK. Additional changes may result in overcorrection, however. Care is similar to that for rigid extended-wear procedures (see Chapter 14). The overnight schedule can be reduced to fewer nights when functional vision is reached during the day. The goal for overnight retainers is the shortest schedule possible.[6] For overnight wear, the highest Dk possible should be fit.[6]
   D. **Follow-up appointments** should be scheduled for every 3–6 months during the use of retainer lenses.

Pearl: *Use several different visual acuity charts to prevent patients from memorizing them.*[9]

VIII. **Troubleshooting OK** may require refitting the patient with another lens.
   A. **With-the-rule astigmatism** may increase during OK. It commonly occurs because the horizontal meridian flattens faster than the vertical meridian. With-the-rule astigmatism can be eliminated with a larger OZD or larger total diameter. It can be induced with superior decentration. The resultant corneal configuration is sometimes known as "rigid-lens-induced keratoconus." Proper centration usually reduces the astigmatism (HJ Marsden, personal communication, 1996).
      1. **Decreased OZD** can help center the lens. Normally, steepening the lens centers a high-riding lens. For a reverse-geometry lens, increasing the width of the secondary curve steepens the lens. This is accomplished by decreasing the OZD.
      2. **Addition of base-down prism** can center a high-riding lens. A common amount is 1.5 prism diopters down, with a secondary curve set at 4 D steeper than the base curve. There may be problems, however, with the increased thickness and visual distortion induced by lens rocking.
   B. **Ghosting and flare** usually accompany decentered lenses. If the lens is already centered, increasing the OZD may be helpful. For the OK series, the OZD can be increased from 6.0 mm to 6.5–7.0 mm. If the lens rides too high, decreasing the OZD or adding prism may work.
   C. **Fluorescein staining** is sometimes apparent with OK patients, usually because the lens is too tight or too dirty. Because of the corneal flattening, lenses can rapidly become too tight. The base curve can be flattened or the diameter reduced. It may be necessary to review or modify cleaning and care procedures with patients with dirty lenses. Patients must be told to keep the lenses clean to avoid tightening[6] (see Chapter 9).
IX. **Corneal topography** is an essential tool when performing OK. Expected changes can be calculated based on **eccentricity values** measured by topography (CD-ROM: OK Topography Gallery: Prefit considerations). Troubleshooting fits are also possible with topography. **Flat and decentered** lenses, **tight fits**, and lenses with too **steep secondary curves** can be detected with maps alone (CD-ROM: OK Topography Gallery).
X. **Fluorescein patterns** differ between **conventional lenses** and **reverse geometry lenses**. A diagnostic lens fitting of both lens types are shown on the CD-ROM. Sometimes, increasing the diameter of reverse geometry lenses improves **centration**, a key factor in OK (CD-ROM: OK: Conventional tricurve lenses; OK: Reverse geometry lenses).

REFERENCES

1. Lakin D, Estes S, Carter W. Reshaping your ideas. CL Spectrum 1995;10(4):25–30.
2. Soni PS, Horner DG. Orthokeratology. In ES Bennett, BA Weissman (eds), Clinical Contact Lens Practice. Philadelphia: Lippincott, 1993(49);1–7.
3. Polse KA, Brand RJ, Keener RJ, et al. The Berkeley orthokeratology study. Part III: safety. Am J Optom Physio Optics 1983;60(4):321–328.
4. Brand RJ, Polse KA, Schwalbe JS, et al. The Berkeley orthokeratology study. Part II: efficacy and duration. Am J Optom Physio Optics 1983;60(3):187–198.
5. Carney L. Orthokeratology. In M Guillon, CM Ruben (eds), Contact Lens Practice. London: Chapman & Hall, 1994;877–888.
6. Winkler TD, Kame RT. Orthokeratology Handbook. Boston: Butterworth–Heinemann, 1995.
7. Marsden HJ, Joe JJ, Edrington TB. The relationship between corneal eccentricity and improvement in visual acuity orthokeratology. Optom Vis Sci 1993;70:139.
8. Carkeet NL, Mountford JA, Carney LG. Predicting success with orthokeratology lens wear: a retrospective analysis of ocular characteristics. Optom Vis Sci 1995;72(12):892–898.
9. Marsden HJ. Common sense orthokeratology. CL Spectrum 1995;10(10):24–32.
10. Harris DH, Stoyan N. A new approach to orthokeratology. CL Spectrum 1992;7(4):37–39.
11. Kerns RL. Research in orthokeratology. Part VIII: results, conclusions and discussion of techniques. J Am Optom Assoc 1978;49(3):308–313.
12. Wlodyga RJ, Bryla C. Corneal molding: the easy way. CL Spectrum 1989;4(8):58–65.
13. Horner DG, Richardson LE. Reduction of myopia with contact lenses. Practical Optom 1992;3(2):64–68.
14. Marsden HJ. Orthokeratology. In CA Schwartz (ed), Specialty Contact Lenses: A Fitter's Guide. Philadelphia: Saunders, 1996;176–183.

PART VI

CD-ROM Chapters

Chapter 22

Rigid Gas-Permeable Fluorescein Patterns

Milton M. Hom, Adrian S. Bruce, and Ronald Watanabe

I. **Fluorescein pattern concepts** are important for visualization of the tear film underneath a rigid lens. Interpretation of **fluorescein patterns** still remains the best clinical way to determine the relationship between a rigid contact lens and the cornea. However, mastering the skill is sometimes difficult because of the many factors affecting the appearance of the pattern.

   A. **Components** that make up the fluorescein pattern (cornea, contact lens, and tear film) are clear, transparent surfaces. Fluorescein is instilled to color the invisible tear layer. The **fluorescence** or **"glow"** properties of fluorescein are used to see what cannot be seen.

   B. **Fluorescein concentration** has a major influence on the appearance of the pattern. The **thickness of the tears** determines the intensity of the fluorescence. The thicker the tear film, the greater the fluorescence.

   1. **Concentration animation** shows the changes of a simulated pattern on a with-the-rule cornea. The animation is based on Young's work.[1] Concentration makes a detectable difference in the pattern appearance. For **higher concentrations**, the **minimum tear layer thickness (TLT)** at which fluorescein becomes visible is **0.012 mm**. For **lower concentrations**, the TLT for fluorescence is **0.028 mm**. **Average concentrations** of fluorescein will fluoresce at TLT of **0.020 mm**.

   2. **Pattern appearance** is simulated at higher, average, and lower concentrations (CD-ROM: Figure 1 RGP fluorescein patterns: Concepts: Concentration simulation: 3 of 7). High concentration fluorescein patterns are shown when the slider is on the left. As the slider is pushed to the right, the concentration of fluorescein is lowered.

   3. **First instilled** fluorescein shows deceptively steeper patterns. This is when the fluorescein is at the highest concentration.

   a. **Having a patient blink** several times and/or **blow his or her nose** can hasten the settling process.

    b. **At lower concentrations**, the pattern looks **flatter** than at normal concentrations. A pattern may have this appearance when the fluorescein runs out.

C. **Static** and **dynamic patterns** are the two types of patterns. **Static patterns** appear when the lens is **centered** on the cornea. When the lens **moves freely** on the eye, the pattern becomes **dynamic**. At any given time, the lens may not be centered on the cornea. To insure a view of the static pattern, the lower lid can be used to position and hold the lens into a centered position. A dynamic pattern often appears very different than a static pattern. The areas of touch and clearance **change in size and location** as the contact lens moves over the cornea. This can be a source of confusion when reading fluorescein patterns.

D. **Bearing** and **clearance** are terms used to describe the different areas of the pattern. Fluorescein enables a **frontal view** of the **cornea-lens relationship** that can be interpreted as a cross-section. Where there are areas of **clearance (vaulting)**, the fluorescein pools under the lens. Where there are areas of **bearing (touch)**, a dark area appears.

    1. **Clearance areas** become increasingly brighter to a certain thickness. After that point, the greater clearance areas do not appear any brighter. This leads to the fact that amounts of **steepness (clearance)** are difficult to quantify.

    2. **Areas of darkness** are not always areas of touch. A dark area within the optic zone indicates a tear layer that has fallen below the **threshold** for fluorescence. Dark areas do not necessarily signify that pressure is applied to the cornea. The area can have a **very thin tear layer**, or an **alignment** relationship.

E. **Pattern reading** should be quantified as **central, mid-peripheral,** and **peripheral**. The central area within the optic zone diameter is considered the **central pattern**. The outer area of the OZ is the **mid-peripheral pattern**. The area under the peripheral curve system is the **peripheral pattern**.

    1. **Movement** and **centering** should also be noted because the pattern is dynamic. Little to no movement usually indicates a steep lens. Excessive movement can indicate a flat lens.

    2. **Two phases** can describe lens movement. The lens is first pulled up by the upper lid in the **rapid phase**. The lens drops back into position in the second **slower phase**. The two phases usually repeat in a cyclical manner with regard to blinking. The positioning of the lens will also vary for different phases in the movement cycle. Attention should be paid to the movement and positioning upon blink and after (post) blink. Too much movement can result in unstable vision.

    3. **Decentered** resting position is a key factor affecting flare and glare. Patients with decentered lenses can experience flare and glare especially at night.

4. A pattern can be read as a **bull's-eye**, noting **centration** and **movement**. For example: central bearing, mid-peripheral clearance, and excessive edge lift; low centration with excessive movement. Specifying these **five factors** will accurately describe a fluorescein pattern.

F. **Eccentricity** plays a large role in pattern appearance. A high shape factor or low eccentricity means there are low amounts of flattening out toward the periphery. Low shape factors or high eccentricity indicates a large amount of corneal flattening toward the periphery. The **animation** (CD-ROM Figure 2 RGP fluorescein patterns: Concepts: Eccentricity simulation: 7 of 7) shows the pattern on a with-the-rule cornea and how it changes with eccentricity. A cornea with high eccentricity **(low shape factor)** is shown when the slider is to the left. A low eccentricity **(high shape factor)** cornea is shown when the slider is on the right. The patterns are variations of with-the-rule alignment and are commonly seen.

G. Sometimes the lens will appear steeper and not aligned when the initial lens is placed on the eye. A **small apex** or the **high corneal eccentricity** will have a steep appearance when fitted on K. Pushing the slider to the right creates this appearance. The fit needs to be adjusted to a flatter lens or a smaller OZ.

II. **Spherical fluorescein patterns.** What is the **optimal** fit? Most practitioners consider alignment to be the goal of RGP fitting. **Alignment** is described as the base curvature that most closely parallels the cornea. There is an evenly thin tear film under the lens. A cross-sectional view reveals the lens and cornea are parallel to each other throughout the entire OZ. There is clearance or edge lift along the periphery.

A. **Alignment patterns** are described in two generally different ways.

1. **Total darkness** throughout the optic zone is one description. Almost an absence of fluorescein under the lens accounts for the large dark area. The area does not fluoresce because the tear layer is very thin. Darkness throughout the OZ is shown in the video (CD-ROM Figure 3 RGP fluorescein patterns: Spherical patterns: Spherical aligned: 2 of 4). There is clearance in the lower mid-peripheral area. The lens is attached to the upper lid and rides in a higher, although acceptable, position.

2. An **even, uniform, light green appearance** of fluorescein over the entire optic zone is another description of **alignment**. Sometimes this appearance is referred to as characteristic **"glow"** under the lens.

3. **Alignment patterns** do not necessarily have total darkness throughout the entire optic zone as shown previously. In some corneas, there are **areas of fluorescence** or **"glow"** within the optic zone for an alignment fit. The fluorescence indicates a tear layer just thicker than the minimum TLT. One rule of thumb is to fit for a **maximum** dark area, rather than total darkness. In the video, the "glow" appears in the lower peripheral area (CD-ROM Figure 4

RGP fluorescein patterns: Spherical patterns: Spherical aligned: 3 of 4). A **with-the-rule cornea** will also contribute to this appearance. The lens centers and moves well with a small amount of lid attachment. Concomitant with an alignment relationship is usually, but not always, good centration and movement.

4. Which is the proper way to describe the **optimal fit**? Darkness or "glow" are both accurate descriptions, depending on the individual eye. **Corneal topography** determines the appearance of the pattern. Unfortunately, alignment does not appear exactly the same from cornea to cornea. Some eyes may have total darkness in the optic zone, while others may display the characteristic glow or small areas of fluorescence. The corneal topography between individuals will vary with the amount of **flattening**, **size**, and **location of apex**. All of these factors will alter the pattern.

Pearl: Amount of flattening, size, and location of the apex alters the appearance of the pattern.

5. **Accuracy** with fluorescein patterns was described in one study[2] as being difficult to achieve. Considering the duplicity in defining an optimal pattern, it is not surprising that such a conclusion was reached. For the most part, patterns are most easily interpreted when static or centered on the cornea.

Pearl: Remember that the appearance of alignment can be different from patient to patient.

B. **Flat** fluorescein patterns usually show touch or bearing on the central area surrounded by clearance. A cross-sectional view reveals central bearing and peripheral vaulting. The tear layer is thicker at the periphery and thins centrally. As opposed to an alignment pattern, the darkness usually indicates **pressure on the cornea**. Smaller dark areas can mean greater degrees of flatness and pressure. By reading the dark areas, **quantifying the amount of flatness** is possible. The smaller the central dark area, the flatter the fit. Peripheral clearance increases with a flatter fit.

   Flat lenses characteristically show large amounts of **movement** and **decentration**. A flat lens is more easily decentered or dislodged with blink. Yawning, laughter, and even a back slap have been known to cause lens loss. **Blinking** brings on much of the lens movement. For lenses that are not lid attached, the lens is pulled up on blink and dropped back into position after the blink. Sometimes, **air bubbles** will appear in the periphery. In the video, the flat lens is pulled up by the upper lid and momentarily attached to the lid (CD-ROM Figure 5 RGP fluorescein patterns: Spherical patterns: Spherical flat: 2 of 2). The lens drops inferiorly after the blink with excessive movement. There is central bearing, mid-peripheral clearance, and edge clearance.

C. **Steep** lenses have a central area of **clearance** in the pattern. Clearance is surrounded by a dark area of touch in the mid-periphery. A cross-section shows clearance in the central area surrounded by touch.

   1. **Lack of lens movement** is a telltale sign of a steep-fitting lens. Steep lenses are noted for initial comfort and can later develop into hazy vision and discomfort at the end of the day. Negative pressure can also build up under a very steep lens and have detrimental effects on the cornea.

   2. **Steep lenses** are usually **well centered**. A steep fluorescein pattern with adequate edge lift is shown on the CD-ROM (CD-ROM Figure 6 RGP fluorescein patterns: Spherical patterns: Spherical steep: 2 of 3). The lens is pushed downward by the upper lid, especially upon blink. There is central clearance, mid-peripheral bearing, and adequate edge clearance.

   3. **Minimal edge clearance** is often displayed with steep lenses. Bright and wide areas indicate a flat peripheral system. Dark and narrow peripheral bands indicate an insufficiently steep peripheral system. In this video, the edge lift is largely inadequate (CD-ROM Figure 7 RGP fluorescein patterns: Spherical patterns: Spherical steep: 3 of 3). The temporal edge shows minimal clearance, while the nasal edge displays virtually no clearance. There is a small central area of clearance, large band of mid-peripheral bearing, and poor edge clearance.

III. **Toric fluorescein patterns** have a distinct appearance. The **steep** and **flat corneal meridians** create two different corneal-to-lens relationships. When combined into one pattern, an alignment fit appears as a **"dumbbell,"** **"doggy-bone,"** or an **"H" type**.

   The lens is aligned with the flatter meridian. The shape of the alignment area usually represents the flattest area of the cornea. **Alignment** is normally obtained with a base curve between the steep and flat meridians. The amount of steepness over the flat K can be anywhere between **one-third to three-quarters the amount of toricity**.

   A. **With-the-rule (WTR) cornea** fitted with an **alignment** lens is shown in the video (CD-ROM Figure 8 RGP fluorescein patterns: WTR toric patterns: WTR aligned: 1 of 2). At the beginning of the video, the lens appears as a clearance fit. When fluorescein is first instilled, the concentration is **high**. The tears need to run out from beneath the lens and lower the concentration before revealing the actual pattern. It may typically take a minute for the lens and tears to settle. In the video, the pattern emerges over time. The lens is also being manipulated with the lids to center on the cornea. This results in an easier to read **static** rather than a more difficult to read **dynamic pattern**.

The lens has **mid-peripheral bearing** along the **horizontal meridian** and **mid-peripheral clearance** along the **vertical meridian**. There is adequate edge lift along the horizontal meridian and excessive edge clearance along the vertical meridian.

The left **"dumbbell"** area is partially obscured with a small area of fluorescein on the front surface. Mucus adheres to the lens quite often. Centering is excellent.

Pearl: Many times, an alignment relationship is the first step in achieving good centration.

B. **Flat WTR fluorescein pattern** is like a flat spherical pattern. It differs only in the shape of the **bearing area**. With a spherical pattern, the bearing area is round. With a WTR pattern, the central bearing area is oval in shape. Since the flatter meridian coincides with the longer axis of the oval, a WTR flat pattern looks like a horizontal band or oval (depending on the **eccentricity**).

1. **WTR flat lens** shown resides between the flat, horizontal meridian and the inferior periphery of the cornea (CD-ROM Figure 9 RGP fluorescein patterns: WTR toric patterns: WTR flat: 2 of 3). An inferiorly positioning lens will show some clearance as it bridges the intermediate zone between the central and lower cornea. Because the clearance area is in the center of the lens, it can be mistaken for apical clearance. The key is recognizing the lower positioning of the lens.

2. **Little to no movement with inferior positioning** sometimes characterizes a flat lens. Normally, poor movement indicates a steep lens. An exception to this is when there is poor movement while riding low. In the video, there is mid-peripheral bearing along the horizontal axis and mid-peripheral clearance along the vertical axis (CD-ROM Figure 9 RGP fluorescein patterns: WTR toric patterns: WTR flat: 2 of 3). There appears to be adequate edge clearance. Centering the lens manually will make the pattern easier to interpret.

3. **Movement** over a with-the-rule cornea (WTR) occurs along the vertical meridian. It is sometimes referred to as **"up and down" movement**. A gap is formed between the lens and cornea at the superior and inferior periphery of the vertical meridian. In the previous video (CD-ROM Figure 9 RGP fluorescein patterns: WTR toric patterns: WTR flat: 2 of 3), the gap appears as the mid-peripheral clearance area along the vertical meridian. As the lens moves along this gap, the lens has a tendency to move up and down. Sometimes, this freedom of movement results in a high or low positioning lens.

4. **Lens movement** may result in the **lens rocking** back and forth on the horizontal axis. The horizontal or flatter meridian can act as a

fulcrum where the lens can teeter or rock. The force of the upper lid can pull the lens up and against the eye, lifting the lower edge of the lens away from the cornea. Rocking motion is more likely seen in **higher toricities**.

C. **Steep WTR fluorescein pattern** appears just like a spherical steep lens in the central area. The entire optic zone will have clearance except for two contact areas in peripheral areas. The two bearing areas are at the 3 and 9 o'clock areas.

    1. **Steep WTR lens** is shown (CD-ROM Figure 10 RGP fluorescein patterns: WTR toric patterns: WTR steep: 2 of 2). Note the low positioning of the lens. This is typical of a WTR lens. There is central clearance, mid-peripheral bearing along the horizontal axis, and mid-peripheral clearance along the vertical axis. There is poor edge clearance with a small amount of movement.

D. **Against-the-rule (ATR) cornea pattern** is characterized by a **vertical band** or **dumbbell.** The pattern resembles a WTR pattern that has been rotated 90 degrees. **Centration** is sometimes difficult to achieve. The lens tends to shift either nasally or temporally on the cornea and lag on horizontal eye movements. A lid-attached larger lens may be needed to keep the lens centered on the eye. Sometimes aspheric lenses are useful. A dark vertical oval is the typical bearing area of a flat lens. A steep lens will show two bearing areas at the 12 and 6 o'clock positions.

REFERENCES

1. Young G. Simulation of fluorescein pattern using a spreadsheet program. ICLC 1996;23:165–171.
2. Bronstein L. The accuracy of fluorescein for determining corneal curvature. Contacto 1959(June):170–171.

Chapter 23

Rigid Gas-Permeable Lens Fitting and Eyelid Geometry

Adrian S. Bruce

I. The hallmarks of a good RGP lens fit are lens-cornea alignment, good centration and comfort. A well-centered lens is important from both an optical and a comfort point of view, as well as to minimize corneal distortion.

II. **RGP Lens centration—patient factors overview**

    A. While the optimal fluorescein pattern may be achieved by considering RGP lens base curves in relation to the keratometry readings, the lens centration is assisted by a number of important patient factors[1]:

        1. **Upper and lower lid positions** (stabilizes lens, reduces sensation)

        2. **Tighter lid tension** (gauge by difficulty of eversion). An example is the Asian eye.

        3. **WTR astigmatism** better than **ATR** (lens doesn't decenter laterally)

        4. **Steeper cornea >45D** (more posterior center of gravity)

        5. **Minus Rx** (more posterior center of gravity)

        6. **Lower Rx** (less lens weight)

        7. **Avoid front surface torics** (similar corneal and refractive astigmatism)

    B. Of these factors, this section will concentrate on the effects of lid position and lens diameter on optimal lens **centration** and **comfort**.

III. **Fitting philosophies—"the lids" or "the cornea"?**

    A. **Diameter and BOZR** can be varied together in a "fitting philosophy." Varying the edge design and in some cases putting on a minus carrier can assist too. The two common fitting philosophies are **"interpalpebral fitting"** and **"lid attachment."**

        1. **Interpalpebral: "fitting the cornea"**

        Small diameter (e.g., 8.2–8.8 mm) well centered with apical clearance (⅓ steeper than flat K, or 0.3 mm). For interpalpebral fit lens diameter = vertical lid aperture less 0.20 mm. Good for steeper corneas, minus Rx, high upper lid.

2. **Lid attachment: "fitting the lids"**
Lens larger diameter (e.g., 8.8–9.6 mm or larger) and flatter (0.25 mm flatter than flat K); possibly lenticular. Thinner edge, more edge lift for more superior movement. Lid attachment is good for lower positioned tighter lid, flatter corneas, and minus Rx or carrier.

3. **Alignment:** moderate lens diameter (e.g., 8.6–9.2 mm), lens aligned with flat K. This philosophy could be considered to be a combination of interpalpebral and lid attachment. The choice of which fitting philosophy to use is based on lid geometry.

IV. **Lid interactions and lens comfort**
A. If either the upper or lower lid hits the lens edge during a blink, then lens comfort will be reduced. This is particularly during the initial adaptation period of 1–2 weeks.

Pearl: Avoid lens edge proximity to lid margin for best comfort.

Try to have the lid either 1 mm or so away from the lens edge, or have the lid overlap the lens edge by a similar amount.

B. **Good comfort** is affected by the lens to lid relationships.
1. **Upper lid** that overlaps the lens and does not hit the edge with each blink is usually comfortable.
2. An area of **clearance** or a **gap** between the lower lid and lens edge also is a good sign to look for with a comfortable lens.

C. **Poor comfort** is also affected by the lens to lid relationships.
1. **Upper lid** that does not overlap the lens and hits the edge with each blink is usually not comfortable.
2. **Lower lid and lens edge** bumping up against each other as the lens drops can indicate an uncomfortable lens.

D. **Good comfort case**
This case shows a first time wearer who experienced good comfort soon after the delivery visit (CD-ROM Figure 45 RGP eyelid geometry: Comfort: 4 of 6).
1. **Lens Parameters**
   BOZR   7.4/8.0 mm
   TD   10.0 mm
   BVP   –4.50/–1.00
   OZ   8.0 mm
   Edge   +0.8 (.6)
            +1.5 (.4)
   Bitoric Tricurve design in Boston ES made by Australian Contact Lenses (Melbourne).
2. **History** is a 16-year-old female wearing lenses for the first time. Comfort was good after the first few days and patient was happy with lenses. Spectacle RX was –0.75/–4.50 × 180.

3. **Fit assessment is** shown in white light to emphasize the lid geometry rather than the fitting pattern (CD-ROM Figure 45 RGP eyelid geometry: Comfort: 4 of 6). Fluorescein pattern was near alignment with good edge lift. Strong lid attachment and the inferior edge did not impact the lower lid.

4. Compare the **normal speed movie** (CD-ROM Figure 46 RGP eyelid geometry: Comfort: 5 of 6), with the **slow-motion version** (CD-ROM Figure 47 RGP eyelid geometry: Comfort: 6 of 6). In the latter, the lid interaction is more clearly seen.

   a. **Normal speed movie** shows the fit looks good and there appears to be minimal interaction with the lower lid.

   b. **Slow-motion movie** shows the interaction with the lower lid is clearly visible.

V. In **assessing lid geometry** both the upper and lower lid positions can be simply evaluated in relation to the adjacent corneal limbus when the eye is in primary gaze.

   A. **Superior lid** covers the limbus slightly (about 1 mm); the positioning would be considered normal or low. If the superior lid is at the upper limbus or above it, it would be "high."

   B. **Inferior lid** assessment is the converse. If the lid margin is adjacent to or below the limbus it would probably be considered normal or low. If the limbus is significantly covered by the inferior lid, then the lid position is high.

   C. **Eyelid geometry** can be thought of in four possible combinations: narrow, ideal, unusual, and wide aperture.

VI. **Lid geometry—choice of lens diameter** is to fit a larger diameter (9.2 mm or larger). Upper lid interaction should be obtained where there is a low or normally positioned upper lid. If the lower lid is also in the normal or lower position, the largest diameter lens is possible in terms of both comfort and centration.

   A. If the **superior lid is high**, then a lid attachment form of fitting may not be possible and an **interpalpebral fitting** will more likely be successful. In this instance a smaller lens diameter may be necessary (< 9.2 mm).

   B. **Diameter** should be greater than 9 mm for **lid attachment**. Diameter should be less than 9.0 mm for **intrapalpebral fit**. Phillips likes to choose 8.70, 9.20, 9.80 diameters.[2]

   C. **Narrow aperture case 1** is characterized by a low upper lid and high lower lid (CD-ROM Figure 48 RGP eyelid geometry: Geometry and diameter: Narrow aperture: 1 of 2).

      1. **Lens Parameters**
         BOZR   7.80 mm
         TD   8.8 mm
         BVP   +7.50 D

OZ   7.2 mm
Edge   +0.7 (.55)
          +1.0 (.25)

Tricurve design in Fluorex 700 made by Australian Contact Lenses (Melbourne).

2. **History** is a first-time wearer with good comfort.
3. **Fit assessment** shows a fluorescein pattern (when lens is centered) with alignment and adequate edge lift. Centration is slight inferior positioning.

D. **Narrow aperture case 2** is characterized by a low upper lid and high lower lid (CD-ROM Figure 49 RGP eyelid geometry: Geometry and diameter: Narrow aperture: 2 of 2).

1. **Lens Parameters**
    BOZR   7.85 mm
    TD   9.0 mm
    BVP   −9.00 D
    OZ   7.0 mm
    Edge   +0.7 (.55)
             +1.3 (.45)

    Tricurve design in Fluorex 700 made by Australian Contact Lenses (Melbourne).

2. **History** is a previous soft contact lens wear. The rigid lens is felt impacting lower lid after blinks.
3. **Fit assessment** shows a fluorescein pattern (when lens is centered) that is aligned to slightly steep with adequate edge lift. Centration changes as the lens tends to drop after a blink. There is a tight Asian upper lid causing inferior decentration of lens resulting in poor lid attachment.

E. **Ideal aperture** is characterized by a low upper lid and low lower lid (CD-ROM Figure 50 RGP eyelid geometry: Geometry and diameter: Ideal aperture: 1 of 1).

1. **Lens Parameters**
    BOZR   8.0 mm
    TD   10.0 mm
    BVP   −3.25 D
    OZ   8.0 mm
    Edge   +0.8 (.6)
             +1.0 (.4)

    Tricurve design in Boston ES made by Nu-Contacts (Adelaide).

2. **History** is a prior lens wearer 26 years old with good comfort.
3. **Fit assessment** shows fluorescein pattern (when lens is centered) that is aligned to slightly flat with adequate edge lift. Centration has a slight inferior positioning. There is strong lid attachment.

F. **Unusual aperture** is characterized by high upper lid and high lower lid (CD-ROM Figure 51 RGP eyelid geometry: Geometry and diameter: Unusual aperture: 1 of 1).

      1. Lens Parameters

        BOZR   7.85 mm

        TD   9.6 mm

        BVP   0.00 D

        OZ   7.4 mm

        Edge   VContour

        PMMA trial lens

      2. History is a first-time wearer with fair comfort.

      3. Fit assessment shows a fluorescein pattern (when lens is centered) as apical clearance with adequate edge lift. Centration is slight inferior positioning.

  G. **Wide aperture** is characterized by high upper lid and low lower lid (CD-ROM Figure 52 RGP eyelid geometry: Geometry and diameter: Wide aperture: 1 of 1).

      1. Lens Parameters

        BOZR   7.65 mm

        TD   9.5 mm

        BVP   −12.25 D

        OZ   7.8 mm

        Edge   +0.7 (.55)

               +1.0 (.30)

      Tricurve design in Equalens II material made by Gelflex Contact Lenses (Perth).

      2. History is a full-time RGP wearer since 1994 and SCL wearer for 15 years previously. Comfort is adequate.

      3. Fit assessment shows a fluorescein pattern (when lens is centered) as apical clearance and mid-peripheral bearing with poor edge lift. Centration is good.

VII. Troubleshooting

  A. **Vary lens diameter** to improve centration.

      1. Use **larger** lenses for lid attachment.

      2. **Flatten base curve** in association with larger diameter.

      3. Use **lenticular** lenses.

      4. Use smaller lenses for narrow lid aperture and to reduce weight if lid attachment is not possible.

  B. **Possible complication** of inferior lens centration is **dessication staining.**

  C. **Possible complication** of superior lens centration is **corneal distortion.**

REFERENCES

1. Bennett ES. Lens design, fitting and troubleshooting. In ES Bennett, RM Grohe (eds). Rigid Gas-Permeable Contact Lenses. New York: Professional Press, 1986;189–220.

2. Phillips AJ. Rigid gas-permeable corneal lens fitting. In AJ Phillips, L Speedwell (eds). Contact Lenses, Fourth Edition. London: Butterworth–Heinemann, 1997;313–357.

Chapter 24

Orthokeratology

Harue J. Marsden

I. **Techniques for orthokeratology (OK)** have existed in some form for several years: from the ancient Chinese with sandbags and palming techniques to the programmed replacement of contact lenses to modify the shape of the cornea. The use of rigid lenses demonstrates notable success in the reduction of myopia and newer lens designs have accelerated the myopia reduction rate. Research has demonstrated that myopia can be reduced by between 2.00 and 3.00 diopters.[1,2] Newer methods report even higher amounts of myopic reduction using advanced OK techniques.[3] Irrespective of the OK technique, rigid lenses can be used to alter corneal topography.

II. **Important steps** to follow:
   A. **Patient selection and education**
      1. Clarify patient motivation.
      2. Frequent visits may be necessary.
         a. Patient must understand financial commitment (no guarantees/no refunds).
         b. Patient must make time commitment for follow-up visits.
   B. **Preliminary testing**
      1. Thorough case history to determine if any contraindications to rigid lens wear or OK exists
      2. Baseline testing
         a. Unaided visual acuity
         b. Corneal curvature measurements
            1. Keratometry
            2. Corneal topography
         c. Objective and subjective refraction
         d. Slit-lamp evaluation
   C. **Diagnostic contact lens fitting**
      1. Lens selection
         a. Conventional lens design
         b. Reverse geometry lenses for accelerated OK
      2. Over-refraction for power determination
      3. Fluorescein pattern assessment for fit (base curve) determination

405

    D.　Contact lens order
- **1.** Conventional tri-curve lens design
- **2.** Reverse geometry lens design

    E.　Dispensing day
- **1.** Lens dispense
  - **a.** Aided visual acuity
  - **b.** Over-refraction
  - **c.** Fit assessment
- **2.** Wear schedule

    F.　Follow-up visit
- **1.** Conventional lens design; one week
- **2.** Reverse geometry lens design; 2–5 days
- **3.** Follow-up testing (with lenses)
  - **a.** Case history (including wear time now and maximum wear time)
  - **b.** Aided visual acuity
  - **c.** Over-refraction
  - **d.** Fit assessment
- **4.** Follow-up testing (without lenses)
  - **a.** Unaided visual acuity
  - **b.** Corneal curvature measurements
    - **1.** Keratometry
    - **2.** Corneal topography
  - **c.** Objective and subjective refraction
  - **d.** Slit-lamp evaluation
- **5.** Lens change

    G.　Retainer lenses
- **1.** Final lens
- **2.** Determine fit
- **3.** Determine wear schedule

III.　Conventional tri-curve lenses are fitted approximately 0.50 mm flatter than an alignment lens. If going through a diagnostic lens fit, you would follow the same procedure to conventionally determine an alignment fit. Centration of the contact lens is important to enhance the effectiveness of the orthokeratology. An over-refraction is necessary to assist in the determination of the contact lens power.

    A.　Example of properly fitting lens in **conventional orthokeratology**.
- **1. Lens: 41.87 D (8.06 mm) BC/9.0-mm OAD**

        Refraction:　　−1.25 DS
        Keratometry:　43.37/42.87 @ 161
        Eccentricity:　0.43

        (CD-ROM Figure 27 Orthokeratology: Conventional tri-curve lenses: 2 of 3)

        Selection of a rigid gas-permeable lens 0.50 D flatter than an alignment lens indicates that a lens with a base curve of 41.87 D

(8.06-mm BC/9.0-mm OAD) should be used. The alignment lens was 42.37 D. The fit of this lens demonstrates a flat, apical bearing relationship with average edge lift. The lens moves freely with the blink facilitating the massaging action of the flat lens on the cornea.

2. **Lens: 41.50 D (8.13 mm) BC/9.0-mm OAD**

   Refraction: −1.25 DS
   Keratometry: 43.37/42.87 @ 161
   Eccentricity: 0.43

   (CD-ROM Figure 28 Orthokeratology: Conventional tri-curve lenses: 3 of 3)

   The flatter lens 41.50 D (8.13-mm BC/9.0-mm OAD) has a smaller bearing area but much greater peripheral edge lift. This fitting relationship can yield problems with centration and subsequent uncontrolled displacement of the corneal apex.

IV. **Reverse geometry lenses** have a unique lens design where the secondary curve is steeper than the base curve (in a conventional tri-curve lens design the secondary curve is flatter). Diagnostic lenses are essential to assess proper fit and centration. Fluorescein analysis is important to ensure that proper centration and adequate tear exchange can occur with moderate central bearing and mid-peripheral pooling. The diagnostic lens base curve can be determined by selecting a lens that is 1.50–2.00 diopters flatter than the flat central K measurement. If patients experience excessive tearing, allow them to blow their nose to eliminate the tears. Check the fit of the lens and be certain to evaluate the lens for adequate movement (1–2 mm) and centration. If these do not exist, corneal health can become compromised and the flattening of the cornea can lead to a displaced visual axis or irregular corneal topography. The fluorescein pattern should demonstrate moderate apical bearing (3–5 mm) and mid-peripheral pooling (2-mm wide band). Once the base curve has been determined, over-refract to determine contact lens power.

A. **Example of OK lens fitting**

   1. **Lens: 8.20 mm/6.0-mm OZ/9.6-mm OAD**

      Refraction: −1.25 DS
      Keratometry: 43.37/42.87 @ 161
      Eccentricity: 0.43

      (CD-ROM Figure 29 Orthokeratology: Reverse geometry: 2 of 16)

      Selecting a lens that is between 1.50 and 2.00 D flatter than flat K indicates that the base curve of the lens should be between 41.37 (8.16 mm) and 40.87 (8.26 mm). For this patient a diagnostic lens of 8.20 mm, a secondary curve that is 3 D steeper, 9.6-mm overall diameter, and 6.0-mm optic zone was selected. In the video, note the central bearing area of the lens to be approximately 4–5 mm. The mid-peripheral pooling area is a ring approximately 2-mm wide with good tear exchange beneath the lens edge. The lens moves freely (1–2 mm) and although the lens tends to ride low, the

upper lid helps to lift the lens. This facilitates the massaging action of the lens to help flatten the cornea.

2. **Lens: 8.10 mm/6.0-mm OZ /9.6-mm OAD**
   Refraction: −1.25 DS
   Keratometry: 43.37/42.87 @ 161
   Eccentricity: 0.43
   (CD-ROM Figure 30 Orthokeratology: Reverse geometry: 3 of 16)
   Using a lens that is slightly steeper (8.10 mm) results in a fit that
   may appear appropriate over the bearing area; however, there are
   tight areas located in the mid-periphery. The dark areas appearing
   nasally and temporally can seal off, resulting in inadequate tear ex-
   change.

3. **Lens: 8.28 mm/6.0-mm OZ /9.6-mm OAD**
   Refraction: −1.25 DS
   Keratometry: 43.37/42.87 @ 161
   Eccentricity: 0.43
   (CD-ROM Figure 31 Orthokeratology: Reverse geometry: 4 of 16)
   A flatter fitting lens (8.28 mm) provides a similar appearing fit to
   the 8.20-mm lens. The central bearing area is smaller and the lens
   tends to position up under the upper lid for a longer duration. Often
   times when a lens rides high, the corneal apex can be displaced in-
   feriorly.

4. **Calculated method of determining the first base curve** for OK
   has been determined by John Mountford. The optimum fitting lens
   is determined by the sagittal depth, determined by the sag of the
   cornea and an allowance for tear layer thickness. The relationship
   has been described by the following formula:

   $$\text{Corneal sag (z)} = \frac{R_0 - \sqrt{R_0^2 - y^2 P}}{P}$$

   where R_0 is the apical radius, P (shape factor) = 1 − e2, and y =
   chord diameter/2 (chord is determined by the total diameter of the
   lens and peripheral curve width). Using this method the optimum
   lens design for the patient in a reverse geometry lens design is a
   base curve of 8.20, a secondary curve that is 4 D steeper with a
   larger overall diameter (11.0 mm) and optic zone (7.0 mm).

5. **Lens: 8.20 mm/6.0-mm OZ /10.0-mm OAD**
   Refraction: −1.25 DS
   Keratometry: 43.37/42.87 @ 161
   Eccentricity: 0.43
   (CD-ROM Figure 32 Orthokeratology: Reverse geometry: 6 of 16)
   Larger diameter lenses can enhance centration, an important
   factor in orthokeratology. Using a lens with a base curve of 8.20
   mm, a 10.0-mm overall diameter, and a 6.0-mm optic zone, the fit

is similar to the 9.6-mm overall diameter. The larger lens appears centered and does not tend to drop inferiorly as the smaller diameter lens. The effective apical relationship is approximately 0.12 D steeper with the larger fit and therefore negligible. The 8.20 mm/6.0-mm OZ/10.0-mm OAD is our ideal lens.

6. **Lens: 8.31 mm/6.0-mm OZ /10.0-mm OAD**
Refraction: −1.25 DS
Keratometry: 43.37/42.87 @ 161
Eccentricity: 0.43
(CD-ROM Figure 33 Orthokeratology: Reverse geometry: 7 of 16)
Flatter lenses may be considered in the larger diameter (8.31-mm base curve and 10.0-mm overall diameter) to account for the sagittal depth difference of the larger lens diameter. One step flatter was placed on the patient's eye. However, the bearing relationship is slightly too flat as indicated by the smaller bearing area in the video. **Corneal topography** with conventional rigid gas-permeable lenses and reversed geometry lenses appears to decrease the **eccentricity** of the cornea, resulting in a more spherical surface.

B. **Dispensing day** is not greatly different from any other rigid lens dispensing. You may feel comfortable rechecking baseline data (unaided VA, keratometry, refraction, and slit lamp evaluation). With the lenses on you should assess aided acuity, over-refraction, and fit.

1. **Application**, **removal**, and **recentration** should be taught as in conventional gas-permeable lens wear. The lens care regimen is the same as that for conventional gas-permeable lenses. If the patient has not previously worn contact lenses, the patient should begin wearing lenses on a limited wear schedule, gradually building up to full-time wear.

2. **Longer wear** results in a greater likelihood for an OK effect to occur. Within the first week, a patient who has never worn lenses should be able to wear the lenses 8–10 hours; maximum full-time wear should be 14–16 hours. As in any lens wear, the patient should be advised that lens wear should be discontinued if any pain or loss of vision occurs. If the patient experiences any irritation (burning, stinging, or scratchiness) or if the lens does not feel like it's moving, the patient should call the office to schedule an appointment for a lens change or modification. You should also inform the patient to expect vision through spectacles to be affected.

C. **Follow-up visits** are scheduled after one week for conventional OK lenses. If the patient is undergoing accelerated OK, the next scheduled visit should be within 3–7 days.

1. **Multiple pairs** of lenses should be ordered so that the lenses can be switched as soon as possible (the recommendation being that the second lens be 0.50–1.00 mm flatter than the first lens). De-

pending on time limitations of you and your patient, you may wish
the patient to wear the lens the first day (or the fitting day) for 2–4
hours. Following lens wear, check aided acuity, comfort, over-refraction, fit, unaided acuity, refraction, keratometry, and corneal
health. If there have been rapid changes, you will want to follow
the patient more frequently.

2. **Patients should be instructed to wear the lenses in.** Aided visual
   acuity and lens fit should be assessed prior to lens removal. If the
   fit has changed (there may be less central bearing), inadequate tear
   reservoir, inadequate movement, or lens adherence, the fit needs to
   be changed. Immediately after lens removal, unaided visual acuity, keratometry, refraction, and corneal health should be assessed.
   With reverse geometry lenses, the rate of corneal change may diminish following the first two weeks. Weekly visits can become
   monthly visits as these changes start to slow down.

3. If the patient **no longer demonstrates change**, going flatter with
   the next lens may provide an additional boost. If the lens has a
   good apical bearing relationship with a good tear reservoir, it may
   be time for the patient to enter into retainer wear. In the case of a
   patient who can obtain 20/20 unaided visual acuity, one should try
   to obtain a refraction of low plus (0.50–0.75) so that the acuity can
   be maintained throughout the day.

D. **Retainer lenses** are needed to maintain the OK effect lenses. They must
   be worn during some periods of the day. There is some discussion as to
   what wear time is appropriate; however, the retainer lens parameters generally are those of the final lens used in the OK procedure. In a conventional tri-curve lens design, the retainer is 0.50 D flatter than the central
   keratometry measurement. In the accelerated OK procedure, it is the last
   lens worn during the OK phase, as long as it provides adequate fit, is
   comfortable, and centers properly.

   1. **Wear time** depends on the desired acuity and length of effect
      needed. Further studies are needed to determine the degradation of
      acuity that occurs when lens wear is ceased. It is recommended that
      the retainer lens be worn until the goal acuity is achieved through-
      out the day. The wear time should be gradually reduced. Most pa-
      tients find it convenient to wear the lenses a few hours in the
      morning and a few hours before bedtime, to maintain the OK effect
      during the day. Patients should chart acuity following lens removal
      to determine the length of time that they can go without lenses.

   2. **Sleeping with retainers** may be successful. You may find that fur-
      ther OK changes can occur during this period, because of the in-
      creased wear time. As an overnight retainer, it is important to
      ensure lens centration and appropriate apical bearing relationship.
      There should also be no lens binding following an evening of

sleeping in the lenses. Many reverse geometry lenses have moderate to high Dk values. In **overnight retainer wear** it is important to use a lens material with a high Dk safe enough for wear during sleep and that maintains the OK effect. The same risks involved with overnight wear of RGP lenses (edema, lens binding, etc.) exist; therefore, the patient should be advised. Aspheric lens designs and fenestrations have been suggested to alleviate the problem of lens binding in overnight wear, but further investigation needs to be pursued.

3. **Regular follow-up** is essential for successful OK (every 3–6 months). Even during retainer wear, it is important to assess corneal health and regression of refractive changes. You may encounter patients who have previously undergone OK, and they feel that their vision with retainer wear is not as sharp as it has been in the past. It has been useful using topography to establish whether further changes can occur and how uniform corneal reshaping has occurred. Reverse geometry lenses may provide additional OK changes and can be used as an effective retainer where conventional tri-curve lenses have allowed regression.

4. In an **orthokeratology practice**, diagnostic fitting is important to ensure proper lens fit, vision, and success. Fee structure varies from practice to practice. This is a time-consuming procedure for the patient as well as the practitioner. Additionally, materials can be very costly depending on number of lens changes. Your fees should reflect costs for professional services and materials so that you and the patient are not uncomfortable with the frequent lens changes (package the material fees as opposed to fee per lens). With accelerated OK, changes occur quickly and frequent office visits are necessary.

V. **Advanced orthokeratology** has been described recently to deal with larger myopic refractive errors and faster results. The lens design is similar to a reverse geometry design rigid contact lens and have no tear reservoirs. The lenses are filled up to 4.00 D flatter than flat K. The patient generally wears the lens overnight and the results are rapid. Corneal topography reveals central flattening, mid-peripheral steepening, and the far periphery appears minimally changed. This topographical shift appears to change the cornea from an oblate surface to a prolate surface.

VI. **Corneaplasty** is the newest application of orthokeratology. An enzyme is injected intrastromally into the cornea. The enzyme is believed to weaken the molecular bonds in the stroma that hold the collagen fibrils together. This creates a malleable cornea that is subsequently fit with a rigid gas-permeable lens to reshape the cornea and decrease a myopic or astigmatic refractive error. A reversing drop is used to allow the cornea to return to a baseline level of structural integrity. This procedure is believed to allow the cornea to maintain the reshaped curvature, eliminating the need for retainer rigid lens wear. Initial clinical trials are being conducted, and the results of those trials may impact the utilization of orthokeratology.

REFERENCES

1. Binder PS, May CH, Grant SC. An evaluation of orthokeratology. Ophthalmology 1980;87(8):729–744.
2. Joe JJ, Marsden HJ, Edrington TB. The relationship between corneal eccentricity and improvement in visual acuity with orthokeratology. J Am Optom Assoc 1996;67:87.
3. Day JH, Rheim T, Bard RD, McGongagill P, Gambino M. Advanced ortho-k using custom lens designs. Contact Lens Spectrum 1997;12(6):34.

SUGGESTED READING

Contex OK Lens for Ortho-K, Contex OK Lens Fitting Guide. Sherman Oaks, CA: Contex, Inc., Oct. 1990.
Cooper MD, Horner DG. Fitting Manual for the OK Lenses. Evansville, IN, July 1991.
Mountford J. Accelerated Orthokeratology. Brisbane, Australia, 1996.

Chapter 25

Orthokeratology Topography Gallery

John Mountford and Harue J. Marsden

I. **Introduction**

There is no doubt that our concepts of corneal shape and how it affects contact lens fitting have changed since the introduction of corneal topography or CCT as it is more commonly known. Similarly, the development of reverse geometry lenses has changed the way we think about orthokeratology (OK).

There are four major uses of corneal topography when it comes to OK:

A. Accurate **pre-fit corneal shape analysis**

B. **Lens effect analysis**

C. **Permanent records** of a course of treatment

D. **Patient education**

The pre-fit evaluation gives valuable baseline information. The data can be used to fit the lenses with a degree of accuracy that is simply not possible with the keratometer.

II. **Pre-fit considerations**

A. **Corneal topography** provides invaluable insight into the chances for OK success. One measure, **eccentricity value**, helps to determine if the cornea will respond well to OK. Normal corneal eccentricity values are 0.40–0.60. This cornea has a low e-value of 0.27, below the normal range (CD-ROM Figure 34 Orthokeratology Topography Gallery: Pre-fit: 1 of 15). Low e-values will usually result in a poor OK response. Higher e-values are more desirable. The expected change in refraction can be found by dividing the e-value by 0.21.

Expected change = 0.27/0.21 = 1.29 D.

For myopia greater than 1.29 D, uncorrected amounts of myopia are expected following OK.

B. **Spherical topographic map** has a low to average e-value of 0.40 (CD-ROM Figure 35 Orthokeratology Topography Gallery: Pre-fit: 3 of 15). The predicted change is calculated to be 1.90 D. Although this cornea is

413

better suited than the previous example, it will not respond well if the refractive error is greater than approximately 2 D.

Expected change = 0.40/0.21 = 1.90 D.

C. **Average e-value** of 0.55 is shown with this cornea (CD-ROM Figure 36 Orthokeratology Topography Gallery: Pre-fit: 5 of 15). The cornea is almost spherical with a low amount of toricity. For refractive errors of around 2.50 or less, this cornea is an excellent OK candidate.

Expected change = 0.55/0.21 = 2.62 D.

D. **E-value** of 0.57 is an average to high amount (CD-ROM Figure 37 Orthokeratology Topography Gallery: Pre-fit: 7 of 15). The calculated expected change is 2.71 D. This is another excellent candidate and should respond well to OK. However, keep in mind that some corneas do not respond well to OK regardless of e-value. Sometimes, corneas with higher e-values are often poor responders. On the other hand, those with an e-value lower than 0.40 may respond better than expected.

Expected change = 0.57/0.21 = 2.71 D.

E. **Steep with-the-rule cornea** with a high to average e-value is shown (CD-ROM Figure 38 Orthokeratology Topography Gallery: Pre-fit: 9 of 15). The expected change is 2.86 D.

Expected change = 0.60/0.21 = 2.86 D.

F. **Average corneal curvature** with **low toricity** has a high e-value of 0.65 in this cornea (CD-ROM Figure 39 Orthokeratology Topography Gallery: Pre-fit: 11 of 15). The predicted change is 3.10 D. This map identifies another cornea that should have a good OK response.

Expected change = 0.65/0.21 = 3.10 D.

G. **High e-value** is shown in this map (e-value of 0.66) (CD-ROM Figure 40 Orthokeratology Topography Gallery: Pre-fit: 13 of 15). A predicted change of 3.14 D is expected. Unfortunately, the high amount of toricity of 3.12 D is likely to result in corneal distortion. An inferior steepening can result in toricities of 2–3 D or more for the with-the-rule corneas. Against-the-rule corneas of 3 D or more usually result in apical displacement following OK.

Expected change = 0.66/0.21 = 3.10 D.

H. **Reverse geometry lenses** are considered for our examples in the gallery. The newer "Advanced Orthokeratology" lenses are obtaining greater magnitude of myopic reduction and what appears to happen is a greater amount of **sphericalization** (e approaching closer to zero) over a smaller surface area. The major disadvantage is that the area of **sphericalization** is 4–5 mm (reverse geometry) vs. 2–3 mm (advanced orthokeratology).

III. **Ideal Response**

(CD-ROM Figure 41 Orthokeratology Topography Gallery: Ideal response: 1 of 2) This is the ideal response for the following reasons:

A. **Significant change in refraction** has occurred. The change in apical corneal power (central reference cross) has a 1:1 relationship to refractive change, so the actual refractive change can be read directly from the subtractive plot and verified either by retinoscopy or the standard techniques. There is a significant reduction in apical corneal power.

B.   **The area of central flattening** is uniform and has an area larger than the pupil outline. One of the most commonly overlooked factors in OK is that the quality of the post-wear vision is not only dependent on the degree of central flattening, but also on the **area of cornea** affected. If the area of flattening is less than the pupil diameter, especially in low illumination, halos, flare, and distortion will adversely affect the vision.

C.   **The mid-peripheral and peripheral areas** show even areas of change. There is an "even" degree of relative peripheral steepening.

D.   **Centration** characterizes the area of flattening with respect to the pupil. There is no distortion in the pupillary zone.

IV.   **Flat/decentered** maps are seen frequently. Lens decentration is the most common problem encountered in OK. If the lens decenters, the area of flattening will not be central and unwanted astigmatism and distortion are induced. The topography plots caused by a superiorly decentered lens are shown (CD-ROM Figure 42 Orthokeratology Topography Gallery: Flat/decentered: 1 of 3).

A.   **Superior positioning** causes superior flattening and relative **inferior steepening**.

B.   **"Smiley face" inferior crescent** of distortion and the off-center flattening of the superior cornea are apparent.

C.   **Unacceptable astigmatism** appears in the pupil zone.

D.   **Flare** would result if the pupil dilates because of the distortion.

E.   **Inferior, nasal, or temporal decentration** will cause similar distortions with the flat area corresponding to the same area as the decentration.

F.   **Further problems** can result with steepening the BOZR. This is associated with a steepening of the Tear Reservoir (TR) or secondary curve as well causing more fit difficulties. For each 0.05 mm steepening of the BOZR, there will be a corresponding increase of 10 microns in the tear layer thickness and vice versa. The wiser alternative is to increase the **lens diameter**, with a corresponding change to the BOZR in order to keep the correct sagittal relationship.

G.   **Tangential periphery** is another alternative. This gives the best results as far as centration control is concerned.

V.   **Tight fit** has three causes:

A.   **BOZR** too steep

B.   **TR or secondary curve** too steep

C.   **Peripheral curve or cone angle** too steep (CD-ROM Figure 43 Orthokeratology Topography Gallery: Tight fit: 1 of 3).

D.   **Base curve** fitted too steep results in the **TR or secondary curve** also being too steep and the **central tear layer thickness** will be greater than 10 microns. The point of contact between the lens and the cornea is the junction between the TR curve and the peripheral curve. A steep lens will cause compression of the cornea in this area. The lens will tighten quickly, and usually adheres to the cornea. This causes the first "tight lens" effect whereby the central cornea flattens but the peripheral cornea steepens prematurely and limits the degree of myopia change. This effect is demonstrated in the topography maps.

E. **Topographic characteristics** of a tight fit are:
1. **Noticeable central steep island**
2. **Paracentral area of corneal flattening**
3. **Signs of peripheral distortion**, especially of the pre-analyzed placido rings
4. **Poor uncorrected vision**

F. **Area of central flattening** is associated with marked peripheral steepening with the tight fit. The mid-peripheral steep area appears to be caused by the "bunching up" of corneal tissue in the TR area. If the central cornea flattens as a result of centrally directed pressure, then there must be an outward movement of corneal tissue towards the periphery. If the BOZR/TR combination is too tight, then peripheral compression at the TR/PC junction will tend to limit the movement of the cornea and cause the peripheral steepening seen here. The solution to the problem is to use a flatter lens and repeat the trial wear period.

VI. **Steep secondary curve** can sometimes be a source of problems (CD-ROM Figure 44 Orthokeratology Topography Gallery: Steep secondary: 1 of 2). The effect of a TR or secondary curve that is too steep is shown on a lens with poor centration.

A. **Area of central flattening** is small when compared to the ideal response. Note that the central flattening area is almost equal to the pupil diameter. This will cause marked flare and halos, especially in dim illumination as the induced corneal shape is similar to a concentric bifocal.

B. **Inferior crescent** is shown.

C. **Peripheral distortion** is shown.

D. **Poor VA** is evident in dim light.

E. **Steepening the TR curve** with respect to the BOZR in order to enhance centration reduces the area of central touch, and is therefore an inadvisable way of overcoming the problem.

VII. **Conclusion**

A. **Post-wear topographical analysis** can be used not only as an aid to more accurate reverse geometry lens design and fitting, but also is invaluable as a means of assessing the corneal response to the trial lens. If the resultant topography plots exhibit the signs of poor fitting outlined above, then remedial steps can be taken prior to dispensing lenses or proceeding with a course of treatment.

B. **Trial and error** characterizes traditional orthokeratology techniques and to a certain extent that is still the case. However, approaching the design, fitting, and prescribing of lenses on the results of post-wear topographical analysis can dramatically reduce the time, number of lenses, and expense involved in the procedure. The time and lens expense savings alone would more than compensate for the cost of the instrument.

C. **Efficacy of OK** can be objectively assessed with topographical analysis. As stated previously, there is a 1:1 relationship between apical corneal power change and refractive change, which can be read directly from the subtractive plots. Also, the area of cornea flattened with respect to the pupil zone and the optical quality of the altered corneal surface can be objectively assessed.

D. **Permanent record** of the effects of various lens design alterations and the corneal changes seen throughout a course of treatment are kept. Being able to explain the changes, whether good or bad, to the patient is an invaluable educational tool.

In conclusion, topographical analysis should be considered an essential instrument for the practice of OK.

Chapter 26

Rigid Gas-Permeable Cases

Milton M. Hom and Ronald Watanabe

I. **Case 1: Glare**
  A. **First lens** (CD-ROM Figure 11 RGP cases: Glare: Case 1: 1 of 3)

    Base Curve/Diameter: 8.00 mm/9.5 mm
    Refraction: −1.75 −0.50 × 180
    K reading: 42.50/43.00 @ 90
    K flat: 7.94 mm

    The first lens (8.00 mm) applied is very close to flat K (7.94 mm). The lens is fitted lid attachment and rides high. The patient complains of symptoms of glare, probably due to superior decentration. The fluorescein pattern appears slightly flat and but close to alignment. There is central bearing and mid-peripheral clearance. The pattern would take a more classical alignment look if centered manually on the eye. There is an incomplete ring of bearing on the superior portion of the lens because of the high positioning. This can be seen best at the end of the video. There is an acceptable larger amount of edge lift seen inferiorly due to the high ride. The lid attachment fit makes the lens move with the lid.

  B. **Second lens** (CD-ROM Figure 12 RGP cases: Glare: Case 1: 2 of 3)

    Base Curve/Diameter: 7.90 mm/9.5 mm
    Refraction: −1.75 −0.50 × 180
    K reading: 42.50/43.00 @ 90
    K flat: 7.94 mm

    The next steeper lens (7.90 mm) was chosen based on positioning and fluorescein pattern. The steeper base curve centers the lens better. The lens rides lower than before because the attachment to the upper lid has been minimized. Sometimes, lid attachment is desirable for centration. In this case, the upper lid force pulling the lens upward was too great with an "on K" fit. Making the lens steeper also increases the centrational forces between the lens and cornea. Symptoms of glare were relieved with the steeper base curve. The fluorescein pattern shows apical clearance surrounded by mid-peripheral bearing. The edge clearance is good, with more clearance inferiorly and nasally than temporally.

   C.   **Third lens** (CD-ROM Figure 13 RGP cases: Glare: Case 1: 3 of 3)

       Base Curve/Diameter: 8.10 mm/9.5 mm

       Refraction: $-1.75 -0.50 \times 180$

       K reading: 42.50/43.00 @ 90

       K flat: 7.94 mm

       A flatter lens (8.10 mm) was applied. The lens positions high and attaches to the lid. The fluorescein pattern appears flat (apical touch). The video shows how the pattern changes over time. When fluorescein is first instilled, the pattern looks steep because of the higher concentration of fluorescein. As the lens settles, the true flat pattern emerges. Blinking helps to flush out the tears and enables better pattern recognition. At the end of the video, the upper lid is lifted out of the way and the flat pattern is more easily identified. The lens shows central bearing, mid-peripheral clearance, and adequate edge lift.

 II.   **Case 2: Flat Feels Bad**

   A.   **First lens** (CD-ROM Figure 14 RGP cases: Flat feels bad: Case 2: 1 of 2)

       Base Curve/Diameter: 7.80 mm/9.5 mm

       Refraction: -3.25 DS

       K reading: 44.50/43.25 @ 87

       K flat: 7.58 mm

       This patient complained of edge awareness. The lid-attached lens (7.80 mm) was fitted flatter than the flat K (7.58 mm). The fluorescein pattern shows apical bearing surrounded by incomplete mid-peripheral clearance (especially apparent in the lower portion of the lens). There is debris on the lens surface. The lens has excellent centration and good movement with the lid.

   B.   **Second lens** (CD-ROM Figure 15 RGP cases: Flat feels bad: Case 2: 2 of 2)

       Base Curve/Diameter: 7.70 mm/9.5 mm

       Refraction: -3.25 DS

       K reading: 44.50/43.25 @ 87

       K flat: 7.58 mm

       A steeper lens was applied (7.70 mm) and the fluorescein pattern improved to alignment. The pattern is dark within the optic zone with a mid-peripheral fluorescent glow more apparent in the lower temporal area. Rather than a prominent clearance, the glow represents a very thin layer of tears characteristic of alignment on some corneas. The lens slowly sinks down to an inferior position after the blink. There is some inferior edge contact with the lower lid. Although the lens positioned better with the previous flatter lens, the constant edge awareness was relieved with the steeper lens.

III. **Case 3: Too Flat**
  A. **First lens** (CD-ROM Figure 16 RGP cases: Too flat: Case 3: 1 of 3)
     Base Curve/Diameter: 8.00 mm/9.2 mm
     Refraction: −4.25 −0.50 × 90
     K reading: 43.75/43.25 @ 80
     K flat: 7.80 mm
     The lens (8.00 mm) is flatter than flat K (7.80 mm). The flat lens decenters significantly after blink, almost rotating around the corneal apex. The lens pivots about the central flat area when disturbed by the blink. The fluorescein pattern shows apical bearing surrounded by mid-peripheral clearance with a great deal of movement and lateral decentration. Throughout the video, inferior clearance characteristic of a flat lens can be seen. The edge lift is also very large inferiorly.
  B. **Second lens** (CD-ROM Figure 17 RGP cases: Too flat: Case 3: 2 of 3)
     Base Curve/Diameter: 7.90 mm/9.2 mm
     Refraction: −4.25 −0.50 × 90
     K reading: 43.75/43.25 @ 80
     K flat: 7.80 mm
     A steeper lens (7.90 mm) was applied. This lens is still flatter than flat K (7.80 mm) and shows apical bearing with more significant mid-peripheral and peripheral clearance inferiorly. The lens is lid attached and demonstrates good centration and movement.
  C. **Third lens** (CD-ROM Figure 18 RGP cases: Too flat: Case 3: 3 of 3)
     Base Curve/Diameter: 7.80 mm/9.2 mm
     Refraction: −4.25 −0.50 × 90
     K reading: 43.75/43.25 @ 80
     K flat: 7.80 mm
     The next steeper lens (7.80 mm) was also equivalent to flat K (7.80 mm). The lens shows an alignment pattern with darkness throughout the optic zone. It is no longer a lid attachment fit. The lens drops low after the blink with an area of clearance in the lower peripheral area. The clearance area is crescent shaped and best seen near the end of the video. The dim area of clearance marks the intermediate zone between the central cornea and the flatter periphery. In this case, a flatter, lid attached lens has better centration than an alignment fit.
IV. **Case 4: Optic Zone Diameters**
  A. **First lens** (CD-ROM Figure 19 RGP cases: OZ: Case 4: 1 of 2)
     Base Curve/Diameter: 7.80 mm/9.2 mm
     Optic Zone Diameter: 7.40 mm
     The next two lenses have identical base curves and diameters. The lenses differ by increasing optic zone diameters (OZD). The first lens (7.40-mm OZD) moves laterally and drops after the blink. The lens has excessive movement. There is darkness throughout the entire OZD, encompassing the central and mid-peripheral areas. The OZD is too small for this

cornea. Small OZD lenses have reduced sag heights and are subsequently flatter fitting.

B. Second lens (CD-ROM Figure 20 RGP cases: OZ: Case 4: 2 of 2)
Base Curve/Diameter: 7.80 mm/9.2 mm
Optic Zone Diameter: 8.00 mm
The second lens has a larger OZD of 8.00 mm. The lens does not ride low after the blink and positions well. The effect of increasing the OZD makes the lens fit steeper. There is darkness throughout the entire OZD. There are also bubbles under the edge of the lens. The lens may benefit from a steeper peripheral curve system to reduce the edge clearance.

V. Case 5: Adhesion
(CD-ROM Figure 21 RGP cases: Adhesion: Case 5 Adhesion: 1 of 1)
A classic case of RGP extended wear adhesion is shown. Adhesion occurs in about 10–15% of patients. Mucous adhesion of the lens is the most accepted theory. Loss of aqueous results in a mucus-rich tear layer that acts like an adhesive. Reduction of lens diameter and widening and flattening of the peripheral system are recommended. Frequent replacement of RGP lenses will also reduce lens binding.

Chapter 27

Translating Bifocals

Rodger T. Kame and Milton M. Hom

I. **Tangent Streak bifocal** is a **monocentric, one-piece, prism-ballasted, truncated, translating lens**. The section "Concepts" is designed to give you insights on how to fit bifocal contact lenses. The "Walk-through" demonstrates an actual bifocal lens fitting.

II. **Tangent Streak concepts** are helpful in fitting **translating bifocal** designs. The lens enjoys a high success rate especially for patients already wearing RGP lenses. The lower lid positioned near the limbus is needed for success.

    A. **Bifocal patient selection** is important for success. For higher add powers, a translating lens is preferred. For lower add powers and a centered corneal apex, an aspheric design may be better. Patients using computers will also benefit from an aspheric design.

    B. **Bifocal fitting tips**

        1. **Low refractive errors** are not ideal candidates. Low hyperopes (1 D or less) will state they see better without any correction. Low myopes (less than 1.25 D) prefer removing their spectacles for near.

        2. Sometimes, **auxiliary glasses** are needed to enhance distance or near vision. Wearing the lenses without an additional spectacle correction 80% of the time is considered successful.

        3. For most problems, checking for an **alignment fit** is the first step.

        4. When fitting the Tangent Streak, expect **nasal rotation**.

    C. **Fitting guidelines**

        1. The manufacturer's **recommended base curves** for the Tangent Streak are:

Corneal Toricity	Base Curve
0	1 D flatter than K
0.50 D	0.50 flatter than K
>1 D	Not steeper than ¼ toricity

        2. The basic **lens parameters** are:

Diameter	9.4/9.0 (truncation)
Prism	2 ½ base down
Base Curve	Alignment (see above)
Add	0.50 D less than refraction data

Segment Height	4.0–4.2 mm
Material	Moderate to high Dk

3. An ideal fit is an **inferiorly positioning lens**, **alignment fluorescein pattern**, and **segment height 1.3 mm below the geometric center of the pupil**. Thirty percent of the pupil can be covered by the segment while looking at distance.

4. **Rotation** (especially nasal) is a common occurrence. Changing the **prism axis** and **increasing prism** helps to stabilize rotation. The prism axis should be changed in the same direction as the rotation. For nasal rotation, the axis is moved in. Sometimes, increasing the prism as little as ¼ prism diopter can make a great difference in stability. If too much upper lid capture is rotating the lens, reducing diameter may be necessary. If the lower lid is at an angle, modifying the **truncation** is helpful.

D. **Evaluation** takes place after the lens is placed on the eye, with special attention paid to **rotation**. The rotation must be evaluated in **primary gaze**, as well as **lateral** and **downward gaze**. Have the patient blink in each direction of gaze tests rotational stability. When the patient looks downward, check the rotation while instructing the patient to give a **light blink** and a **full blink**. Finally, translation can be checked by lifting the upper lid on downgaze. The superior portion of the lens should move over the superior limbus.

E. **Key fitting points**

1. **Center of gravity** needs to be taken into consideration with the Tangent Streak. The monocentric optics are derived with a one-piece bifocal having a slab-off near add. However, the slab-off configuration requires a thicker lens and also raises the center of gravity of the lens. Thus, the higher the segment height, the higher the center of gravity. This factor can be offset with increased prism ballast (as little as ¼ prism) to stabilize the lens from unwanted rotation or torque.

2. **Design versatility** is a plus. Tangent Streak design can be made with both front and back toric curves to address toric corneas. Refractive astigmatism, as well as difficult internal astigmatism, can be managed. The lens is also available in trifocal design. The main pitfall is that the required additional thickness due to slab-off sometimes increases the discomfort of the lens.

3. **Blink considerations** are important. **Full blinking** tends to torque the lens nasally due to the action of the lower lid. The inward or nasal thrust is absent or minimal with a **light** or **partial blink**. As mentioned previously, evaluate the lens with both a full blink and a light blink.

Pearl: Have your patient perform the two types of blink when evaluating a translating bifocal: light blink and full blink.

4. **Enhanced depth of focus** should be taken into consideration when prescribing. Increased thickness of the lens creates a plus lens effectivity. The required add power is usually +0.50 D less, providing an enhanced depth of focus.

5. **Modification** of lenses can be done by the practitioner. Lenses are easily modified in-office. With diagnostic fitting, the modifications needed are minimal.

III. **RGP bifocal walk-through** is a step-by-step fitting of a Tangent Streak bifocal.

A. Our patient has K readings of 44.75/46.00. The first lens applied is flat (CD-ROM Figure 22 Translating bifocals: Walk-through: 1 of 5). The central bearing area indicates a flat fitting lens on a with-the-rule cornea. There is a large amount of edge clearance. The appearance changes as the lens moves on the eye. At first, the lens looks stable with no significant rotation. After the patient is instructed to look laterally and blink, nasal rotation becomes apparent. Both the segment line and truncation indicates the rotation. Blinking helps the lens to settle back, but the nasal rotation still returns.

B. **With-the-rule steep pattern** is clearly shown with the second lens (CD-ROM Figure 23 Translating bifocals: Walk-through: 2 of 5). The two bearing areas are at the 3 and 9 o'clock positions on the eye. After one hard blink, the lens rotates nasally and never recovers.

C. **Flat fluorescein pattern** is shown. (CD-ROM Figure 24 Translating bifocals: Walk-through: 3 of 5). There are excessive movement and decentration. The lens rotates nasally in all fields of gaze.

D. **Prism axis** was moved in 10 degrees nasally for the next lens (CD-ROM Figure 25 Translating bifocals: Walk-through: 4 of 5). Although the lens has a steep with-the-rule pattern, it shows good mobility. At first, the lens nicely recovers from any rotation with **light blinking**. **Full blinking** on downgaze, however, causes nasal rotation. Even with light blinking, the lens does not recover well.

E. **Alignment lens** maintains good stability and recovery in all fields of gaze (CD-ROM Figure 26 Translating bifocals: Walk-through: 5 of 5). The pattern shows a steeper inferior cornea as compared to the superior quadrant. After looking laterally and blinking, the lens has no significant rotation. When the upper lid is lifted, the lens shows adequate translation. Notice the lens has translated over the superior limbus. On downgaze, the lens does rotate with full blinking. However, **light blinking** at primary position brings back full recovery. This was the diagnostic lens used for the final order.

Chapter 28

Newer Designs for Keratoconus

Shelley I. Cutler

I. **Keratoconus** has always been a challenge to even the most experienced of contact lens fitters. Throughout the years, many excellent designs, including patented, trademarked, and other proprietary material have become available for our use. No one design will work for all corneas; otherwise the need for the other designs would not exist. In choosing a lens design to fit a particular cornea, it helps to think in **three dimensions**. Knowledge of the many lens designs available is extremely helpful, as some designs are more appropriate for a given cone or specific shape than others are.

A. **Corneal topography** can be an excellent aid for a starting point. It establishes the position of the cone apex in the keratoconic patient and the basic surface pattern in both. A topographical map can also assist the practitioner in deciding whether warpage from a previous fit exists.

B. **What constitutes a successful fit?** The criteria for a successful fit in a keratoconic cornea is really no different than for a standard RGP lens. The lens should be **comfortable**, wearing time should be all waking hours (if possible), vision needs to be acceptable, as does the post-wear biomicroscopy, and the lens needs to stay on the eye. Obtaining these are the challenge.

1. **Complications** are a factor when working with keratoconic patients. These patients seem to be much more **sensitive** than the average patient. Many times there is an allergic history that may complicate management. **Dry eye** complaints are very common in this population, especially in those patients with corneal grafts.

2. **Vision**, even with contact lenses, may not improve to 20/20. The bottom line: is the final acuity satisfactory for this patient's needs?

3. **Health of the cornea** is most important and relates to lens wearing time. Keratoconus is a progressive disease, even with no lens wear. Some feel that a poorly designed lens can cause **scarring** and facilitate this progression. There have been debates as to the optimum

cornea/lens relationship, with the best relationship being that of total alignment. This will rarely happen with a keratoconic or grafted cornea. With the grafted patient, if a lens does not satisfy physiological needs, the irritation may stimulate a rejection.

4. **Optimal fitting relationship** is when the weight-bearing forces of the contact lens are as evenly distributed as possible over the cornea. For the keratoconic cornea, a light **"kissing" touch** over the cone is preferred. It seems to provide maximum acuity for these patients. For the grafted cornea, this is a greater challenge. Due to the difference in surgical techniques, there are many peaks and valleys that make equal weight distribution impossible.

5. Let the **fluorescein pattern** be your guide. Most of the time, the shape of the cornea will not allow a "pretty" or perfect fluorescein pattern. Many times, whether the fit is acceptable can only be answered with time.

II. **Corneal ectasia** seen in keratoconus results in a thinned protrusion usually decentered off of the visual axis.

A. Historically, **three topographical keratoconic patterns** have been established. They are a **nipple cone** (the steepest dioptric value is smaller in shape and somewhat central in location), an **oval or sagging cone** (the steepest dioptric portion of the cone is larger, inferior, and decentered somewhat nasally) and **keratoglobus** (the majority of the cornea is thinned and steep in its dioptric values). With the advent of the topographer, many patient variations are now seen. In fact sometimes it can be difficult to decide exactly what the cone should be described as. No eye is exactly the same and the steepest part of the cornea can vary in its location.

B. Designing a contact lens to contour appropriately, allowing a good physiological response and maximum visual acuity, has frustrated many a practitioner. One of the many objectives of the **CLEK (Collaborative Longitudinal Evaluation of Keratoconus)** study is to evaluate, over time, whether the ideal fit is **apical clearance, apical touch,** or **3-point touch**.

III. There are many **keratoconic fitting sets** available today. You can design your lens using **multicurve sets** with specific parameters. It is suggested to make the base curve approximately equal to the optic zone. The **secondary and tertiary curves** should be **progressively flatter** to align the cornea as best as possible. There are some authors who have given their philosophies in detail. This can be very effective in fitting cones for the experienced practitioner.

A. **The Soper Cone** was introduced in the mid-1970s. This is a bicurve contact lens. The two posterior curves are separately cut and polished. The fitting philosophy is based on sagittal depth. As the curvature of the central posterior curve (base curve) is increased for a given diameter or the diameter of a given curve is increased, the vaulting effect of the lens is also increased.

1. **Peripheral curve** is 7.50 mm unless the central base curve is flatter than 6.49 mm. Then the peripheral curve is 7.85 mm. This allows for intermediate curve(s) to be added by standard techniques, if necessary.
2. **The trial set** consists of 10 lenses. They are named by the letters: A–H. There are three groups of a given diameter/optic zone relationship. The steep central posterior curvature varies in order to fit the cone.

B. **The McGuire keratoconic lens system** was introduced in 1978. It is a modification of Soper's design. There are three groups. They are labeled the **Nipple cone** (D/OZ 8.1/5.5), the **Oval cone** (D/OZ 8.6/6.0), and the **"Globus" cone** (D/OZ 9.1/6.5). There are a series of four peripheral curves. They should be well blended to create an almost aspheric relationship. The secondary curve is 0.5 mm flatter than the central base curve (width of 0.3 mm). The third curve is 1 mm flatter than the secondary curve (width of 0.3 mm). The fourth curve is 1.5 mm flatter than the tertiary curve for a width of 0.3 mm, and the fourth and final peripheral curve is 2 mm flatter than the tertiary curve for a width of 0.4 mm.

C. **Aspheric Contact Lenses**. There are a few labs that make true aspheric lenses designed specifically for the keratoconic cornea. The posterior apical radius needs to be very steep in some cases and sometimes this can be a limiting factor with this design. Because plus power in the periphery is the nature of an aspheric lens, presbyopic keratocones may find this lens preferable if the fit is acceptable.
1. **KAS** by GBF Contact Lens, Inc. is an aspheric lens. It has a paraboloidal ocular surface geometry with a spherical front surface. The edge lift would be considered hyperboloidal. Diameters can range from 7.5–10.0 mm. The lens furnishes up to a +2.25 add by the nature of the design.
2. **Contex, Inc.** has eight aspherical designs available with varying eccentricity (E) values. The less severe the cone, the lower the recommended e-value. The aspheric-20 is the most common for keratoconus. It has a hyperbolic design. Larger diameters (10.2 mm) are recommended and varying edge lifts are available.

D. **Spherical OZ with aspheric posterior peripheral curves** are similar to the true aspheric lens in its philosophy but with a spherical optic zone. Visual acuity is many times sharper and more stable.
1. **ComfortKone** ™ by Metro Optics is a triaspheric lens with a 4.0-mm optic zone. The lens flattens into the aspheric "A" curve, which is considered the fitting curve. The greater the "A" value, the greater the change from the base curve to the peripheral fitting curve. The fitting set consists of 24 lenses. The diameter is either 8.5 or 9.0 mm. There is a choice of base curves of several "A" val-

ues: 5, 10, 15, or 20. By diagnostic fitting, one can specify any "A" curve from 3–20.

2. **Infinity Cone** by Infinity Optical, Inc. fits on the sagittal value principle. Larger diameters are used (9.0, 9.5, 10.0, and 10.5 mm). The optic zone is 1.5 mm less than the diameter. The goal is to fit the periphery of the lens on the peripheral area of the cornea as far away from the cone protrusion as practical. A 26-lens trial set is available. Each base curve has either 2 or 3 diameters included. There is a standard edge lift of a proprietary nature but it can be made flatter or steeper as needed. The fitter has the option to vary the base curve, diameter and/or edge lift to maximize the fit.

3. **Valley K** by Valley Contax is a unique design modified after the McGuire lens. Instead of the four blended peripheral curves, there are computer-lathed curves halfway in between the basic McGuire curves. It is very reproducible. The peripheral curve system can be modified as needed by making the curves flatter or steeper for a given base curve. The trial set consists of 12 lenses. The optic zone is standard at 5.0 mm. The diameter is 9.0 mm for the flatter base curves and 8.5 mm for the steeper base curves.

E. **Custom designs** have appeared in recent years.

1. **Rose K** is a lens design with a complex, computer-generated peripheral curve system that resulted after several hundred fittings by Paul Rose. There is a trial set with the standard peripheral curve system. This claims to fit about 60% of the patients. The ideal edge lift is 0.8-mm wide. Flatter combinations are available 1.0, 1.5, 2.0, 2.5, and 3.0 flatter than the standard peripheral curve system to obtain this. A steeper peripheral curve system is available in 0.5 and 1.0 steeper than the standard edge lift. The decision to alter the peripheral curve system is made after the fluorescein pattern of the standard edge lift is observed. The optic zone decreases as the base curve steepens. Toric curves are available on both the front and rear surface, as well as peripherally.

2. **NiCone Lens**, patented in 1986, is available from Lancaster Contact Lens, Inc. It is described as a multiple back surface vaulting system designed with scientific formulas.

   a. Each lens has **three "base curves"** and a **peripheral curve of 12.25 mm**. There are three fitting sets (the #1 cone for mild keratoconus, #2 cone for the average cone, and #3 cone for advanced keratoconus). These are designations of curvatures between the Numbers 1, 2, and 3 base curves, depending on the selection of the primary base curve. Each time the central posterior radius is changed, regardless of whether it is a Number 1, 2, or 3 cone, all of the formulas of the second and third base curves change as well.

   b. **The second base curve** acts as a buffer between the diseased
   and non-diseased areas of the cornea. It is a 0.3-mm transi-
   tional zone for lens diameters up to 10.5 mm. A diameter
   larger than 10.5 can have a second base curve of 0.4 mm, 0.5
   mm, or greater.

   c. **Lens diameter and optic zone** may vary. They are not standard. All base curves of these lenses are lathe-cut and optically
   polished, and, thus, according to the manufacturer, do not create optical distortion that is present in grounded curvatures.

3. **Menicon** makes a keratoconic lens that has a decentered optic
   zone. The central base curve is the fitting curve; however, there is a
   back surface reverse annular which seems to line up with the visual
   axis. The best candidates are those with cones decentered below
   the midline of the eye. The initial lens design can be determined
   by their standard trial set (D/OZ 9.2/7.0; Secondary 7.5/0.6; Intermediate 9.5/0.3; Peripheral 12.0/.2). Prism increases as the base
   curve steepens and more minus power is needed. Initial lens selection is the base curve that corresponds to about the keratometric
   reading if the patient is looking up or from the topographical map.
   The recommended procedure would be to locate the cone; the base
   curve should be around the ring that corresponds to the base of the
   cone. If you choose not to go with the standard optic zone, the OZ
   should be about 1 mm larger than the cone and should be fairly
   close to the base curve. At the time of this writing, Menicon has
   suspended business in the U.S. market.

4. **The Porus K**™ is made by Lens Mode. This is a smaller lens
   diameter that fits over the apex of the cone. It strives for total alignment. The average diameter is 8.0 mm but can vary between
   7.7–8.4 mm. The steeper the cone, the smaller the diameter. The
   flatter the cone, the larger the diameter. There are 5 curves that are
   all computer lathed. There is a complex trial set with curves known
   only by the manufacturer. Parts of one lens can be combined with
   another for a custom fit.

5. **Computer-assisted** contact lens designs are available from some
   laboratories. Because they are designed from corneal topography,
   and the keratoconic cornea can have changes in curvature that are
   too detailed for the corneal map to reveal, this type of design may
   or may not work when the lens is placed on the eye and interacts
   with the ocular environment.

IV. **Fitting keratoconus** is more efficient with a topographical map. Once the
   shape and location of the cone are noted, an initial lens design and lens need
   to be selected. Experienced keratoconic fitters may prefer to design their own
   lens from a multicurve trial set. This allows for every curve to be specified
   by the fitter. Specific areas of the contact lens can be altered by remakes or

modification. Some expert fitters may even question why these specialty sets exist. For the less experienced fitter, using today's proprietary sets can be a method to gain the knowledge to move on. Others have done the "dirty work," making the specific design after years of their own experience. An experienced fitter may like these specialty designs as it can minimize the chair time for the final successful result. **Suggested initial lens selection** for specialty design selection is as follows:

A.   **Nipple** type cones are smaller, steeper, and more central. Spherical OZ with an aspheric periphery, the Rose K, the Porus K, or possibly an **aspheric design** are considered for an initial lens. The apex of these cones is just minimally off the visual axis. Centration is usually good since lenses tend to center over the steepest part of the cornea. The limitation of these designs is usually not the final fluorescein patterns, but vision. Smaller diameter/optic zone combinations may not be large enough to maintain sharp, stable vision. If this occurs, a larger OZ is needed. The Infinity lens, with its larger diameter/optic zone might be an ideal choice in this situation. The Nicone lens is also a good lens of choice if a larger optical zone is needed (CD-ROM Figure 53 Keratoconus: Cone Nipple: 3 of 7).

B.   **Oval, sagging cones** present a more difficult situation. Because the contact lens will center over the steepest part of the cornea, these lenses ride low. Vision can be variable or compromised altogether if a smaller lens and optic zone are used, as the patient is usually viewing through a junction zone.

   1.   **Larger lenses with larger optic zones** may be successful if contoured appropriately. Another alternative is to attempt to fit over the more normal superior cornea and attach the lens to the lid. Care needs to be taken to be certain excessive pressure on the cone does not occur.

   2.   **Menicon's decentered** optic zone works well for inferior displaced cones. Even though the visual axis is through the secondary curve, acuity can be exceptionally good. The Nicone design also will work well with a sagging cone. The optic zone can be made larger to vault the cone as well as cross the visual axis. The larger diameter Infinity lenses can also be successful with these larger sagging cones due to the larger optic zone (CD-ROM Figure 54 Keratoconus: Cone Oval: 5 of 7).

C.   **Keratoglobus** or large cones are difficult to fit. Recommended lenses are Infinity Cone or Nicone (CD-ROM Figure 55 Keratoconus: Cone Globus: 7 of 7).

V.   **Assessment** of trial fit starts with the cone itself. How is the base curve/optic zone diameter combination housing the cone? If there is too much bearing, more vaulting needs to occur. This can be accomplished by making the base curve steeper for a given OZ diameter (the easiest way if working with one trial set of standard parameters). If fitting sets with variable OZ diameters (such as the Infinity Cone, Nicone, or Porus K) are available, diameters can be increased while maintaining the base curve. The Rose K decreases the optic zone as the base curve steepens so you may have to make changes of larger increments to accomplish what you want.

A. **When is the base curve correct?** One good suggestion is to continue to steepen the base curve until there is apical clearance and then work backward. There should be just enough touch to maximize vision. Striving for a light feather or "kissing" touch seems to be ideal. Sometimes a steeper lens will not work. The optic zone diameter may need to be altered. A design switch maybe merited.

B. **Air bubbles** may exist in the pooling around the cone although there is a good base curve–cone relationship. The best way to eliminate them is to decrease the optic zone. To maintain the same sagittal depth and fluorescein pattern, steepen the base curve also. Be aware that the smaller optic zone may interfere with the visual acuity.

C. **Paracentral** or **mid-peripheral area** under the contact lens should be examined. The goal is to strive for alignment. In theory, this should not be exceptionally difficult, especially if the curves of the contact lens are known. Be prepared to be disappointed. There are corneas that no matter how the curves are altered, the ideal alignment pattern never seems to appear. Accept this. However, do not accept heavy bearing that allows for seal off. Tears need to be exchanged. If proprietary sets are used, you are somewhat at the mercy of the labs as you can only request flatter or steeper curves. Many times this works out just fine.

D. **Peripheral portion** of the lens can be viewed by looking at the edge lift. There needs to be enough to allow good tear pumping under the lens but not too much to cause the patient discomfort. Too little edge lift will predispose the adjacent corneal area to desiccation as well as poor tear exchange.

E. Once you have what you think looks like an **acceptable fit**, dispense the lens and begin following the patient, closely at first. It is often the rule, rather than the exception, that a few changes or modifications in lens design will occur during the fitting process. Alert your patient to this possibility.

F. **Follow-up** patients at least twice a year if it seems they are doing well. Remind the patient that keratoconus is a progressive ectasia. What is an acceptable fit now could change. Patient signs and symptoms are decreased vision, decreased comfort and/or wearing time, increased difficulty in removing the lens, removal of lenses becomes much too easy, or lens dislocation or ejection from the eye (assuming that it was not a problem before). Along with any complications of routine contact lens wear, any of these problems should alert the patient to see you sooner.

G. **Changes** can be detected at routine follow-ups. If you see a change in the fluorescein pattern or corneal picture, a refit will most likely be necessary. If you review the patient's history, some subjective signs might be there but the patient really didn't feel it was relevant.

VI.   Keratoconus Cases: Patient #1

    A.   History

A 41-year-old white female presented for a routine check of her lenses. She had been fit and followed yearly by a practitioner who moved out of the area. She wore her lenses 8–9 hours a day. She would remove them for an hour or two if she needed to wear them in the evening. This was acceptable to her. She used the Boston System for cleaning and disinfecting and an enzyme soak every 1–3 weeks. Visual acuity was 20/25 OD and OS.

    B.   Lens Parameters

Fluoroperm 30

	BC	BVP	D/OZ	2nd (width)	PC (width)
OD	7.10	–5.75	8.6/7.0	8.50 (.4) mm	10.50 (.4) mm
OS	6.90	–8.50	8.4/6.8	8.50 (.4) mm	10.50 (.4) mm plus lenticular edge

    C.   OD

        1.   Topography

This is a large nipple cone. It appears to be temporal and slightly inferior in location (CD-ROM Figure 56 Keratoconus cases: Patient 1: Topography: 2 of 6).

        2.   Video

The base curve of the lens corresponds to the light green ring (47.50 D/7.10 mm). The optic zone is almost identical to the base curve. The lens centers over the cone, which is now obviously inferior and temporal. There is a light kissing touch over the apex. The mid-peripheral region seems totally aligned with good peripheral edge lift. This fluorescein pattern is probably the closest example of alignment that can be seen in a keratoconic fit. The lens doesn't appear to have much movement; however, on close observation movement and tear exchange are evident (CD-ROM Figure 57 Keratoconus cases: Patient 1: Video: 3 of 6).

The patient only is comfortable for 8–9 hours of continuous wear. To try and improve upon that, a change in material will be made in the future (a higher Dk) when it is time for lens replacement. The addition of liquid enzyme will also be introduced at that time. However, since the fluorescein pattern appears optimal, no change was deemed necessary.

    D.   OS

        1.   Topography

This is also a nipple cone, located temporal, and slightly inferior to the optical axis. Note, it is relatively larger than the cone in the right eye (CD-ROM Figure 58 Keratoconus cases: Patient 1: Topography: 5 of 6).

        2.   Video

The base curve of this lens falls between the yellow and green ring (about 49.00 D/6.90 mm). The optic zone is again, almost the same as the base curve. There is a large area of bearing over the cone. This is not unexpected considering the size of the cone. There is an area of pooling surrounding the cone, which is very common in most keratoconic lens fits. The bearing in the mid-peripheral region is acceptable; however, a more aligned relationship would be ideal. The edge lift is acceptable (CD-ROM Figure 59 Keratoconus cases: Patient 1: Video: 6 of 6).

At the moment, no changes will be made since vision and wearing time are acceptable and there are no adverse physiological responses.

When these lenses need to be replaced, certain changes will be made. Along with a higher Dk material, the base curve will be made steeper. Although the bearing is light, an attempt for less bearing will be made. A change in the optic zone might have to occur. The important factor is that the touch is and remains light. An attempt will be made to have a more aligned relationship in the mid-peripheral area. This could be accomplished by adding one or two more peripheral curves or using a design that has an aspheric periphery.

VII. Keratoconus Cases: Patient #2

A. History

A 48-year-old white male presented for a routine checkup of his present lenses. This pair was a little over a year old. Care regimen consisted of various gas permeable daily cleaners (Boston, Miraflow, Optifree) and Boston Conditioning solution. Daily cleaning was performed in the evening and overnight storage in the conditioning solution. He used an enzyme soak weekly. Wearing time was 16 hours a day but his complaints were of a greasy feeling with comfort and vision decreased at the end of the day. The clinical picture was almost identical OU. Only the left eye will be presented.

B. Video

The lens centers. There is a light central touch. However, note the small air bubble in the area of clearance around the cone. When this is observed, it is usually an indication that the optic zone is too large. Due to the photography without a wratten filter, the bearing in the mid-peripheral is actually heavier than that displayed. The edge lift is acceptable, bordering on excessive. Visual acuity was 20/50+. Note how the light reflex breaks up, indicating poor wettability. The scratches on the front surface also aid in the non-wetting. There was minimal 3:00 and 9:00 staining with no scarring over the apex (CD-ROM Figure 60 Keratoconus cases: Patient 2: Video: 2 of 19).

C. Lens Parameters

SGPII   Plus edge lenticular carrier

BC	BVP	D/OZ	2nd (width)	3rd (width)	PC (width)
6.85	−11.00	9.5/6.6	8.5 (.5) mm	9.5 (.5) mm	11.0 (.45) mm

These lenses were polished and the patient was put on a lid hygiene regimen to improve his symptoms during the refitting process.

D. Topography

The topography reveals a classic nipple cone. There are several choices of lens designs that might be ideal for this eye. When assessing the present (quad-curve) lens, a more aspheric periphery might be in order to attempt alignment in the mid-peripheral region. This could be accomplished with a true aspheric lens (especially since the patient is a presbyope) or a lens with a spherical base curve having an aspheric periphery. KAS by GBF labs attempted the aspherics first (CD-ROM Figure 61 Keratoconus cases: Patient 2: 4 of 19).

E. Trial Fittings

1. Video

KAS by GBF labs

BC 6.58 mm   D 8.75 mm   BVP –5.50 D

Aspherics need to have a central base curve significantly steeper than flat K. The philosophy is to vault the apex of the cornea and have alignment over the mid-peripheral cornea (CD-ROM Figure 62 Keratoconus cases: Patient 2: Video: 5 of 19).

The lens drops inferiorly post blink and remains with light blinks. In this inferior position, the central area reveals heavy bearing, mid-peripheral pooling, and an area of arcuate bearing when the lens rests on the inferior cornea. If you look closely, after a hard blink you can see what appears to be an aligned pattern but for only a minisecond. In the inferior position, this lens appears too flat. If centration could be improved, the overall performance of this lens design should improve as well. Good endpoint acuity was not obtainable.

2. Video

KAS by GBF labs

BC 6.40 mm   D 8.8 mm   BVP –4.5 D

This steeper lens was chosen to try to improve centration. As the patient moves his eye and blinks, the lens does center better than the previous one. Note the light central touch when centered. Like the previous lens, this one also drops inferiorly and prefers that position. In this inferior position the central bearing and mid-peripheral pooling can be seen. Of significance is the heavy bearing peripherally, indicating that this lens is much too steep or tight in that area. Again, a good consistent endpoint acuity was not achieved (CD-ROM Figure 63 Keratoconus cases: Patient 2: Video: 6 of 19).

In order to continue to improve centration, vision, and the overall performance of this aspheric design, the base curve radius needs to be steeper and the diameter smaller, probably to about 8.0–8.3 mm. This would maintain the proper sagittal depth and prevent peripheral seal off.

The patient's pupils dilate significantly in dim illumination. Because of the large pupil, the small lens diameter would not be acceptable. A spherical base curve with an aspheric periphery was selected next.

3. **Video**

From the fluorescein pattern of the patient's own lens (light central touch with an air bubble in the area of clearance around the cone), a smaller optic zone will be used. Since the touch over the cone seems appropriate, a slightly steeper base curve will be chosen in an attempt to maintain this relationship (CD-ROM Figure 64 Keratoconus cases: Patient 2: Video: 7 of 19).

Valley K lens by Valley Contax

BC 6.75 mm   D/OZ 9.0 mm/5.0 mm   BVP –8.00 D

This lens design was chosen first because the optic zone is slightly larger than the ComfortKone by Metro Optics (4.0 mm). Note the light central touch surrounded by pooling. The mid-peripheral to peripheral bearing of this lens is much too wide and heavy. This is not acceptable. Edge lift might be considered less than optimum.

A flatter base curve was not trialed because the amount of central bearing is the maximum amount that is acceptable. If requested, a flatter peripheral curve system is available (of proprietary information) for any base curve in the trial set. This is what was ordered. Over-refraction yielded 20/30+ acuity, which delighted the patient.

4. **Video**

This is the dispensed Valley K lens

BC 6.75 mm with a flatter peripheral curve system   D/OZ 9.0 mm/5.0 mm Boston ES   BVP –11.75 D

The lens centers nicely. There is a light central touch over the cone with an area of pooling around the apex. The mid-peripheral area reveals more bearing than is preferred, but the edge lift appears to allow adequate tear flushing with the blink. Acuity is 20/30. The patient was instructed to use both the Boston cleaner and conditioning solutions. In addition, SupraClens was to be used every night in the conditioning solution. He was also to remain on his daily lid hygiene routine (CD-ROM Figure 65 Keratoconus cases: Patient 2: Video: 8 of 19).

5. **Video**

One-week follow-up

Patient reports the lens is comfortable and vision is excellent. Wearing time is all waking hours. Cleaning regimen is being followed correctly. He confesses that he is only doing the lid hygiene every other day (CD-ROM Figure 66 Keratoconus cases: Patient 2: Video: 9 of 19).

The lens continues to center well. Today the central area of bearing seems a little heavier than on the day of dispensing. An area of fluorescein pooling surrounds the apex of the cone. The area of mid-peripheral bearing seems slightly larger, but as the patient blinks, it is clear that tear exchange does occur under that area. The tears seemed to have more debris in them than usual. Some of this can be visualized on the lens surface.

Although the patient was happy with the vision and wearing time, the fluorescein pattern was not optimum. In my opinion, the mid-peripheral bearing was a little excessive.

In order to try to improve on this, the ComfortKone lenses by Metro Optics were now trialed.

6. **Video**

ComfortKone

BC 6.70 mm   A5   D 9.0 mm   BVP –6.00 D

A slightly steeper base curve compared to the Valley K lens was initially selected because the ComfortKone has a slightly smaller optic zone.

This lens centers well. Centrally there is a light touch over the cone. The pooling surrounding the cone is evenly distributed. The bearing in the mid-peripheral region is excessive. There is minimal edge lift. Over-refraction yielded 20/30– acuity (CD-ROM Figure 67 Keratoconus cases: Patient 2: Video: 10 of 19).

7. **Video**

ComfortKone

BC 6.80 mm   A10   D 8.5 mm   BVP –5.00 D

The A value needs to be increased. The A10 peripheral system in the 9.0-mm diameter needed to be trialed. However, there were no A10s in the 9.0-mm diameter available in the fitting set. The 6.80 BC A10 8.5 D lens was applied to justify ordering the A10 peripheral system.

This lens centers well. Centrally there is a little more bearing. This is expected as the base curve is slightly flatter than the previous one. Also, the smaller diameter will reveal an overall flatter fit. Interestingly enough, the central bearing doesn't seem excessive. The mid-peripheral region and edge lift look much better. Note the light touch and excellent tear exchange. This lens was not as comfortable as the 9.0-mm diameter, probably due to the increased edge lift. At this point it looks like the 6.70-mm or even a 6.75-mm base curve with an A10 peripheral curve system will work (CD-ROM Figure 68 Keratoconus cases: Patient 2: Video: 11 of 19).

A few more lenses were trialed just to give more information to support this decision. A range of A values in the 6.70–6.90-mm base curves were available.

8. **Video**

   ComfortKone

   BC 6.70 mm   A15   D 8.5 mm   BVP –6.00 D

   This was the next lens that was available. The significantly increased A value, along with the smaller diameter, clearly makes this lens too flat, even though the central base curve should be correct. Notice the superior position of the lens. Because of this displacement, there appears to be a central-nasal bearing with mid-peripheral pooling and excessive edge lift (CD-ROM Figure 69 Keratoconus cases: Patient 2: Video: 12 of 19).

9. **Video**

   ComfortKone

   BC 6.90 mm   A8   D 9.0 mm   BVP –1.75 D

   This lens was applied to determine the performance of the A8 peripheral curve with a flatter base curve. As expected, there is central bearing over the cone. The mid-periphery of this lens has a nice even distribution of weight. The fluorescein pattern reveals alignment in this area. There is good peripheral edge lift that allows for excellent tear exchange. The information gleaned from this trial lens suggests that a flatter value would be needed with a steeper based curve to find what base curve would be considered too steep (CD-ROM Figure 70 Keratoconus cases: Patient 2: Video: 13 of 19).

10. **Video**

   ComfortKone

   BC 6.50 mm   A15   D 8.5 mm   BVP –7.00 D

   A smaller diameter was evaluated with a steeper base curve. The A15 was the only A value available in the fitting set. Clearly the central fluorescein pattern is that of apical clearance. Note the central pooling along with the small air bubble. The mid-peripheral area under this lens appears to have a relatively aligned pattern. The edge lift might be considered a little excessive. The patient commented that this was not a comfortable lens (CD-ROM Figure 71 Keratoconus cases: Patient 2: Video: 14 of 19).

   After diagnostic fitting, this lens, was ordered:

   ComfortKone

   BC 6.75 mm   A10   D 9.0 mm   BVP –11.75 D

11. **Video**

   Dispensed ComfortKone

   BC 6.75 mm   A10   D 9.0 mm   BVP –11.75 D

   This lens centers and moves well. Comfort was fine. There is a light touch over the cone with fluorescein surrounding the apex. The mid-peripheral portion exhibits an alignment to light bearing relationship. Edge lift is adequate, allowing for good tear exchange.

Visual acuity was 20/30 with an extra +1.00 over refraction. The patient commented that there was not good contrast compared to the original Valley K lens. The patient was allowed to wear this lens. Upon return for follow-up, the over-refraction was incorporated and the A value increased slightly (CD-ROM Figure 72 Keratoconus cases: Patient 2: Video: 15 of 19).

The following lens was ordered:
ComfortKone
BC 6.70 mm   A13   D 9.0 mm   BVP –11.00 D

12. **Video**

Dispensed ComfortKone
BC 6.70 mm   A13   D 9.0 mm   BVP –11.00 D

The lens centers and moves well. The minimally steeper base curve produces a lighter touch over the cone with fluorescein pooling surrounding the apex. There does not seem to be heavy bearing in the mid-peripheral area and the edge lift is good. Actually, the edge lift might be considered a little too much, but the patient was comfortable and there seemed no reason to change anything (CD-ROM Figure 73 Keratoconus cases: Patient 2: Video: 16 of 19).

Although the fluorescein pattern was excellent, the vision was unacceptable to the patient. He had 20/30 acuity but didn't like "what the real world looked like." He wanted to know why he couldn't go back to the original (Valley K) lens.

This lens was returned to him. He was to wear this lens and return for follow-up in one month.

13. **Video**

One-month follow-up of Valley K
BC 6.75 mm flatter PC   D 9.0 mm Boston ES   BVP –11.75 D

The lens centers appropriately, especially as the patient moves his eyes laterally, but seems to be in a more inferior location than on previous examination. Notice how the central bearing seems heavier and in a more superior position than previously noted. The mid-peripheral portion under the lens seems more aligned than before. Edge lift is adequate, although a little more would be preferred (CD-ROM Figure 74 Keratoconus cases: Patient 2: Video: 17 of 19).

Vision is excellent, a sharp 20/30 +1. Wearing time is all waking hours. With the exception of a few scattered SPK on the cornea, physiological response seems excellent.

Comments

This is an interesting case. Almost before our eyes, the fluorescein pattern of the dispensed Valley K lens changed over time. Why? It has been established in the past that an apical clearance fit lens can exhibit light touch after a 10–20 minute adaptation as the tear film thins. Is this an extreme variation? Is the keratoconus progressing or is the cornea molding to this lens, secondary to pressing in the mid-peripheral region? If there is a little molding, is this detrimental?

This could have been one of those examples where the fluorescein pattern does not exhibit a "perfect" pattern, but something just seemed wrong. After questioning, the patient revealed he had switched lenses. Returning the lenses to their correct eye, the fluorescein pattern looked very similar to that of the one-week follow-up.

F. Follow-up

Six months later, Patient 2 returned for follow-up. He had no complaints. Vision and comfort were acceptable. The lens continues to center and move well. There is a light central touch over the cone with an area of pooling around the apex. The mid-peripheral area reveals an alignment-type relationship. The edge lift appears to allow good tear flushing with the blink. Acuity is 20/30. Post-wear physiology is excellent (CD-ROM Figure 75 Keratoconus cases: Patient 2: Video: 19 of 19).

Comments

Many times when fitting a more complicated situation, it is easy to compromise, especially if the patient appears to be doing well. If something just doesn't seem right, pursue a reason. Your instincts are usually correct.

VIII. Keratoconus Cases: Patient #3

A. History

A 50-year-old white male came in wearing his most recent pair of lenses. They were 4 years old, however, he was wearing his spare pair, beginning 3 months ago. His complaints were that of decreased wearing time (uncomfortable at the end of the day, although wearing time continues to be 14 hours), vision seemed "warped" (OD 20/30+, OS 20/25−), and the lenses seemed to pop out much easier than before. Past records were unavailable. He uses the Boston cleaning regimen with weekly enzyme soaking. Only the right eye will be presented.

B. Lens Parameters

Verified:

	BC	BVP	D/OZ	PCs
OD	6.52 mm	−10.00 D	9.3 mm/7.8 mm	unavailable

C. Video

The video depicts the patient's present lens. Note the large, heavy bearing centrally and pooling in the mid-peripheral area. There is minimal edge clearance from at 8:30 to 1:00 and excessive edge lift in the remainder of the lens periphery (CD-ROM Figure 76 Keratoconus cases: Patient 3: Video: 2 of 15).

Impression

There is too much central bearing, uneven distribution of weight-bearing forces, and excessive inferior edge lift. Essentially, this fit is too flat.

D. Topography

The topography of the patient's eye reveals an extremely large cone. Looking carefully at the dioptric values of the blue and green colors, you'll note that they are in the 50's and 60's range. Although the auto alignment feature of the topographer was on, this was a very difficult map to capture. The Y and Z axes are off from zero, so it may be difficult to determine whether this is an extremely large nipple or a sagging variety, as one seems to flow into the other.

Note the flatter areas in the center region. These correspond to the scarring areas present at the cone apex (CD-ROM Figure 77 Keratoconus cases: Patient 3: 4 of 15).

E. Refitting procedure

The cone can be classified as either nipple or sagging. The Rose K was trialed initially. The trial set has an 8.7-mm diameter with a proprietary peripheral curve system. Knowing that his own lens of 6.52-mm BC was significantly too flat, a 6.10-mm BC for the Rose K was initially selected. This, along with a 6.00 mm, was much too flat. The clinical picture was not that different than his present lenses and not captured on video.

   1. Video

Rose K

BC 5.80 mm   D 8.7 mm   BVP –16.00 D

The next lens trialed (shown in clip) after the 6.10-mm and 6.00-mm BC was 5.80-mm BC. As the patient blinks, there is a nice even distribution of weight over the apex of the cone. Tear exchange reveals a kissing type of touch even though the area is large. The area superior to the cone is total clearance, but no air bubbles are present. There really doesn't seem to be a definitive mid-peripheral pattern. When the superior lid is raised, the bearing in the superior quadrant becomes evident. A flatter peripheral curve system could be considered, but might create too much edge lift inferiorly. Over-refraction revealed an excellent endpoint visual acuity of 20/25+ (CD-ROM Figure 78 Keratoconus cases: Patient 3: 5 of 15).

   2. Video

Rose K

BC 5.60 mm   D 8.7 mm   BVP –18.12 D

Another steeper lens was tried to find the place where the base curve is too steep. In this example, notice as the patient blinks, there seems to be an even distribution of bearing forces until the post-blink. Carefully watching the fill behind the lens, especially in the central and mid-peripheral portion of the lens, a vaulting sensation can be appreciated. It seems that on the blink, the cornea molds to the posterior curves, only to have the lens vault afterward (CD-ROM Figure 79 Keratoconus cases: Patient 3: 6 of 15).

3. **Video**

Rose K

BC 5.70 mm   D 8.7 mm   BVP –17.00 D

Going slightly flatter reveals a similar vaulting appearance. This suggests that this base curve is also too steep (CD-ROM Figure 80 Keratoconus cases: Patient 3: 7 of 15).

A Rose K lens with a 5.80-mm BC, standard peripheral curve system was ordered. The fluorescein pattern was identical to the trial fitting. Comfort was excellent. The patient could wear the lens all waking hours but didn't. Vision was so variable that he actually preferred his original pair. The measured optic zone was 6.5 mm, which was not unreasonably small. Part of the reason for this variable vision may have been due to some vaulting with this base curve.

Here is an example where the fluorescein pattern (and probably post-wear health) might be acceptable, but the vision was not. So, an alternative design needs to be used.

4. **Video**

ComfortKone

BC 5.80 mm   A20   D 8.5 mm   BVP –10.00 D

The Infinity lens (the larger OZ of all the designs with spherical OZ and aspheric peripheries) would have been my first choice for this design but the trial set was not available. The Valley K would have been the next choice since its OZ (5.0) is larger than the ComfortKone's (4.0), but this was not available either. Therefore, the ComfortKone was fitted (CD-ROM Figure 81 Keratoconus cases: Patient 3: Video: 8 of 15).

The first ComfortKone chosen was the closest base curve to the best fitting Rose K lens. Note the central area. Although the entire weight of the lens is concentrated in the center, it would not be considered heavy bearing. In fact, it could be described as aligned centrally. The paracentral and peripheral portion reveals extreme pooling. The patient was not comfortable with this lens. Endpoint acuity was a variable 20/25–. The periphery of this lens is too flat and needs a smaller A value.

5. **Video**

ComfortKone

BC 5.70 mm   A15   D 8.5 mm   BVP –11.00 D

This lens was trialed because of the smaller A value. The lens centers well. The central area in this lens also supports all the weight of the lens. Again, it is more of an aligned pattern as opposed to the heavy bearing seen in his original lens. The mid-peripheral portion of this lens also seems more aligned. The edge lift is excessive. Although the A15 edge lift is better than that of the A20, it is still uncomfortable to the patient. Endpoint acuity was 20/25– (CD-ROM Figure 82 Keratoconus cases: Patient 3: Video: 9 of 15).

Comments

This lens would not work for this patient. There is a good possibility that a lower A value (an A10, for example) might have given an acceptable peripheral pattern and improved comfort, but the limitation would be the acuity.

At this point, it was clear that a larger optic zone would be needed to match the clear, consistent acuity of his present lenses.

6. **Video**

Menicon

BC 5.72 mm   D 9.2 mm   BVP –19.00 D

The next design tried was Menicon's Decentered optic zone for keratoconus. Since it appears that the cone might be a large sagging one, this might be the optimum design. The standard fitting set has a 9.2-mm diameter, with a 7.0-mm optic zone. The secondary curve is 7.5 mm (0.6) for most base curves. The flattest base curve has an 8.0-mm secondary curve (0.6). The intermediate curve is 9.5 mm (0.3) and the peripheral curve is 12.0 mm (0.2).

This lens centers, but movement has to be questioned. It's actually difficult to view tear exchange. There is a small air bubble in the pooling surrounding the apex of the cone. Even though there is no heavy bearing centrally, this central base curve is a little too steep. The mid-peripheral bearing and low edge lift support this.

Movement is minimal. The mid-peripheral portion still seems to have too much bearing. With the proper over-refraction, vision was clear (20/20–), but variable. A flatter lens of the same design was needed (CD-ROM Figure 83 Keratoconus cases: Patient 3: Video: 10 of 15).

7. **Video**

Menicon

BC 5.82 mm D 9.2 mm   BVP –18.00 D

This lens centers well. Adequate movement and tear exchanged are observed. The central area over the cone displays almost an alignment pattern over the cone. There is a small area of pooling around the large apex and an alignment pattern in the mid-peripheral region. Good edge lift is seen until the superior portion of the lens (under the lid) is observed. Although the edge lift is not ideal, there is an alignment relationship in that area. This pattern reveals excellent distribution of weight-bearing forces (CD-ROM Figure 84 Keratoconus cases: Patient 3: Video: 11 of 15).

The lens is comfortable and does not dislodge during eye movement. Endpoint acuity is clear, but again, very variable.

8. **Video**

   Menicon

   BC 5.92 mm   D 9.2 mm   BVP −17.00 D

   The next flatter base curve was trialed for comparison. Looking at the fluorescein pattern over the cone, there is more touch, although it clearly remains light. A small air bubble appears in the clearance over the superior mid-peripheral region. The remainder of the mid-peripheral region and periphery reveals pooling, suggesting this lens may be too flat (CD-ROM Figure 85 Keratoconus cases: Patient 3: Video: 12 of 15).

   If this design was to be ordered, the 5.82-mm base curve appears to be the best; however, it's clear that the patient appreciates the secondary zone and is not satisfied with the visual result.

   The Nicone lens will now be tried. Although the design is proprietary, there is some control of lens parameters.

9. **Video**

   Nicone #2

   BC 5.80 mm   D/OZ 9.3 mm/7.0 mm   BVP −11.00 D

   The 5.80-mm base curve seems to be the appropriate curve for this cone apex for several designs and was also chosen for the Nicone design. Unfortunately all of the lenses available in the fitting set had significantly larger diameters than preferred. Three-dimensional thinking is needed to look at selected areas. The central area over the cone is fairly aligned. This is a large cone, but there doesn't seem to be any heavy bearing. The scarring at the cone apex is evident. The intermediate area or mid-peripheral area is bearing too much. In time there could be seal off even though the edge lift seems to be adequate. With proper over-refraction the acuity was a clear, consistent 20/20− and the patient was thrilled. Not knowing the second and third zones or base curves for this lens, since it is proprietary information, lens diameter and optic zone were decreased to achieve a more aligned peripheral relationship (CD-ROM Figure 86 Keratoconus cases: Patient 3: Video: 13 of 15).

   The following lens was ordered:

   Nicone #2

   Material OP3

   BC 5.80 mm   D/OZ 8.7 mm/6.5 mm   BVP −15.00 D (Peripheral curve information is proprietary.)

F. **Follow-up**

   1. **Video**

      One-week follow-up visit

      Nicone #2

      Material OP3

BC 5.80 mm   D/OZ 8.7 mm/6.5 mm   BVP –15.00 D (Peripheral curve information is proprietary.)

Centrally, note the even weight distribution over the cone. There is a large kissing area of touch as evidenced by the light tear exchange with the blink. In the mid-peripheral portion of the lens, there is a balance of weight distribution. There may be a little too much touch in the superior quadrant than desired but this is where compromises are made. Peripherally there is adequate edge lift for tear pumping action. The patient's acuity is 20/20–. Wearing time is 16 hours/day and comfortable throughout the entire wearing schedule (CD-ROM Figure 87 Keratoconus cases: Patient 3: Video: 14 of 15).

The patient's vision and comfort remain acceptable to date. The lenses are polished at the office visit.

This is an example where perseverance and patience ultimately produced a successful result. Although the Rose K and Menicon decentered OZ lenses fit well from the practitioner's viewpoint, the vision was not acceptable, and therefore did not satisfy the criterion of a successful fit.

IX. Keratoconus Cases: Patient #4
A. History
A 50-year-old white male presented for a contact lens evaluation. Although he was to be followed every 6 months, his last visit had been over 3 years ago. His complaint was decreased vision, both distance and near, for about 6 months. Comfort OS was excellent. Wearing time was all waking hours. He was using the Boston cleaning system with enzyme weekly.

Distance acuity was 20/50, near acuity was J2. Acuity could not be improved with over-refraction. He had been wearing the following lens parameters successfully for 6 years. This lens was 3 years old.

B. Lens Parameters
KAS design SGP II

BC (posterior apical radius)	BVP	D/OZ
OS 6.18 mm	–11.00 D	8.6 mm/7.9 mm

At the last visit, acuity in the left eye was 20/30+ at distance and J1 at near. The lens centered, revealed light bearing over the cone with areas of bearing in the mid-peripheral region allowing the weight of the contact lens to be more evenly distributed over the cornea. Other than minimal 3 and 9 staining, post-wear biomicroscopy was unremarkable.

C. Video
His present KAS lens centers and moves appropriately. There is a large area of light bearing centrally, surrounded by pooling. Bearing is also present in the mid-peripheral region, inducing **corneal wrinkling** underneath the lens. Note the area of 9:00 staining. Higher magnification views are on the next screens (CD-ROM Figure 88 Keratoconus cases: Patient 4: Video: 2 of 12).

D. Topography

This cone is very large and has a slightly inferior-temporal location. Since the X, Y, and Z coordinates are not quite zero, one must realize the location is not exact. This cone could probably be described as a nipple cone, as opposed to a low sagging one, but due to the size it's not definite. A clue would be the fluorescein pattern of his present lens. The position of the cone seems to be more centrally located. This would enforce the description of a nipple-type cone (CD-ROM Figure 89 Keratoconus cases: Patient 4: 6 of 12).

E. Design considerations for refitting

This patient had been wearing an aspheric design successfully for many years. Now that vision is reduced, one has to ask if it is just the age of the lens, or the fact that the cone changed a little.

A design change was made in an attempt to maximize the distance vision and fluorescein pattern. With a multifocal lens, vision can be slightly compromised, even if the patient does not have keratoconus. The patient understands that his presbyopia will truly manifest itself, now that the multifocal will be removed. Having to wear reading glasses for close work no longer presented a problem as he wanted vision to be as sharp and stable as possible.

The first design trialed was a spherical base curve with an aspheric periphery. This seemed to be the logical choice after years of aspheric wear. Both the Valley K and ComfortKone have spherical OZs and aspheric peripheries. The Valley K was first trialed.

1. Video

Valley K

BC 6.25 mm standard PC system   D 8.5 mm   BVP –12.00 D

Upon immediate evaluation, it can be seen that this lens is too steep. There is apical clearance centrally with a large air bubble. The bearing in the mid-periphery is excessive with little edge lift. There is minimal to no movement. The lens maintains an inferior position. Comfort was poor (CD-ROM Figure 90 Keratoconus cases: Patient 4: Video: 8 of 12).

2. Video

Valley K

BC 6.49 mm standard PC system   D 8.5 mm   BVP –10.00 D

A flatter Valley K was placed onto the eye. This lens centers and moves well. There is excellent tear exchange. Note the light, kissing touch over the cone. The remainder of the central area is clearance but not excessive. The mid-peripheral bearing appears to be a little too heavy. This did not present a problem since a flatter peripheral curve system can be requested. There is a possibility that the topography of his present cone would change now that the heavier bearing was no longer present with the KAS lens (CD-ROM Figure 91 Keratoconus cases: Patient 4: Video: 9 of 12).

This lens was extremely comfortable. With the proper over-refraction, acuity was a stable 20/25−, which thrilled the patient. A flatter peripheral curve system was tried to alleviate the heavy mid-peripheral bearing.

3.   Video

Valley K

Boston ES

BC 6.49 mm flatter PC system   D 8.5 mm   BVP −9.75 D

This lens centers and moves well. The central fluorescein pattern is almost identical to the trial lens, a light, kissing touch over the cone, surrounded by an area of clearance. The mid-peripheral relationship exhibits light touch with acceptable edge lift. There is excellent tear exchange overall. Acuity is 20/25 with excellent comfort. The patient was instructed to substitute this lens for his present lens, wearing and caring for it as before (CD-ROM Figure 92 Keratoconus cases: Patient 4: Video: 10 of 12).

4.   Video

One month later, the patient is wearing this lens all waking hours. The lens is comfortable and acuity remains 20/25. He continues using the Boston care system. The fluorescein pattern looked identical to the day it was dispensed. Post-wear biomicroscopy was excellent. In fact, the 9:00 staining that was present with his old lens was no longer there (CD-ROM Figure 93 Keratoconus cases: Patient 4: Video: 11 of 12).

Although the mid-peripheral area might look steeper than one might like, this pattern probably indicates more of an alignment relationship; otherwise the physiological response would not be as good as it is.

Comments

Since it appears that the cone is stable, one might consider that the age of the patient's presenting lens was the reason vision was reduced. This might very well have been the case, but with the newer keratoconic designs available, an attempt was made to find a lens to satisfy criteria with a more satisfactory fluorescein pattern. If one looks carefully at the central area over the cone, the corneal wrinkling which was present in the KAS lens has been eliminated.

X.   Keratoconus Cases: Patient #5

A.   History

A 36-year-old white male presented to me for a contact lens evaluation. He had tried rigid lenses once before in an optometrist's office. He did not feel his vision was improved with the contact lenses. He would like to try again to improve his vision. There was no information as to what type of rigid lenses had been attempted before. Only the right eye will be evaluated.

Visual acuity was OD 20/30 with manifest refraction of +0.75 –2.75 × 15.

B. Topography

This pattern could be described as a lower, sagging-type of cone (CD-ROM Figure 94 Keratoconus cases: Patient 5: 2 of 4).

Comments

Because this cone is in a lower position than the classic nipple type of cone, a first choice was a lens that could be made in a larger diameter/optic zone combination. A Nicone lens was first trialed. The final vision was 20/40+. There was no improvement in acuity. The next design tried was Menicon's decentered optic zone for keratoconus. Unfortunately, Menicon has suspended business in the U.S. market at the time of this writing.

C. Video

Menicon Z material

BC 6.62 mm   D/OZ 9.2 mm/7.0 mm   BVP –6.25 D

Remainder of parameters standard for this design.

The base curve of this lens corresponds to the darker green ring of the topography map. This is approximately the base of the cone. Notice that this lens maintains an inferior position. This should be expected because of the prism that is standard with this design (as well as centering over the steepest area of the cornea, the cone). In this inferior location, it can be appreciated that the patient is almost looking through the flatter annular zone that surrounds the decentered optic zone. If this lens remains in a static position, it could compromise acuity, but as the patient blinks and moves his eye, the lens floats nicely over the entire cornea. Visual acuity is a crisp 20/25 (CD-ROM Figure 95 Keratoconus cases: Patient 5: Video: 3 of 4).

During the blink, as the lens moves to a more central location, a light touch over the cone can be appreciated. Interestingly enough, with the fluorescein pattern, it should be noted that the apex of the cone is not quite as inferior as one would have expected from topography. The intermediate area of the fluorescein pattern varies with the location of the contact lens on the eye. Because of the decentered optic zone, this paracentral light bearing is a horseshoe pattern. As the lens is pushed to a more superior location (that might simulate downgaze) there seems to be more bearing throughout the entire lens surface. This should be expected since the superior cornea is significantly flatter than the inferior cornea.

The weight distribution of this lens for this cornea is excellent through most positions of gaze. Even though there may be too much bearing when the eye is in extreme downgaze (i.e., the lens is in a very superior position), this is not the majority of the time. Also the hyper-DK value allows for oxygen transmissibility during these moments. At the time of this writing, Menicon has suspended business in the U.S. market but is expected to resume.

Chapter 29

Post-Penetrating Keratoplasty

Shelley I. Cutler

I. **Approximately 20%** of patients who undergo a penetrating keratoplasty will benefit from a contact lens correction. Even in the hands of the most skilled surgeon, there may be an irregular surface or high corneal astigmatism as a result of the surgery. Anisometropia may also exist, which necessitates contact lens correction.

   A. **Several factors** that have nothing to do with the surgery itself may complicate the fitting process. Included are physiology of donor cornea, existing host corneal disease and/or neovascularization (pre- or post-surgery), and tear film abnormalities.

   B. **Corneal lenses** are the optimal choice. Sometimes this is not possible and alternatives, including soft lenses, piggyback fits (soft lenses in combination with a rigid corneal lens), scleral RGPs, and hybrid lenses may be the only successful option. The focus will be on corneal lenses.

   C. **Graft rejection** can be precipitated by contact lens wear. It is important to be able to recognize the signs and symptoms. These signs also occur as routine contact lens wear complications and could cause confusion to the practitioner. Subjective complaints can include ocular discomfort or pain, redness, tearing, and reduced vision.

   D. Rejection can involve the **entire cornea** or the **epithelium**. For an epithelial rejection, an elevated line might be seen across the cornea and/or sub-epithelial infiltrates. Endothelial rejection, which is a far more serious situation, can present with a significant anterior chamber reaction, including keratic precipitates, or can display corneal edema and stromal thickening if endothelial function is disrupted.

II. **Topographic maps** can maximize efficiency and minimize time when fitting post PK corneas. Once a shape factor is decided, an initial lens design and lens can be selected. Several surface patterns can be found following a transplant. Tripoli et al.[1] has designated different topographies after the sutures are removed. Regular astigmatism can be seen as both a **prolate shape** (steeper

451

centrally and flattening peripherally) or **oblate pattern** (flatter centrally and steepening peripherally). There can be a combination butterfly pattern of a **mixed prolate oblate** within the donor cornea. **Asymmetric astigmatism** may be seen in which the two steep semi-meridians are not aligned along a single meridian. Resulting from uneven suturing or healing, the surface pattern can be seen as a steep red area on one side and becoming progressively flatter toward the other side **(steep to flat)**. Finally, every once in a while a cornea gives a similar appearance to that of a **keratoconic pattern**. There is inferior steepening with a more normal appearance superior.

III.   **Lenses** available for fitting the graft are available to address the grafted cornea. Larger diameters usually work better than smaller ones. Standard lens designs as well as **aspheric, biaspheric lenses (the Boston Envision)**, and **bitoric lenses** should all be considered. Two companies make lens designs specifically for penetrating keratoplasties.

    A.   **The POST PK** by Lens Dynamics consists of two basic designs. The first is a 10.4 diameter with a 9.0-mm fixed optic zone. The second is a 10.4-mm diameter with a floating optic zone. The OZ decreases as base curve steepens. There are proprietary sets of peripheral curves that flatten from the BC to fit the outer portion of the cornea (the host) prior to surgery.

    B.   **The PSC (Post Surgical Cornea)** is a lens by Infinity Optical. It is fit on the sagittal value principle and has the same basic concept as their keratoconic lenses. The difference is that these lenses are larger in diameter and flatter in base curve. The periphery of the lens should rest on the peripheral area of the cornea as far away from the surgery as practical. The optic zone is spherical and 1.5 mm smaller than the diameter of the lens. The peripheral curve system is aspheric with three edge lift values available. The trial lenses will be in the standard lift.

    C.   **Reverse geometry designs** can address the idiosyncrasies of the post-PK cornea. This is where the secondary curve is steeper than the base curve of a lens, creating a plateau shape. Some of the proprietary designs are:

        1.   **The PK Bridge** by Conforma Labs. This lens has a secondary curve that is a reverse aspheric surface. It progresses from the center towards the paraperipheral region with no hard zone. The targeted amount of steepening is about 3 diopters. The peripheral curve is an aspheric flattening. The downside of this lens is that it induces some cylinder when verified on radioscope and lensometer.

        2.   **The NRK** by Lancaster Contact Lens is a patented design, which follows scientific formulas to produce a contact lens that is steeper in the periphery than the central base curve. Diameters are usually 10.0 mm or larger with an 8.0-mm optic zone, but these can be altered by the fitter as needed. Final design parameters are suggested after a trial fitting.

        3.   **The OK series** by Contex offers a lot of variety as far as reverse geometry designs are concerned. The second steeper curve is des-

ignated by the name on the lens: OK-3 (3 diopters steeper than the base curve); OK-4 (4 diopters steeper than the base curve); OK-6 (6 diopters steeper than the base curve); etc. The secondary steeper curve can be spherical or aspheric. The peripheral curve is aspheric. Larger diameters are recommended. A good starting point is a 10.2-mm diameter, an 8.0-mm optic zone, with the OK-3 design.

4. **The Plateau Lens** by Menicon, USA, is a proprietary design consisting of a spherical base curve, a secondary curve steeper than the BC (usually around 3 diopters but as high as 7 diopters) and an aspheric peripheral curve system. All parameters can be designated by the fitter; however, the standard lens has a 10.0 mm/8.0 mm (D/OZ) and a secondary curve that will be 3 diopters steeper than the designated base curve.

IV. **Initial Lens Selection** will vary depending on the surface patterned revealed from corneal topography. Tripoli et al. has designated different topographies after the sutures are removed.[1]

A. **Prolate pattern** has a steeper central area and a flatter periphery. This is seen in 31% of the corneas. The donor cornea is almost protruding out. Sometimes, a donor button that is too large will cause this type of topography after the graft is in place. Using corneal topography as a guide, several lens designs could be trialed initially. A large diameter sphere, aspheric, or biaspheric (the Boston Envision) lens would be a good initial choice. Depending on the amount of toricity, a toric base or bitoric lens would be a reasonable choice. On occasion, depending on the location and the size of the toric portion of the graft, a keratoconic design might be the optimum choice (CD-ROM Figure 96 Penetrating keratoplasty: Prolate Graft: 2 of 7).

B. **Oblate pattern** is plateau shaped. This is seen in 31% of the corneas. The flatter donor cornea is surrounded by steeper host cornea. A reverse geometry is ideal for this type of pattern. Depending on the amount of astigmatism present, a toric basic curve or bitoric reverse geometry design might allow for better weight distribution. On occasion, a standard design (be it spherical, aspheric, or toric) might be successful if there is good lens/eyelid interaction but usually there is too much edge lift and central bearing (CD-ROM Figure 97 Penetrating keratoplasty: Oblate Graft: 3 of 7).

C. **Mixed Prolate Oblate Pattern** has a flat side and a steep side of the cornea. There is a roughly symmetrical astigmatism present. This is seen in 18% of the corneas. A toric base curve or bitoric design proves to be the most successful in these cases (CD-ROM Figure 98 Penetrating keratoplasty: Mixed Graft: 4 of 7).

D. **Asymmetric Astigmatism** is a combination of all patterns and can be seen in this pattern. The cornea looks irregular and distorted. This is seen in 9% of the corneas. Large biaspheric (Boston Envision) or standard design works well for these patterns. An attempt to fit the peripheral host cornea as best as possible is a good goal to strive for. On occasion a toric base curve (or bitoric design) will distribute the weight of the lens more appropriately. The post-PK or PSC designs might be a good choice in these situations (CD-ROM Figure 99 Penetrating keratoplasty: Asymmetric Graft: 5 of 7).

E.   **Steep to Flat** is steep on one side, flat on the other side. It is like a mixed prolate oblate pattern without the symmetrical astigmatism. This is seen in 13% of the corneas. This by far is the most difficult pattern to fit. The lens wants to center over the steepest part of the cornea. This often leads to a decentered lens onto the sclera. Large diameters are needed so the optic zone will cross the visual axis. One could start with a large sphere, aspheric, or biaspheric (Boston Envision) design. Good lid interaction is needed for stabilization. The PSC or post-PK might be an optimal choice as an initial lens selection (CD-ROM Figure 100 Penetrating keratoplasty: Steep Graft: 6 of 7).

F.   **Keratoconic** is when the cornea protrudes a great amount, a keratoconic pattern will appear. If this pattern results, a keratoconic design could be a good starting point. An attempt to fit a large, high riding lens would also be a reasonable option (CD-ROM Figure 101 Penetrating keratoplasty: Keratoconic Graft: 7 of 7).

V.   **Evaluation** of the fit begins with insertion of the selected lens on the eye and allow the patient to adapt. Instill fluorescein and evaluate the lens position and pattern. Thoughts vary as to whether the optic zone should be within the donor button or larger and vaulting it. One needs to be flexible when fitting the grafted cornea. What is an optimal fit for one graft will be totally inappropriate for another. The important point to remember is to try to distribute the weight bearing forces of the contact lens as evenly as possible.

A.   **Observe the center** of the graft. Is there too much bearing? Then using standard methods, attempt to vault the area more. Is there an obvious toricity? Would toric base curves be stabler? Or is the reverse observed? Is there an air bubble present, suggesting too much vaulting and a steep pattern? Use standard methods to flatten the relationship.

B.   **Observe the paracentral** or **mid-peripheral area** of the lens. This usually directly relates to the graft-host junction. It is most important to try to align this area the best you can. Many times it is most difficult to nearly impossible. This is where you may need to try several different designs to see which one centers the best, moves, and distributes the weight most evenly.

C.   **Observe the periphery** of the lens. There should be adequate edge lift to promote good tear exchange. In some situations, there is excessive lift due to a sharp junction where the host and donor corneas meet. Do your best to minimize desiccation on the underlying cornea. Sometimes this is impossible.

    D. **Some situations are beyond your control.** A "pretty" fit may not be possible. There are occasions, in which the contour of the cornea does not allow what the majority of practitioners would even label as an acceptable fit. You may have followed all of the normal fitting protocols and rules of rigid contact lenses and all lenses have ejected out of the eye. In these cases, one must strive to get something to stay in the eye. Attempting to fit a lens that rides high with the eyelid usually yields the best success. (The alternative after this is piggyback, scleral lenses, hybrids, etc.) Use your knowledge of maximizing eye-to-lid forces and lens edge carriers to accomplish this.

    E. **A successful fit** may include a fluorescein pattern that may look excessively flat to you or appear blatantly ugly. Under normal circumstances you might try something else. Under these circumstances, be grateful something is staying in the eye, and follow the patient. If all goes well, this may end up being a successful fit. If it doesn't, then continue the fitting process.

VI. Penetrating Keratoplasty Cases: Patient A

    A. **History**

        An 81-year-old white male presented for a contact lens fit of his left eye. He had undergone penetrating keratoplasty to improve vision secondary to pseudophakic bullous keratopathy 2 years previously. Ocular history after the transplant included an episode of conjunctivitis, an IOP spike, and an early graft rejection. Entering acuity was 20/300 with a correction of plano to –0.75 D.

    B. **Video**

        The surface irregularity and edema of the cornea can be seen in the host cornea. The graft, however, is clear. Until the topography is viewed, one might question why the vision is so poor (CD-ROM Figure 102 Penetrating keratoplasty cases: Patient A: Video: 2 of 15).

    C. **Topography**

        The surface pattern is one of an oblate high (about 7 D) astigmatic pattern. There is a figure-eight butterfly shape, flatter in the center than in the periphery. This irregularity could be the explanation of decreased acuity and this patient should see clearer with a rigid contact lens (CD-ROM Figure 103 Penetrating keratoplasty cases: Patient A: Topography: 4 of 15).

        General Thoughts

        Many experts advocate large, flat lenses for fitting a graft. This is a good starting point, but a more ideal goal would be to contour a lens to the cornea as best as possible. The first lenses attempted will be reverse geometry lenses. This makes sense considering the oblate shape of the cornea. The NRK from Lancaster is a reverse geometry lens. Base curves, diameters, and optic zones can be altered, but the rest of the design is proprietary.

    D. **Trial Fittings**

        1. **Video**

           NRK

BC 8.05 mm   D/OZ 10.5 mm/8.0 mm   BVP +0.75 D

This base curve was selected because this was the closest lens available in the fitting set to his flat K reading. If you look at the Sim K reading (43.50), the 8.05 BC might be considered excessively flat, but if you then look at the minimum K (41.52), the BC is just minimally steeper than this. Sometimes you just have to try what you have, evaluate the fluorescein pattern, and go on from there (CD-ROM Figure 104 Penetrating keratoplasty cases: Patient A: Video: 6 of 15).

This lens positions superior and somewhat temporally. The bearing over the central cornea is evident, but appears somewhat nasal due to the overall location of the lens. There is pooling in the mid-peripheral area, most noted temporally. The excessive pooling and edge lift is obvious by the little air bubble seen around 5:00.

This lens is overall too flat. Now we know that the Sim K reading is more appropriate. More NRK loaner lenses with base curves between 7.70 mm and 7.90 mm were requested.

2. **Video**

NRK#1

BC 7.74 mm   D/OZ 10.3 mm/8.0 mm   BVP +0.25 D

This was the next trial lens used. It was the closest of the loaner lenses available to the flat Sim K reading. This lens maintains a superior lid-attached position. On a rare occasion, not captured on film, it does release as the patient moves his eye around. Note the overall central bearing. It's not a heavy bearing and might be described as an aligned to flat relationship. The mid-peripheral area varies with the corneal topography. There are areas of pooling and areas of bearing. If you look closely in the peripheral portion of the lens, there is subtle light touch where the flat portion of the cornea is in close proximity to the lens edge (CD-ROM Figure 105 Penetrating keratoplasty cases: Patient A: Video: 7 of 15).

The upper lid was elevated to get an appreciation of the overall relationship without lid forces. One can see the typical flat pattern. The overall fit is reminiscent of a Korb or lid-controlled fit. Over-refraction yielded 20/40 acuity. For comparison, the other loaners were trialed.

3. **Video**

NRK#1

BC 7.78 mm   D/OZ 10.5 mm/8.0 mm   BVP +1.75 D

This lens is very similar to the previous one. The diameter is a little larger and the base curve is minimally flatter. The overall appearance is not that much different, a lid-attached lens that is fit flatter than K. There is more clearance in the periphery as noted by the air bubble. As the patient blinks, there appears to be too much mass in general, pressing harder on the cornea. The smaller diameter is preferred (CD-ROM Figure 106 Penetrating keratoplasty cases: Patient A: Video: 8 of 15).

4. **Video**

NRK

BC 7.82 mm   D/OZ 9.9 mm/6.5 mm   BVP +0.25 D

This lens has a slightly flatter base curve, as well as a smaller diameter. The sagittal depth is reduced and renders this lens too flat. Note the decentered position nasally. The lens even extends over the nasal limbus. The bearing is evident in the central area of the cornea, which is the temporal area of the lens, surrounded by mid-peripheral and peripheral clearance (CD-ROM Figure 107 Penetrating keratoplasty cases: Patient A: Video: 9 of 15).

5. **Video**

SPE Bitoric

BC 7.95 mm/7.35 mm   D/OZ 9.6 mm/7.7 mm   (delta K = 3D)

BVP PL −3.00 D × flat meridian

For comparison, some bitoric lenses were trialed to see if a flat toric base curve might align better with the cornea. For the few moments that the lens raises with the lid, the fluorescein pattern looks very aligned, centrally, mid-peripherally, with acceptable edge lift. However, the lens would not stay attached to the lid, once the patient adapted. Note in this inferior position, the heavy bearing as the lens presses against the inferior quadrant of the host cornea. With a heavy blink, an air bubble is induced (CD-ROM Figure 108 Penetrating keratoplasty cases: Patient A: Video: 10 of 15).

6. **Video**

SPE Bitoric

BC 8.23 mm/7.62 mm   D/OZ 9.6 mm/7.8 mm   (delta K = 3.25)

BVP PL −3.25 D × flat meridian

A flatter base curve was attempted to improve the fit. This lens does maintain a longer lid attached position with the blink, but only initially. When held up by the lid, note the overall flat pattern (central bearing with mid-peripheral and peripheral pooling) and excessive edge lift inferiorly. The lens has a tendency to release from the eyelid, preferring the inferior position. In this position, the central bearing and mid-peripheral pooling is still present as well as the inferior arcuate bearing as the lens presses against the inferior quadrant of the host cornea (CD-ROM Figure 109 Penetrating keratoplasty cases: Patient A: Video: 11 of 15).

A minus edge carrier could be placed on the lens to help maintain a superior position, but the reverse geometry design offered a better fit. The NRK looked like a better fit over the bitoric.

The following lens was ordered:

NRK #1

BC 7.75 mm   D/OZ 10.3 mm/8.0 mm   BVP +0.75 D

7. **Video**

NRK #1

BC 7.75 mm   D/OZ 10.3 mm/8.0 mm   BVP +0.75 D

This is the ordered lens on a 2-week progress visit. The patient has limited wearing time to 8 hours, as instructed. He is using the Boston System, no enzyme at this point. Visual acuity with a –1.00 D over-refraction was 20/40.

The lens centers fairly well. It stays in place on lateral movement. Most of the time it is tucked under the upper eyelid, but will release on occasion. There is heavy central bearing, mid-peripheral, and peripheral pooling. This a flat fit (CD-ROM Figure 110 Penetrating keratoplasty cases: Patient A: Video: 12 of 15).

8. Video

In grafts, flat fits are acceptable if the eye remains healthy. Although hard to see in this video, there was some superficial punctate staining that developed under the area of bearing. It was followed for a few weeks and was not acceptable (CD-ROM Figure 111 Penetrating keratoplasty cases: Patient A: Video: 13 of 15).

9. Video

NRK

BC 7.80 mm   D/OZ 9.5 mm/7.8 mm   BVP –1.00 D

A marginally flatter but considerably smaller in diameter lens was tried in an attempt to reduce the staining. Decreasing the diameter of a lens, as well as flattening the base curve, should produce an overall flatter relationship by reduction of sag. However, there was an overall decrease in lens mass to allow a looser, lighter fit. The position is under the eyelid in a central temporal location. This is only in primary gaze. As the patients looks laterally the lens moves freely and does not dislocate. There is a central area of bearing; however, the weight seems to be distributed more than the previous 7.75-mm BC.

There is mid-peripheral and peripheral pooling, indicative of the flat fit; however, as the patient looks laterally there is light contact of the peripheral curves with the host cornea. The lens is comfortable and the patient doesn't really notice any difference in acuity than the previous one. Over-refraction is +0.50 D 20/40. The patient was released with this lens (CD-ROM Figure 112 Penetrating keratoplasty cases: Patient A: Video: 14 of 15).

When the patient returned 2 weeks later, the lens position and movement remained the same. The SPK was no longer present. The same parameters were ordered with a –0.50 power. He is presently appreciating 20/40 vision, wearing the lens all waking hours, and very happy.

This is an example where the fluorescein pattern may not be pretty or perfect, but it satisfies criteria. In the future, toric base curves with the reverse geometry configuration may be considered.

VII. Penetrating Keratoplasty Cases: Patient B

A. History

A 79-year-old white male presented for a contact lens fitting of his left eye. He had a penetrating keratoplasty secondary to bullous keratopathy

9 years previously. Visual acuity with a manifest refraction of + 0.50 −6.00 × 90 was 20/50.

B. Topography

This is an interesting surface pattern. The pattern appears to be a mixed prolate oblate pattern. Centrally there are approximately 6 diopters of against-the-rule astigmatism, which is present in the refraction. There is an obvious steepening in the inferior nasal quadrant (from about 5:00 to 10:00) that will be the challenge of this fit (CD-ROM Figure 113 Penetrating keratoplasty cases: Patient B: 2 of 6).

Fitting Considerations

With the against-the-rule astigmatism over the visual axis, a bitoric lens was first attempted. The approach was treating the eye as a routine toric cornea. If relatively high position of the lens is maintained, inferior lens-cornea interaction may be avoided where the cornea is relatively steep.

C. Trial Fittings

1. Video

SPE Bitoric

BC 7.50 mm/7.03 mm (45.00/48.00)   D/OZ 9.6 mm/7.5 mm

BVP PL −3.00 D × flat meridian

A flat K, slightly steeper than the flat Sim K, was chosen. Looking carefully at the topography, it can be noted that the Sim K value is a very small area. The dioptric value is surrounded by an area that is slightly steeper in value. This was the flat meridian on the chosen lens.

The lens centers and has a central, superior, central type of movement. When the lens rises under the eyelid, the fluorescein pattern reveals a more even distribution of bearing forces. The light bearing centrally over the flat area of the cornea is evident, which is at the lower position of the lens. The paracentral area in the superior cornea shows light clearance. The edge lift is adequate.

When the lens releases from the lid and falls, the bearing now appears in the superior quadrant of the lens. The light paracentral pooling is displayed in the mid-peripheral region. Light bearing areas can be seen anterior to the peripheral curve. Overall there is a good weight distribution of lens, but a more constant superior position is preferred (CD-ROM Figure 114 Penetrating keratoplasty cases: Patient B: Video: 3 of 6).

To maximize lid grab, a minus edge lenticular carrier will be ordered. The diameter was made slightly larger as well. In an attempt to contour the cornea a little better, a steeper base curve in both meridians will be the trialed. Over-refraction yielded 20/50 acuity.

2. Video

SPE Bitoric

Boston ES

BC 7.42 mm/6.96 mm (45.50/48.50)   D/OZ 9.8 mm/7.5 mm

BVP +0.50 −3.00 × flat meridian

The steeper lens centers and the larger diameter help keep it in a more superior position, but it continues to release from the eyelid. In the superior position a more aligned pattern can be seen; however, as the lens drops the flat meridian becomes more evident. The bearing is not heavy, so this is acceptable. There is a little more bearing in the mid-peripheral area just anterior to the peripheral curve than preferred, but only when the lens is in the lower position. There is excellent tear exchange. The patient appreciates 20/50 vision and is very happy (CD-ROM Figure 115 Penetrating keratoplasty cases: Patient B: Video: 5 of 6).

The patient built up wearing time conservatively and is now wearing the lens for all waking hours. The Boston care system was dispensed. Post-wear biomicroscopy remains unremarkable. This lens satisfies the criteria for a post-penetrating keratoplasty fit. Decreased lens diameter to the original trial size may be considered in the future to minimize some of the bearing anterior to the peripheral curve.

VIII. Penetrating Keratoplasy Cases: Patient C

A. History

An 87-year-old white female was referred for a contact lens post penetrating keratoplasty OS secondary to pseudophakic bullous keratopathy. Refraction OS was −6.50 −1.00 × 35 yielding a visual acuity of 20/60+. She had a great positive attitude about her ability to handle a contact lens, even though she had never worn lenses before.

B. Topography

This topography demonstrates what would be considered a flat to steep shape. If one looks at the simulated keratometic readings and the refraction, it does not appear as if there is a lot of astigmatism. This is the beauty of corneal topography. One can see on closer inspection that indeed there is more present, as evidence of the minimum K reading. Note that the X and Y axes are not aligned at zero. The real cylinder is probably just off the visual axis. The central findings are only a minimal part of this picture (CD-ROM Figure 116 Penetrating keratoplasty cases: Patient C: Topography: 2 of 3).

Comments

Both a reverse geometry lens and regular design of the same base curve were attempted at approximately the same diameter. There was no appreciable difference. There was significant bearing in the central region of the lens with pooling in the mid-peripheral and peripheral region. The fluorescein pattern of the standard design seemed to bear more evenly across the center than the reverse geometry lens. A 3 D toric base curve was trialed but this decentered inferiorly. A large diameter aspheric lens was tried in the hope that a lens can be found to fit the eye.

C. Video

Achievement lens from Art Optical

Boston 7 material

BC 7.75 mm   D 9.4 mm   BVP PL

With a steep to flat topographical configuration, one never knows how a given design is going to respond on an individual's eye until it is tried. Lenses will center over the steepest area of the cornea. Many times it is not at a desirable position. With a large and flat lens, the lid interaction can significantly change an unsuccessful attempt to a successful one. The patient has an extremely ptotic eyelid. Other designs were attempted but this standard design seemed to stay on her eye and give her the most consistent vision of all those tried. The lens fulfilled two important criteria: the lens stayed on the eye and it remained centered. Although the pattern appeared significantly flat in the center with a large amount of edge lift, the fit was acceptable. Final acuity was 20/40 (CD-ROM Figure 117 Penetrating keratoplasty cases: Patient C: Video: 3 of 3).

REFERENCE

1.   Tripoli NK, Ibrahim OS, Coggins, JM, et al. Quantitative and qualitative topography classification of clear penetrating keratoplasties. Invest Ophthal Vis Sci 1990;30(Suppl):480.

Appendixes

Appendix A Extended Keratometer Range with +1.25 D and −1.00 D Lenses

Actual Drum Reading	Extended Value	Actual Drum Reading	Extended Value
+1.25 D lenses			
43.00	50.13	47.62	55.53
43.12	50.28	47.75	55.67
43.25	50.42	47.87	55.82
43.37	50.57	48.00	55.96
43.50	50.72	48.12	56.11
43.62	50.86	48.25	56.25
43.75	51.01	48.37	56.40
43.87	51.15	48.50	56.55
44.00	51.30	48.62	56.69
44.12	51.44	48.75	56.84
44.25	51.59	48.87	56.98
44.37	51.74	49.00	57.13
44.50	51.88	49.12	57.27
44.62	52.03	49.25	57.42
44.75	52.17	49.37	57.57
44.87	52.32	49.50	57.71
45.00	52.46	49.62	57.86
45.12	52.61	49.75	58.00
45.25	52.76	49.87	58.15
45.37	52.90	50.00	58.30
45.50	53.05	50.12	58.44
45.62	53.19	50.25	58.59
45.75	53.34	50.37	58.73
45.87	53.49	50.50	58.88
46.00	53.63	50.62	59.02
46.12	53.78	50.75	59.17
46.25	53.92	50.87	59.31
46.37	54.07	51.00	59.46
46.50	54.21	51.12	59.61
46.62	54.36	51.25	59.75
46.75	54.51	51.37	59.90
46.87	54.65	51.50	60.04
47.00	54.80	51.62	60.19
47.12	54.94	51.75	60.33
47.25	55.09	51.87	60.48
47.37	55.23	52.00	60.63
47.50	55.38		

Appendix A   *(continued)*

Actual Drum Reading	Extended Value	Actual Drum Reading	Extended Value
−1.00 D lenses			
36.00	30.87	39.12	33.55
36.12	30.98	39.25	33.66
36.25	31.09	39.37	33.77
36.37	31.20	39.50	33.88
36.50	31.30	39.62	33.98
36.62	31.41	39.75	34.09
36.75	31.51	39.87	34.20
36.87	31.62	40.00	34.30
37.00	31.73	40.12	34.41
37.12	31.84	40.25	34.52
37.25	31.95	40.37	34.63
37.37	32.05	40.50	34.73
37.50	32.16	40.62	34.84
37.62	32.27	40.75	34.95
37.75	32.37	40.87	35.05
37.87	32.48	41.00	35.16
38.00	32.59	41.12	35.27
38.12	32.70	41.25	35.38
38.25	32.80	41.37	35.48
38.37	32.91	41.50	35.59
38.50	33.02	41.62	35.70
38.62	33.13	41.75	35.81
38.75	33.23	41.87	35.91
38.87	33.34	42.00	36.02
39.00	33.45		

Source: Adapted from ES Bennett, VA Henry. Appendix 3: Extended Keratometer Range with +1.25 D Lens. In ES Bennett, VA Henry (eds), Clinical Manual of Contact Lenses. Philadelphia: Lippincott, 1994;488–489.

Appendix B   Vertex Conversion Table of Plus and Minus Powers

Spectacle Lens Power	8 mm	9 mm	10 mm	11 mm	12 mm	13 mm	14 mm	15 mm
Plus power								
4.00	4.12	4.12	4.12	4.12	4.25	4.25	4.25	4.25
4.50	4.62	4.75	4.75	4.75	4.75	4.75	4.75	4.87
5.00	5.25	5.25	5.25	5.25	5.25	5.37	5.37	5.37
5.50	5.75	5.75	5.75	5.87	5.87	5.87	6.00	6.00
6.00	6.25	6.37	6.37	6.37	6.50	6.50	6.50	6.62
6.50	6.87	6.87	7.00	7.00	7.00	7.12	7.12	7.25
7.00	7.37	7.50	7.50	7.62	7.62	7.75	7.75	7.75
7.50	8.00	8.00	8.12	8.12	8.25	8.25	8.37	8.50
8.00	8.50	8.62	8.75	8.75	8.87	8.87	9.00	9.12
8.50	9.12	9.25	9.25	9.37	9.50	9.50	9.62	9.75
9.00	9.75	9.75	9.87	10.00	10.12	10.25	10.37	10.37
9.50	10.25	10.37	10.50	10.62	10.75	10.87	11.00	11.12
10.00	10.87	11.00	11.12	11.25	11.37	11.50	11.62	11.75
10.50	11.50	11.62	11.75	11.87	12.00	12.12	12.25	12.50
11.00	12.00	12.25	12.37	12.50	12.75	12.87	13.00	13.12
11.50	12.62	12.87	13.00	13.12	13.37	13.50	13.75	13.87
12.00	13.25	13.50	13.62	13.87	14.00	14.25	14.50	14.62
12.50	13.87	14.12	14.25	14.50	14.75	15.00	15.25	15.37
13.00	14.50	14.75	15.00	15.25	15.50	15.62	16.00	16.12
13.50	15.12	15.37	15.62	15.87	16.12	16.37	16.62	16.87
14.00	15.75	16.00	16.25	16.50	16.75	17.12	17.50	17.75
14.50	16.50	16.75	17.00	17.25	17.50	17.87	18.25	18.50
15.00	17.00	17.37	17.75	18.00	18.25	18.62	19.00	19.37
15.50	17.75	18.00	18.25	18.75	19.00	19.37	19.75	20.25
16.00	18.25	18.75	19.00	19.37	19.75	20.25	20.50	21.00
16.50	19.00	19.37	19.75	20.25	20.50	21.00	21.50	21.87
17.00	19.75	20.25	20.50	21.00	21.50	22.00	22.25	22.87
17.50	20.50	20.75	21.25	21.75	22.25	22.75	23.25	23.75
18.00	21.00	21.50	22.00	22.50	23.00	23.50	24.00	24.62
18.50	21.75	22.25	22.75	23.25	23.75	24.50	25.00	25.62
19.00	22.50	23.00	23.50	24.00	24.75	25.25	26.00	26.50

Appendix B   *(continued)*

Spectacle Lens Power	8 mm	9 mm	10 mm	11 mm	12 mm	13 mm	14 mm	15 mm
Minus power								
4.00	3.87	3.87	3.87	3.87	3.87	3.75	3.75	3.75
4.50	4.37	4.37	4.25	4.25	4.25	4.25	4.25	4.25
5.00	4.75	4.75	4.75	4.75	4.75	4.75	4.62	4.62
5.50	5.25	5.25	5.25	5.12	5.12	5.12	5.12	5.12
6.00	5.75	5.62	5.62	5.62	5.62	5.50	5.50	5.50
6.50	6.12	6.12	6.12	6.00	6.00	6.00	6.00	5.87
7.00	6.62	6.62	6.50	6.50	6.50	6.37	6.37	6.37
7.50	7.12	7.00	7.00	6.87	6.87	6.87	6.75	6.75
8.00	7.50	7.50	7.37	7.37	7.25	7.25	7.25	7.25
8.50	8.00	7.87	7.87	7.75	7.75	7.62	7.62	7.50
9.00	8.37	8.37	8.25	8.25	8.12	8.00	8.00	8.00
9.50	8.87	8.75	8.62	8.62	8.50	8.50	8.37	8.37
10.00	9.25	9.12	9.12	9.00	8.87	8.87	8.75	8.75
10.50	9.62	9.62	9.50	9.37	9.37	9.25	9.12	9.12
11.00	10.12	10.00	9.87	9.75	9.75	9.62	9.50	9.50
11.50	10.50	10.37	10.37	10.25	10.12	10.00	9.87	9.87
12.00	11.00	10.87	10.75	10.62	10.50	10.37	10.25	10.12
12.50	11.37	11.25	11.12	11.00	10.87	10.75	10.62	10.50
13.00	11.75	11.62	11.50	11.37	11.25	11.12	11.00	10.87
13.50	12.25	12.00	11.87	11.75	11.62	11.50	11.37	11.25
14.00	12.62	12.50	12.25	12.12	12.00	11.87	11.75	11.50
14.50	13.00	12.75	12.62	12.50	12.37	12.25	12.00	11.87
15.00	13.37	13.25	13.00	12.87	12.75	12.50	12.37	12.25
15.50	13.75	13.62	13.50	13.25	13.00	12.87	12.75	12.62
16.00	14.25	14.00	13.75	13.62	13.50	13.25	13.00	12.87
16.50	14.50	14.37	14.12	14.00	13.75	13.62	13.50	13.25
17.00	15.00	14.75	14.50	14.25	14.12	14.00	13.75	13.50
17.50	15.37	15.12	14.87	14.75	14.50	14.25	14.00	13.87
18.00	15.75	15.50	15.25	15.00	14.75	14.62	14.37	14.12
18.50	16.12	15.87	15.62	15.37	15.12	14.87	14.75	14.50
19.00	16.50	16.25	16.00	15.75	15.50	15.25	15.00	14.75

Source: Adapted from CA Schwartz. Appendix 6. In Schwartz CA (ed), Specialty Contact Lenses: A Fitter's Guide. Philadelphia: Saunders, 1996;319.1

Appendix C   Keratometer Conversion (Diopter to Millimeters)

Diopter	Milli-meters	Diopter	Milli-meters	Diopter	Milli-meters	Diopter	Milli-meters	Diopter	Milli-meters
36.00	9.37	40.12	8.41	44.25	7.63	48.37	6.98	52.50	6.43
36.12	9.34	40.25	8.38	44.37	7.61	48.50	6.96	52.62	6.41
36.25	9.31	40.37	8.36	44.50	7.58	48.62	6.94	52.75	6.40
36.37	9.27	40.50	8.33	44.62	7.56	48.75	6.92	52.87	6.38
36.50	9.24	40.62	8.30	44.75	7.54	48.87	6.91	53.00	6.36
36.62	9.21	40.75	8.28	44.87	7.52	49.00	6.89	53.12	6.35
36.75	9.18	40.87	8.25	45.00	7.50	49.12	6.87	53.25	6.34
36.87	9.15	41.00	8.23	45.12	7.48	49.25	6.85	53.37	6.32
37.00	9.12	41.12	8.20	45.25	7.46	49.37	6.84	53.50	6.31
37.12	9.09	41.25	8.18	45.37	7.44	49.50	6.82	53.62	6.29
37.25	9.06	41.37	8.16	45.50	7.42	49.62	6.80	53.75	6.28
37.37	9.03	41.50	8.13	45.62	7.40	49.75	6.78	53.87	6.26
37.50	9.00	41.62	8.10	45.75	7.38	49.87	6.77	54.00	6.25
37.62	8.97	41.75	8.08	45.87	7.36	50.00	6.75	54.12	6.23
37.75	8.94	41.87	8.06	46.00	7.34	50.12	6.73	54.25	6.22
37.87	8.91	42.00	8.03	46.12	7.32	50.25	6.72	54.37	6.21
38.00	8.88	42.12	8.01	46.25	7.30	50.37	6.70	54.50	6.19
38.12	8.85	42.25	7.99	46.37	7.28	50.50	6.68	54.62	6.18
38.25	8.82	42.37	7.96	46.50	7.26	50.62	6.67	54.75	6.16
38.37	8.79	42.50	7.94	46.62	7.24	50.75	6.65	54.87	6.15
38.50	8.76	42.62	7.92	46.75	7.22	50.87	6.63	55.00	6.13
38.62	8.73	42.75	7.89	46.87	7.20	51.00	6.62	55.12	6.12
38.75	8.70	42.87	7.87	47.00	7.18	51.12	6.60	55.25	6.10
38.87	8.68	43.00	7.85	47.12	7.16	51.25	6.58	55.37	6.09
39.00	8.65	43.12	7.82	47.25	7.14	51.37	6.57	55.50	6.08
39.12	8.62	43.25	7.80	47.37	7.12	51.50	6.55	55.62	6.07
39.25	8.59	43.37	7.78	47.50	7.10	51.62	6.54	55.75	6.05
39.37	8.57	43.50	7.76	47.62	7.08	51.75	6.52	55.87	6.04
39.50	8.54	43.62	7.74	47.75	7.06	51.87	6.50	56.00	6.03
39.62	8.51	43.75	7.71	47.87	7.05	52.00	6.49		
39.75	8.49	43.87	7.69	48.00	7.03	52.12	6.47		
39.87	8.46	44.00	7.67	48.12	7.01	52.25	6.46		
40.00	8.43	44.12	7.65	48.25	6.99	52.37	6.44		

Source: Adapted from CA Schwartz. Appendix 6. In CA Schwartz (ed), Specialty Contact Lenses: A Fitter's Guide. Philadelphia: Saunders, 1996;320.

Index

Note: Page numbers in *italic* indicate figures; page numbers followed by t indicate tables.

About the CD-ROM

CD-ROM CONTENTS

Using animation and morphing to illustrate important concepts, the **RGPDisc software** featured on this companion CD-ROM presents different aspects of fitting RGP contact lenses. The self-contained program runs entirely on the CDR; however, you must have **Quick-Time 4** installed on your computer to access the various sample movies contained within the program. See **Readme.txt** file on the disc for installation.

The CDR also features the content of the *Manual of Contact Lens Prescribing and Fitting with CD-ROM, Second Edition* in an interactive **Adobe Acrobat PDF** interface. There's also an **interactive index** (in PDX format) that's been generated from the chapter PDFs. To access all of these files, you must use **Adobe Acrobat** or **Reader 4** or higher. You can run Reader directly from the CDR or install the software onto your computer's hard drive. See the **Readme.txt** file on the disc for access and installation instructions.

WELCOME.PDF

To make surfing the contents of the CDR even easier, we've linked all the files to a single Acrobat PDF file. Once you've installed all the required software, simply open **Welcome.pdf**. All the contents of the CDR are linked within this PDF file.

Macintosh Users

Mac users can simply double-click on the **Welcome.pdf** icon; this will open the file within Acrobat Reader on the CDR.

Windows Users

Windows users will first need to launch Acrobat Reader, and then open the **Welcome.pdf** file found in the route folder of the CDR.

To run Acrobat Reader from the CDR, run **D:\Software\AcroRead\Reader\ AcroRd32.exe** (where "**D**" is the designation of your CD drive.) Then, from within Reader, go to the File pull-down menu and open, **D:\Welcome.pdf**.

TECHNICAL SUPPORT INFORMATION

Beyond providing replacements for defective discs, Butterworth-Heinemann does not provide technical support for the software programs included on this CD-ROM. For replacement of a defective disc, address your questions via email to **techsupport@bhusa.com**, call 1-800-366-2665, or write to Butterworth-Heinemann, Customer Service Dept., 225 Wildwood Avenue, Woburn MA 01801-2041. Be sure to reference item number **CD-72153**.